RESEARCH ORIENTED
MEDICAL EDUCATION

RESEARCH ORIENTED MEDICAL EDUCATION

THE ESSENTIALS

Editors

Madhav G. Deo
Renu Bharadwaj
Rita Mulherkar

White Falcon Publishing
www.whitefalconpublishing.com

MOVING ACADEMY OF MEDICINE AND BIOMEDICINE
Pune-411067, India

Research Oriented Medical Education - The Essentials
Madhav G. Deo, Renu Bharadwaj, Rita Mulherkar

www.whitefalconpublishing.com

First Edition, 2023

Cover design by White Falcon Publishing, 2023
Cover image source freepik.com

Requests for permission should be addressed to
deo.madhav@gmail.com, rmulherkar@gmail.com,
renu.bharadwaj@gmail.com

ISBN - 978-1-63640-814-9

Table of Contents

Authors: Addresses, Affiliations and Contact Information

Sr. No	Authors and Their Details
1.	**Dr Renu Bharadwaj, MD** Past President Indian Association of Medical Microbiology, Consultant Microbiologist, Professor & Head of Department of Microbiology (Retired), BJ Medical College, Pune, India renu.bharadwaj@gmail.com Mob: +91-9372465940
2.	**Dr Arun Bhatt, MD** Consultant – Clinical Research & Drug Development, Mumbai, India Email: arun_dbhatt@hotmail.com Mob: +91-9820190311
3.	**Dr Narendra Chirmule, PhD** Symphony Tech Biologics, Philadelphia, USA Email: chirmule@gmail.com Mob: +91 9538777099
4.	**Dr Avinash Deo, MD** Consultant, Medical Oncology, Raheja Hospital, Mumbai, India Email: avinashdeo@gmail.com Mob: +91- 9821025517
5.	**Dr Madhav Deo, MD, PhD** President, Moving Academy of Medicine and Biomedicine; Former Director, Cancer Research Institute Mumbai; Ex-Professor of Pathology, AIIMS, New-Delhi, India Email: deo.madhav@gmail.com Mob: +91-9922403266
6.	**Dr Amitab Gaur PhD** Innovative Assay Solutions, San Diego, CA, USA Email: agaursd@gmail.com Mob: +1 (858)735 2907

Sr. No	Authors and Their Details
7.	**Dr Vikram Gota, MD** **Professor of Pharmacology** ACTREC, Tata Memorial Centre, Navi Mumbai, India Email: vgota@actrec.gov.in Mob: +91- 7715019117
8.	**Dr Nikhil Gupte, PhD** Director, Biostatistics and Data Management, Centre for Clinical Global Health and Education, Johns Hopkins University, Baltimore, MD, USA Email: ngupte1@jhmi.edu Mob: +91- 9822070853
9.	**Dr Nilima Kshirsagar, MD, PhD** Emeritus Scientist, Former National Chair ICMR, Chairperson Academic Council AIIMS Delhi, Ag VC MUHS, Director ME, H Dean HOD & Professor Clinical Pharmacology, GS Medical College, KEM Hospital Mumbai, India Email: kshirsagarna@yahoo.in Mob: +91-9821036616
10.	**Dr Shreerang Joshi, MS** Prof and Head of Dept of Orthopaedics, BKL Walawalkar Hospital, Dervan, Distt Ratnagiri, Maharashtra, Consultant, Ratna Memorial and Joshi Hospitals, Pune, India Email: joshishreerang@yahoo.in Mob: +91-9823042591
11.	**Dr Megha Joshi, MD, FCAP** Medical Director and Associate Staff Pathologist, WICU and FCM Laboratories, Beth Israel-Lahey Health, Winchester Hospital, Winchester, MA, House of Delegates Steering Committee Member and Council of Accreditation (CAP). Email: meghascarff@yahoo.com
12.	**Dr Manjunath Nookala Krishnamurthy** Associate Professor Department of Clinical Pharmacology Advanced Centre for Treatment, Research and Education in Cancer Sector-22, Kharghar Navi Mumbai – 410210 Maharashtra, India Email: nk.manjunath@gmail.com> Tel: 022 2740 5130 Authors: Addresses, Affiliations and Contact Information B xiii Sr. No Authors and Their Details

Sr. No	Authors and Their Details
13.	**Dr. Sharath Kumar** Oncotherapeutics Fellow Department of Clinical Pharmacology Advanced Centre for Treatment, Research and Education in Cancer Sector-22, Kharghar Navi Mumbai – 410210 Maharashtra. India Email: <sharathkumarhj@gmail.com> Tel: 022 2740 5130
14.	**Dr P Manickam,** Scientist E, ICMR-National Institute of Epidemiology, Chennai, India Email: manickamp@gmail.com
15.	**Dr Prashant Mathur,** MD Director, ICMR-National Centre for Disease Informatics and Research, Bengaluru, India Email: director-ncdir@icmr.gov.in Mob: +91-9482347643
16.	**Dr Roli Mathur,** PhD Scientist F & Head, ICMR Bioethics Unit, Consultant, WHO Collaborating Centre for Strengthening Ethics in Biomedical and Health Research, National Centre for Disease Informatics and Research, Bengaluru, India Email: rolimath@gmail.com Mob: +91-9810539489
17.	**Dr Rita Mulherkar, PhD, FNASc** Professor and Scientific Officer 'H' (retired), ACTREC, Tata Memorial Centre, Mumbai Presently Director, Samarthakrupa Lifesciences Pvt Ltd, Pune, India Email: rmulherkar@gmail.com Mob: +91-8369077085
18.	**Dr Avani S Nadkarni, MBBS** Anesthesia Resident, Sumandeep Vidyapeeth, Vadodara, Gujarat, India Email: avani.nadkarni97@gmail.com
19.	**Dr Shubha Phadke** MD [Pediatrics], DM [Medical Genetics] Professor & Head, Department of Medical Genetics, Sanjay Gandhi Postgraduate Institute of Medical Sciences, Lucknow, India, 226014 Email: shubharaophadke@gmail.com Mob: +91- 91522 2494325

Sr. No	Authors and Their Details
20.	**Dr Priyanka Raipur** B. J Govt. Medical College-Johns Hopkins University Clinical Research Site, B J Govt Medical College & Sassoon General Hospitals, 1st Floor, ENT Department, PGP Hall, Jai Prakash Narayan Road, Pune - 411001, India E-Mail: dr.priyanka.a.k@gmail.com Phone: +91-8806844997
21.	**Dr K Satyanarayana** Former Sr Deputy Director-General & Chief Editor, Indian Journal of Medical Research, Indian Council of Medical Research, New Delhi Email: kanikaram_s@yahoo.com
22.	**Dr Madhuri Somani, MD** Consultant Microbiologist 1402 Ashoka Enclave Plot 9a, Sector 11 Dwarka New Delhi 110078 Tel: 9644355582 Email: madhurikm9@gmail.com
23.	**Dr Vani Srinivas, MD** Scientist E, ICMR-National Centre for Disease Informatics and Research, Bengaluru, India Email: vani.srinivas@icmr.gov.in Mobile: + 91 92434 21822
24.	**Dr Madhuri Thakar, PhD** Scientist G, Dept of Immunology and Serology, ICMR-National AIDS Research Institute, Pune, India Email: mthakar@nariindia.org Mob: 9423583340

Foreword

As a student, I hardly had any exposure to medical research. The training was more focused on clinical disciplines and my teachers encouraged me to pursue postgraduate training in a clinical speciality. Diagnoses were made on the basis of clinical features and laboratory investigations were rarely prioritized. As students, we neither heard the word research, nor were we exposed to any basic sciences. However, things changed in the West with Abrahams Flexner's report, which made science an integral part of medical education, resulting in identifying a breed of medicos equally interested in science - the "physician-scientists". It also marked the dawn of evidence-based medicine, where laboratory investigations could not be ignored in patient management. Special programs were developed to promote research, the mother of new knowledge. Looking at the status of medical research globally, it is clear that the prioritization of topics and funding allocations are made by high income countries, often ignoring the local public health priorities of lower income ones. This book will hopefully promote a research culture in developing countries, which have lagged behind.

All editors of this book are globally acclaimed Bio-medical Investigators. Dr. MG Deo, one of the editors was a Professor of Pathology at the All-India Institute of Medical Sciences, New Delhi, the Country's premier medical institute. He retired as director of the Cancer Research Institute, Mumbai. He is the incumbent President of the Moving Academy of Medicine and Biomedicine. Dr Renu Bharadwaj was Professor and Head, Department of Microbiology, BJ Medical College, Pune, a leading institute in India. Dr Mulherkar, a Biologist, was a Professor and Chief of Molecular Genetic Laboratory in Advanced Center for Treatment, Research and Education in Cancer, which is the first Cancer Research Institute in India. She is also Vice President of the Moving Academy of Medicine and Biomedicine.

About ten years ago, Dr Deo developed the concept of Researcher-Oriented Medical Education (ROME), which essentially consists of hosting in medical colleges in different parts of India, mobile, short duration, in-study workshops on cutting-edge research topics, taking new knowledge to students' doorsteps. I have personally witnessed these workshops which are extremely useful to medical students and help to kindle latent research passion in them.

The book opens with a short account of the concept of ROME. It covers the principles used in Laboratory and Clinical Research such as Study Designs, Statistics, Ethics in Medical Research, commonly used Laboratory Technologies in Molecular Biology and Immunology and implications of Information Technology which has pervaded almost all Biomedical Research. There are chapters on good Clinical and Laboratory Practices, Informed Consent, Development of a Clinical Protocol, especially for non-communicable disorders, Medical Writing and writing a grant application for a research project. The book also deals with some topics of general interest like Genetic Disorders, Molecular Medicine and Gene Therapy, Drug and Vaccine Development and the Indian Regulatory System. Often even the best researchers flounder on the presentations of their data. There is a special chapter on Platform Presentation. The chapters are very brief and succinctly highlight the essential points.

The book is a grammar for biomedical research and will be an asset for students with research aptitude in developing nations that lack financial and manpower resources. It is expected to will promote a research culture that will hopefully lead to a new generation of physician-scientists in more countries. Students of the dual degree MD-PhD program may also find the book handy. All in all, a welcome addition to a medical students reading list!

Soumya Swaminathan, MD, FMedSci
Chief Scientist, WHO
Geneva, Switzerland

Preface

Advances in medicine often originate from discoveries in basic sciences, which lead to new concepts with implications to all disciplines - preventive, diagnostic and therapeutic. A good example is the discovery of the microscope which enabled humans to see objects beyond the naked eye. This led to the discovery of bacteria and their diversity. It was soon recognised that different classes of organisms were causally associated with different types of diseases, creating a new field of infectious diseases. Laboratory methods were developed to grow the organisms in controlled conditions and manipulate their physiology at will. These advances enabled Alexander Fleming to discover Penicillin which completely transformed the impact of bacterial infections on human health. Globally, the life expectancy at birth has increased from 47 to 70 years between 1950 and 2020, resulting in a change in the disease pattern. Infectious diseases are now replaced by Non-Communicable Disorders (NCD) like cardiovascular diseases, cancers, chronic obstructive respiratory diseases and diabetes as the leading causes of mortality. Today, NCDs account for 71% of mortality globally.

Despite the evident impact of basic science discoveries, from time immemorial the practice of medicine at its core has remained an 'art of healing', based primarily on the doctor's opinion and experience. For these reasons medical training often consisted of an apprenticeship with a 'practising' doctor. Things changed in 1910 with Abraham Flexner's report that made science an integral part of medical education. In the process, the report created two streams of medical professionals - one inclined to investigative medicine and the second in medical practice.

The second world war was highly destructive but it also saw tremendous growth in both physical and life sciences which had a major impact on medical education and practice. Medicine could no more be practised simply as an 'art of healing'. Medical practice became more evidence-based. Laboratory investigations were crucial and could no longer be ignored in patient management. Discoveries occurred at an unprecedented fast rate. There was urgency to transform them for patient care. The concept of the bench to bedside became a buzzword in medicine. A new discipline of 'translation medicine' was born. Its main aim was to facilitate the application of basic research to clinical medicine. Translational research required physicians who were interested in research, the so-called Physician-Scientists. Most physicians are not trained in basic sciences, which they find difficult to grasp. With the result there was a progressive decline in the number of Physician-Scientists which in turn adversely affected medical research globally.

A number of programs were developed, especially by the NIH, USA, to promote research culture in physicians. It was with this idea that the combined MD-PhD programs were launched 60 years ago. Today, 100 out of 155 US medical schools offer the program which is also offered in many other countries, including India. Despite inducement (tuition waivers plus a stipend) offered to matriculants, the course is not very popular. In 2021, the number of applicants was just 3.7% of those seeking admission to the conventional MD program. The program was launched 60 years ago. Despite time-to-time bolstering,it has not met the expectations of the scientific world. The number of Physician-Scientists has remained stable. It is necessary to develop other approaches to promote research culture in physicians.

The MD-PhD program needs considerable infrastructure and human and financial resources. Developing nations are perpetually short of funds even in providing basic health services. Their medical school/medical colleges have limited infrastructure even for routine teaching; in such a setting, research is a 'luxury'. The overall research performance of medical colleges in India has been low. More than 90% of the medical colleges in the States, especially private colleges, published no publications in major peer-reviewed journals during 2011-2014. Despite this sorry state, it is necessary that these nations develop their own cost-effective disease-control strategies to meet the challenges posed by the changing health scenario and not depend exclusively on the West.

In 2001, a group of 13 globally acclaimed Indian physicians and scientists established a new organization, Moving Academy of Medicine and Biomedicine, to meet these challenges. The Academy soon developed a program - Research-Oriented Medical Education (ROME). The principles of the program were:

(a) Short duration *in-study* mobile hands-on workshops on research methodology,
(b) Held in medical colleges in different parts of India,
(c) Being *in-study* did not affect routine,
(d) Participation was voluntary, and
(e) There was no inducement or reward, except an attendance certificate.

The last two features ensured that only those interested in research actually participated in the workshops.

This book emanates from instructions provided as a part of the ROME program. It contains general research topics such as Designs of Clinical and Epidemiological Research, Data

Analysis, Biostatistics, Ethics in Medical Research, commonly employed Laboratory Procedures, Development of Clinical Protocols, Drug and Vaccine Development, Regulatory Scenario in India, Medical Writing and Drafting of a Grant Application.

The purpose of this book is to provide an introduction to Biomedical Research, ranging from bench to bedside. In other words, the book is a sort of grammar for Biomedical Research. Each chapter is a primer on topics on which otherwise there are separate books and symposia. It is hoped that a student interested in a specific topic would later take time off and attend a regular advanced workshop/symposium.

I am deeply grateful to all authors for contributing chapters to this book which would not have been possible without the help of two co-editors - Dr Rita Mulherkar and Dr Renu Bharadwaj. My special thanks to Dr Aruna Kukarni for her help in the language editing of the chapters.

Nobel Laureate Madame Curie once said, “One never notices what has been done, one can only see what remains to be done”. The future of medicine is bright and lies in the hands of the current trainees. It is to these trainees that we dedicate this roadmap.

Madhav G. Deo

Abbreviations

ADE	Antibody-Dependent Enhancement
ADME	Absorption, Distribution, Metabolism and Excretion
AI	Artificial Intelligence
ANA	Anti-Nuclear Antibodies
APA	American Psychological Association
AYUSH	Ayurveda, Yoga, Unani, Siddha, Homeopathy
BIRAC	Biotechnology Industry Research Assistance Council
CD	Cluster Of Differentiation
cDNA	Complementary DNA
CDSCO	Central Drugs Standard Control Organization
CEA	Carcino-Embryonic Antigen
CECHR	Central Ethics Committee on Human Research
CEPI	Coalition for Epidemic Preparedness Innovations
CIOMS	Council of International Organisations of Medical Sciences
CIT	Community Intervention Trial
CLIA	Clinical Laboratory Improvement Amendments
CLIAs	Chemi-Luminescent Immuno-Assays
CMO	Chief Medical Officer
CQA	Critical Quality Attributes
CRF	Case Record Form
CSIR	Council of Scientific and Industrial Research
CTA	Clinical Study Agreement
CTRI	Clinical Trial Registry India

CVD	Cardiovascular Disease
DAB	(3, 3′) Diaminobenzidine Tetrahydrochloride
DBT	Department of Biotechnology
DHR	Department Of Health Research
dNTPs	Deoxyribonucleotides
DOH	Declaration of Helsinki
DOI	Digital Object Identifier
DRA	Data Recovery Agent
DSMB	Data Safety Monitoring Board
DVT	Deep Vein Thrombosis
EHR	Electronic Health Record
ELISA	Enzyme-Linked Immuno-Sorbent Assay
EQA	External Quality Assessment
FDA	Food and Drug Administration
GCP	Good Clinical Practice
GISRS	WHO Global Influenza Surveillance Response System
GITC	Guanidium Isothiocyanate
GMP	Good Manufacturing Practice
HBsAg	Hepatitis B Surface Antigen
HCV	Hepatitis C Virus
HMSC	Health Ministry Screening Clearance
HRP	Horseradish Peroxidase
IB	Investigator's Brochure
ICD	Informed Consent Document
ICF	Informed Consent Form
ICH	International Council for Harmonisation
ICH-GCP	International Council of Harmonization-Good Clinical Practice Guidelines
ICMR	Indian Council of Medical Research
IEC	Institutional Ethics Committee
IHC	Immunohistochemistry
IND	Investigational New Drug/Product

IP	Investigational Products
IPC	Indian Pharmacopoeia Commission
IQC	Internal Quality Control
IRB	Institutional Review Board
LAR	Legally Acceptable Representative
MEDLARS	Medical Literature Analysis and Retrieval System
MEDLINE	MEDLARS Online
MIoT	Medical Internet of Things
MOCF	Ministry Of Chemicals & Fertilizers
MOHFW	Ministry Of Health & Family Welfare
MOP	Manual Of Procedures
MTD	Maximum Tolerated Dose
NCC-PvPI	National Co-Ordinating Centre-Pharmaco vigilance Program of India
NCD	Non-Communicable Diseases
NDHM	National Digital Health Mission
NGS	Next-Generation Sequencing
NLP	Natural Language Processing
NOEL	No Observed Effect Levels
PBS	Population-Based Screening
PCR	Polymerase Chain Reaction
PHR	Personal Health Record
PIS	Patient Information Sheet
PNH	Paroxysmal Nocturnal Haemoglobinuria
PRC	Project Review Committee
PSA	Prostate-Specific Antigen
PT	Proficiency Testing
PvPI	Pharmaco vigilance Program of India
QA	Quality Assurance
QC	Quality Control
RCT	Randomized Clinical Trial
RE	Restriction Enzymes

RIA	Radioimmunoassay
RMA	Rapid Meta-Analysis
ROME	Research-Oriented Medical Education
RT	Reverse Transcriptase
RT-qPCR	Reverse Transcriptase - Quantitative Polymerase Chain Reaction
RWD	Real-World Data
S&T	Science and Technology
SAE	Serious Adverse Events
SCID	Severe Combined Immunodeficiency
SCP	Specific Call for Proposals
SDS-PAGE	Sodium Dodecyl-Sulfate - Poly-Acrylamide Gel Electrophoresis
SERB	Science and Engineering Research Board
SMART	Specific, Measurable, Achievable, Relevant and Time-Based
SMC	Safety Monitoring Committee
SOP	Standard Operating Procedures
TMG	Trial Management Group
TPP	Target Product Profile
TRIPS	Trade-Related Aspects of Intellectual Property Rights
TSC	Trial Steering Committee
UNESCO	United Nations Educational, Scientific and Cultural Organisation
US NIH	United States National Institutes of Health
VLP	Virus-Like Particle
WHO	World Health Organisation
ZIKV	Zika Virus

CHAPTER

1 Research-Oriented Medical Education

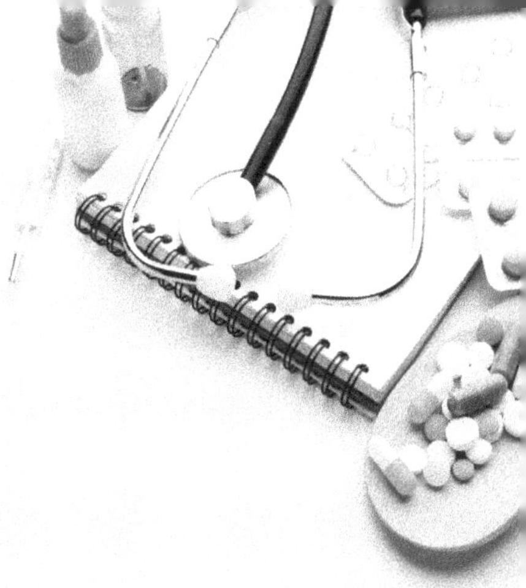

Madhav Deo

1. Introduction

Research is a highly neglected field in developing Nations as they are perpetually short of funds, even for routine health services. Yet, they must promote research to develop their disease control strategies and not depend on 'Parachute' research. On the assumption that research-oriented students are evenly distributed, these Nations would have a good potential to conduct research, provided the manpower is suitably trained. The much publicised, very long duration MD-PhD course that requires considerable resources is not suitable for them. This chapter briefly describes a short, in-service mobile workshop module that exposes interested students to the grammar of biomedical research. The program needs modest infrastructure and should be suitable for developing Nations.

2. Physician-Scientists and MD-PhD

Abraham Flexner's report, published in 1910, is a landmark publication that permanently transformed the medical education system both in the US and Canada [1]. The report recommended close integration of science and medicine and, in a way, resulted in identification of two breeds of physicians interested in

(a) only eeeeeeee practice of medicine and
(b) both in medicine and science, especially in applying discoveries to medicine - the physician-scientists. There is a global concern about the progressive decline in the number of physician-scientists. To arrest the trend, research culture must be promoted at all levels of medical education.

With this objective a number of programs have been developed, especially by the NIH (USA). As early as 1956-57, it developed an Experimental Training Program (ETP), which involved summer research experiences for medical students. STS (Short Term Studentship) of the Indian Council of Medical Research (ICMR) is more or less a similar program. The ETP was a forerunner of the - double-degree MD-PhD program launched seven years later [2].

Today, the combined degree course is offered by 100 out of the 155 medical schools in the US and many medical colleges/schools in other parts of the globe. To attract students, matriculants are offered inducements such as fees waiver and stipends.

Despite the inducement, the course is not very popular. The number of applicants, matriculants and graduates has increased but it still remains smaller than the projected workforce needed. In 2021, there were only 750 matriculants for the MD-PhD degree, which was 3.3% of those seeking admission to the regular MD. One of the consequences of this gross imbalance is that the matriculants of the program often suffer from the Imposter Syndrome. Despite bolstering from time-to-time the program has not met its expectations since it was launched. The number of double degree graduates is below its projected requirements. What is equally bothering is the observation that even their research performance is no better than the research-oriented combined residency-fellowship program students. The NIH group appointed to study the impact found that the total number of physician-scientists has remained stable over the past few decades but declined as the percentage of the total biomedical research workforce. There is a need to develop alternative strategies, especially for the money-starved developing Nations.

The program was based on the assumption that inducement should attract bright students to the course. This would ordinarily have been true but not always. Students can be *extrinsically or intrinsically* motivated to take the research path. The former category uses research to promote his/her career opportunities. The latter participates out of interest and enjoyment and in the long run, they become, in the true sense, pillars of research. None of the categories needs any inducement. However, some students may not be interested in research but find the course attractive because of the inducement that makes medical education, otherwise expensive, cheap. Also, compared to the conventional MD, the course is less competitive.

3. MD-PhD and Developing Nations

A big deterrent to adapting the MD-PhD program is its longer duration of 3-4 years compared to the conventional MD. The program needs a large infrastructure and human and financial resources. Therefore, it is not suitable for developing nations that lack funds even for routine health and medical services. Their medical schools/medical colleges have abysmal infrastructure even for routine teaching. The training is geared more toward producing practising doctors to meet social obligations of providing human resources for health services. Research is considered a 'luxury' [3]. It is often carried out as 'parachute research' where the economically poor host Nations are simply used as sample providers. It should be a matter of concern that in a random survey most 'parachute research' publications had no researcher even as a co-author from the host Nation. It is necessary that these Nations develop their cost-effective disease-control strategies and do not depend on the "West." This can only be done through research, the mother of new knowledge. It is challenging to spot students with a research aptitude. However, research aptitude would show a normal (Gaussian) distribution like all physiological functions. Irrespective of caste, creed, or geographic location even developing societies should have motivated research students. Maybe, they need to be nurtured through short-term Research-Oriented Educational Programs.

4. Moving Academy of Medicine and Biomedicine

It is recognised that medical curricula worldwide are very heavy and there is a need to develop modules of short-term, cost-effective, in-study Research Training Programs without disturbing everyday routines. In October 2001, a group of 13 globally acclaimed physicians and scientists established the **Moving Academy of Medicine and Biomedicine,** Pune, India to meet these challenges. This was the basis for establishing the ICMR-funded program, the 'RESEARCH ORIENTED MEDICAL EDUCATION (ROME).' It was essentially a mobile workshop conducted even in remote, difficult to access medical colleges, taking knowledge to students' doorsteps [4].

5. Research-Oriented Medical Education (ROME)

The ROME program has been conducted all over India (Figure 1.1). The host institute provides minimum infrastructure such as a lecture hall/room. There is no financial burden on the colleges. The entire cost of the workshop is met out of the ICMR grant. The program has also been internationalised. A **"Foundation Workshop on Clinical and Laboratory Medicine Research"** was conducted for UGs from medical colleges in the nations under the South Asian Forum for Health Research (SAFHeR). The member countries of SAFHeR include Bangladesh, Bhutan, Maldives, Nepal, Pakistan, Sri Lanka, Thailand and India.

General features

The course contents are broadly categorised into:

1. **Interactive lecture sessions** on basic concepts in biomedical research with emphasis on clinical and epidemiological research.
2. **Clinical research protocol development** is the last lecture of the first day. The participants are then divided into groups of 10 - 12and each group is given a specific topic to develop the protocol. Libraries are kept open upto midnight to facilitate the development of protocols that are discussed in the presence of experts in the afternoon session of the second day.
3. **Lab medicine** consists of demonstrating the latest laboratory procedures to a small group of 8 - 10students. The session is held on the last day.

In addition, at every workshop a few lectures are delivered by experts on current topics such as Trends in cancer research, HIV-Tb, stem cell biology, Swine-flu, Covid-19 pandemic etc.

The first two days are devoted to Clinical and Epidemiological research. Lab medicine demonstrations are held on the last day. Special lectures are held at the convenience of the experts. Wherever possible, the participants are also exposed to a bird's eye view of the research spectrum of the host institute.

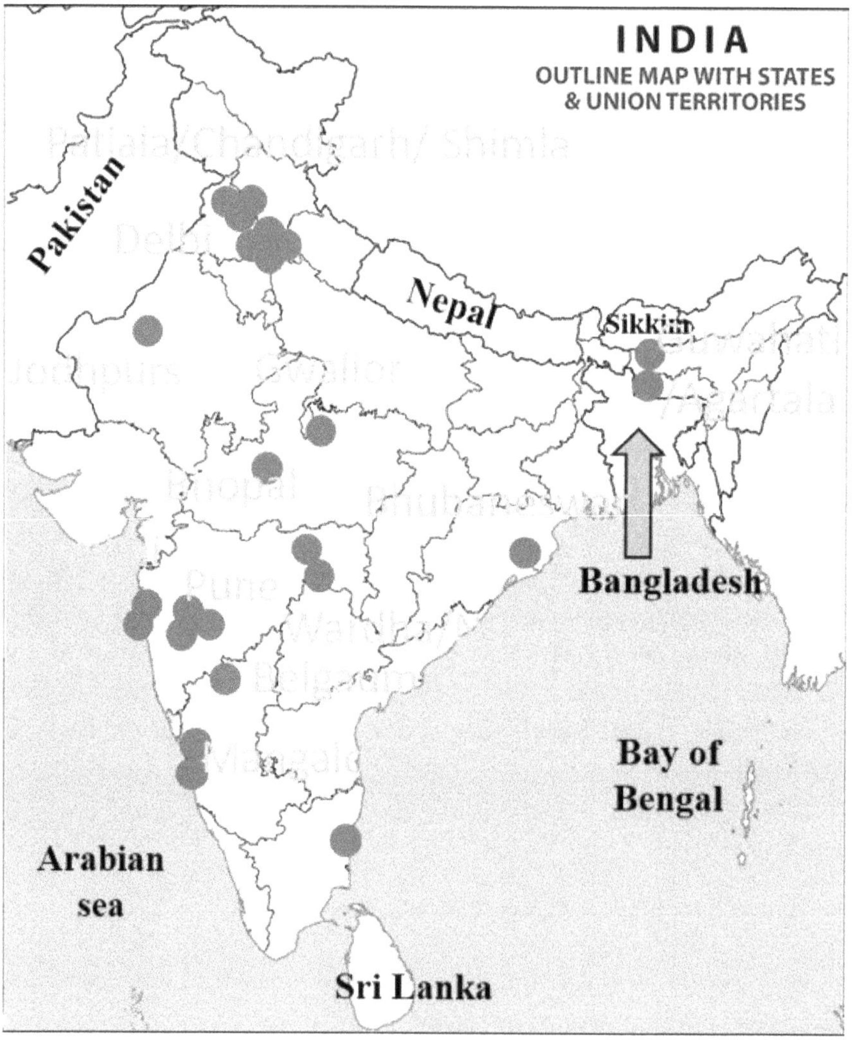

Figure 1.1: Towns (names shown in light shade) where the ROME has been conducted

Lectures

Lectures are very interactive and cover the following topics:

1. Types of research (basic, clinical, translational, observational/ interventional)
2. Study designs (Case reports, case-control studies, cross-sectional, cohort)
3. Medical ethics including formulation of Informed Consent

4. Biostatistics highlighting commonly used procedures such as mean, median, mode, ranges, standard deviation, standard error, Testing hypotheses (null hypothesis), the p-value, Chi-square, level of significance, t-test (one or two-tailed), degree of freedom, confidence intervals, Type I and Type II errors and Sampling
5. Data and Data Analysis
6. Use of commonly used computer software for statistical packages such as SPSS
7. Good Clinical Practice (GCP) and Good Clinical Laboratory Practice (GCLP)
8. Elements of clinical protocol development with emphasis on issues such as primary and secondary objectives, inclusion and exclusion criteria, study design, sample size, methodology details, clearance from the institutional review board, informed consent
9. Elements of Epidemiological Research
10. Randomised Controlled Trials (RCT) and drug development including clinical phases of drug/vaccine trials
11. Formulation of a research question
12. Communication skills, writing of reports and papers for publication
13. Submission of research proposals to funding agencies such as the ICMR

Group Activities

Participants are divided into groups each containing 10-12 students and given topics to design clinical research protocols at the end of the first day. The protocols are discussed by experts at a special session held in the afternoon of the second day. The following were some topics of protocol development:

1. Assess the relative bioavailability of Fe (Iron) from the powdered supplement marketed by a pharmaceutical company and the traditional Fe tablet in pregnancy
2. Compare the immune responses and safety of a licensed and new candidate for Influenza Vaccine in Children
3. Investigate the relative incidence of acute pancreatitis associated with Exenatide (Byetta) and other anti-diabetics
4. Measure the prevalence of hypertension in adults in the Tribal populations

Lab Medicine

The last day starts with a lecture on basic principles of commonly used molecular medicine technologies. The students are then divided into small groups that are rotated at suitable intervals. Demonstrations are held on the commonly used molecular medicine techniques mentioned below:

1. Isolation and purification of tissue proteins
2. Protein Electrophoresis (PAGE & SDS PAGE)
3. DNA Extraction
4. Agarose Electrophoresis

5. PCR, RT-PCR
6. Restriction Enzyme Digestion
7. ELISA
8. Immunoperoxidase
9. Cytogenetics, and
10. Demonstration of special types of equipment (FACS, Confocal microscopy, EM etc) and techniques (DNA microarrays) that are available at the host institute.

6. Impact of Workshops

The workshop's impact was assessed by administering pre-and post-workshops with multiple-choice single-answer questions (MCQ) related only to the course. Pre-workshop MCQs have 40 questions that can be broadly classified as clinical research including protocol development (10), RCT and drug development (6), biostatistics (7), and writing skills including discussion on the submission of grant applications to funding agencies (3)_, medical ethics (3) and lab medicine (11). The post-workshop MCQs have all the pre-workshop MCQs plus 30-40 additional questions. For assessing the knowledge impact of the workshop, the performance of a student in respect to the questions common to both pre-and post-workshop tests is used. Results are submitted for statistical analysis using paired, two-tailed, Students' t-test. P-value of < 0.05 is considered significant.

Depending on the MCQ scores, students are arbitrarily placed in the following categories: Students scoring 50-59%, 60-69%; 70-79% and ≥80% are graded as Pass, B (satisfactory), A (good) and A+ (excellent), respectively. There is no negative marking. The minimum pass percentage is kept at 50%. The results are shown in **Figure. 1.2**.

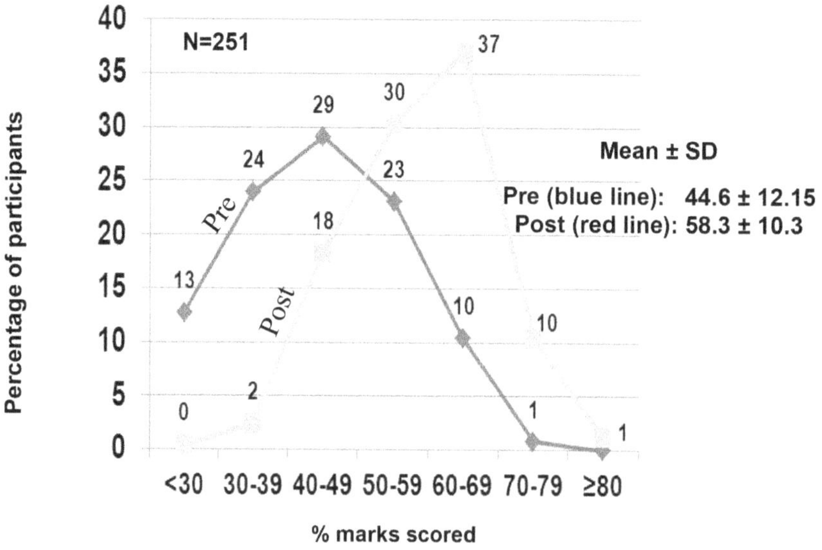

Figure 1.2: Pre-and post-workshop scores of participants

Briefly, there were no differences in the participants' performance at different centres. **Figure. 1.2** gives the pre and post-workshop performances of students at the last five workshops. A total of 279 students participated in these workshops. The pre and post-workshop assessment could be performed only on 251 (90%) students. Others could not be included in the analysis because they had not taken the pre or post-workshop tests. The average scores ± SD in the pre-and post-workshop tests was 44 ± 12.1 and 58 ± 10.3, respectively. The number of students who obtained less than 50% marks was 66% and 20% in the pre and post-workshop tests, respectively. The picture was reversed in students who scored A grades (>70% marks). Only 1.0% of students could make the A grade in the pre-workshop test. This number increased 11-fold in the post-workshop tests **(Figure. 1.2)**. Statistically, the differences are highly significant.

7. Participants' Feedback

Anonymous feedback was obtained using a simplified questionnaire in which the participants were asked to comment on whether the workshop had been beneficial to them and, if so, whether they would like to have workshops on some specific topics. They were also asked to comment on the course content, the quality of lectures and the reading material. Comments were obtained on the duration of the workshop in three broad scales - optimal, too long or too short. Finally, to get some quantitative ideas of their overall perception, participants were asked to rate the workshop quantitatively on an ascending scale of 0 to10. The results are shown in **Figure 1.3**. The average grading was 8.3 which is an indication that the participants liked the program very much.

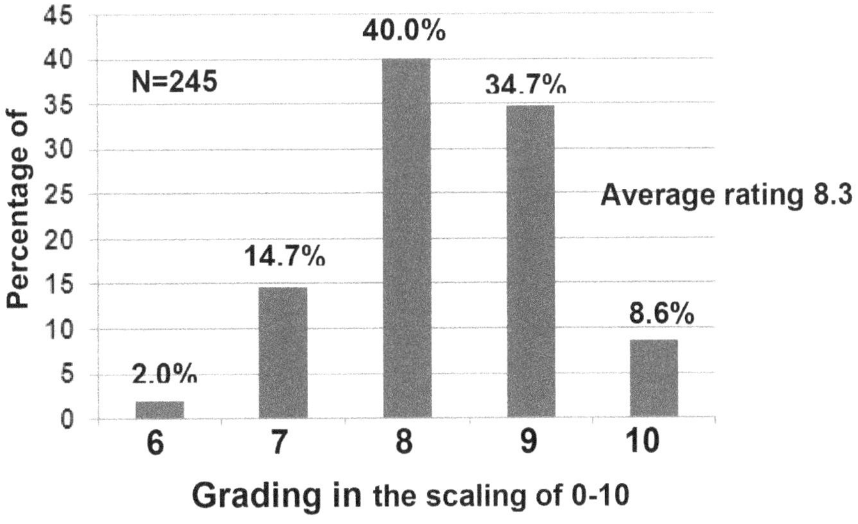

Figure 1.3: Feedback grading on an ascending scale of 0-10

(Figures on the top of each bar denote the percentage of participants in that category)

Conclusion

This article briefly describes a short-duration, in-study mobile workshop program in research procedures. The program, named ROME (Research-Oriented Medical Education), needs only modest infrastructure. Therefore, it is highly suitable for developing Nations.

References

1. **Duffy, TP**
   The Flexner Report — 100 Years Later
   Yale J Biol Med. 2011; 84: 269–276.

2. **Harding, CV, Akabas MH.; Harding, V**
   History and Outcomes of Fifty Years of Physician-Scientist Training in Medical Scientist Training Programs
   Acad Med. 2017; 92:1390–1398.

3. **Deo MG**
   Research training for medical students in developing nations
   Medical education 2012; 46:1124-1125.

4. **Deo MG**
   Mobile Research-Oriented Medical Education for Graduate Medical Students
   Natl Med J (India) 2013; 26: 169-73.

CHAPTER

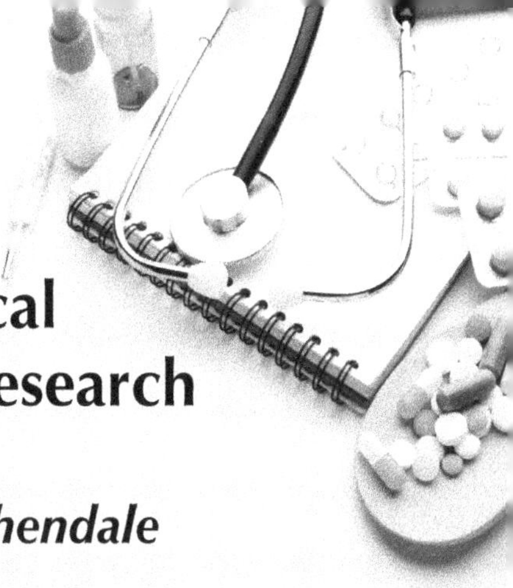

2 Study Designs in Clinical and Epidemiological Research

P Manickam and Sanjay Mehendale

1. Introduction

There is a perceived need to improve the quality and quantity of clinical research [1]. There is also a growing emphasis on evidence-based medicine and increasing expectations from policymakers and program managers to provide robust data to formulate policies and programs. Therefore, it has become critically important to build public health system's capacity and undertake high-quality research studies among health care providers. It has also been widely realized that a research mind-set might make doctors more humane, logical and non-judgmental in their approach and pragmatic in providing patient care. Thus, it is prudent to teach basic principles and practices in biomedical and health research to medical students, nurses and students of other supporting disciplines.

Many systematic reviews have pointed out the need to strengthen methodological aspects in the conduct of clinical research. It is essential to design scientifically sound research studies that can provide insights into the prevention, treatment and control of diseases and other health-related conditions. A reliable yardstick for the quality of a research proposal is the ability of researchers to get it funded; and a good quality research study is the ability of researchers to publish their findings in high-quality peer-reviewed journals. As reviewers of medical journals or research project proposals, we often come across documents with fundamental methodological errors in addition to other commonly observed problems related to the content, presentation and language (Table 2.1).

Table 2.1: Commonly identified missing elements in clinical research protocols

Key missing elements	*Explanatory note*
1. Strong rationale	No clarity on what is known and not known in terms of interventions or research topics for specific disease/health condition
2. Research objectives	Use of incorrectly defined or imprecise action verbs (e.g., 'study' or "assess") that do not indicate whether it is a descriptive or analytical study; primary objective/s not quantitatively stated and lack of distinction between primary and secondary objectives

Key missing elements	*Explanatory note*
3. Inclusion and Exclusion Criteria	Inclusion and exclusion criteria lack specificity
4. Operational definitions	Not using standard operational definitions (as per National/ International guidelines or classical texts) for disease conditions/ measurement of covariates and outcomes, and also while defining new terms
5. Drug/Intervention (s)	No details are given about the interventions to be implemented [preventive, therapeutic, or programmatic]
6. Standard Protocol Guidelines	The proposals do not make use of specific guidelines available and recommended for various study designs
7. Clinical Trial/s or Research Registration	Failing to comply with the national regulations like lack of registration of clinical trials with the Clinical Trials Registry of India (CTRI)
8. Ethical Issues	Ethical issues specific to the nature of the study are not adequately spelt out, and the patient information sheet does not provide relevant and critical details to research participants (disease, drugs/ interventions) in the common man's language
9. Referencing/Citation	Non-adherence to standard recommendations for providing citations/references (ICMJE guidelines-www.icmje.org)
10. Comprehensible Write-up	Writing without verbs and bullet points is inappropriate [and sometimes incomprehensible] for research proposals or papers

Various guidelines have evolved that serve as reference sources for research scientists, registered medical practitioners, manufacturers and health authorities. The government of India has issued the Indian Good Clinical Practice (GCP) Guidelines[2]. The purpose of these guidelines is to improve the quality and value of clinical research. The principles of GCP are not only meant for clinical trials but also for the entire paradigm of clinical research [Table 2.2].

Table 2.2: Key principles of Good Clinical Practice

1.	Any clinical trial should be conducted following ethical principles in accordance with the Declaration of Helsinki (ICMR)
2.	Before initiating any trial, possible risks and inconveniences to participants should be weighed against possible benefits to participants and society
3.	Rights, safety & well-being are the most important principles and should prevail over the interests of science & society
4.	Adequate information to be available on investigational products to support the proposed clinical trial
5.	Clinical trials should be scientifically sound and clearly described in a detailed protocol

6. The protocol should be approved by the Institutional Review Board (IRB) or Institutional Ethics Committee (IEC)
7. Medical care should be provided and decisions made only by qualified Study Physicians
8. Each investigator should be qualified with respect to education, training & experience
9. Informed consent should be obtained from every participant prior to the trial/research study participation
10. All study information should be recorded, handled and stored carefully to allow subsequent scrutiny and verification
11. The confidentiality of study participants should be protected, and their records archived as per regulatory requirements
12. Investigational products should be manufactured, handled and stored in accordance with good manufacturing practice
13. Systems and procedures that can enhance the quality of every aspect of the trial should be implemented

As indicated earlier, it is necessary to design clinical research protocols in compliance with GCP principles. This would invariably result in mitigating the deficient or missing elements in protocol design and make them ethically and scientifically stronger. The qualifications, experience and competency of the investigators are pivotal for the success of clinical research. Hence, formal training and strict adherence to GCP in clinical research are being increasingly institutionalized. Researchers must learn to adapt their research concepts to well-known epidemiological study designs while designing clinical research protocols.

2. Research Question, Hypothesis and Objectives

Research entails careful and systematic investigation or exploration in a particular area to ultimately improve the health and well-being of the people. Formulation of research objectives should follow a three-step process:

(a) Spelling out a research question
(b) Conceptualizing an appropriate research hypothesis
(c) Stating clear study objectives

3. The Life-cycle of Research

The life-cycle of research begins with identifying the knowledge gap in a particular area that needs to be translated into a research question. Following this, study objectives are formulated and a plan of analysis is decided. Using data collection instruments designed for the study, data is collected and analyzed as per the plan, which is decided *a priori*. Conclusions are drawn based on the research objectives and recommendations are shared with stakeholders to take appropriate action. This process ends by identifying another uncertainty or need which may begin the research cycle once again.

Research is never-ending.

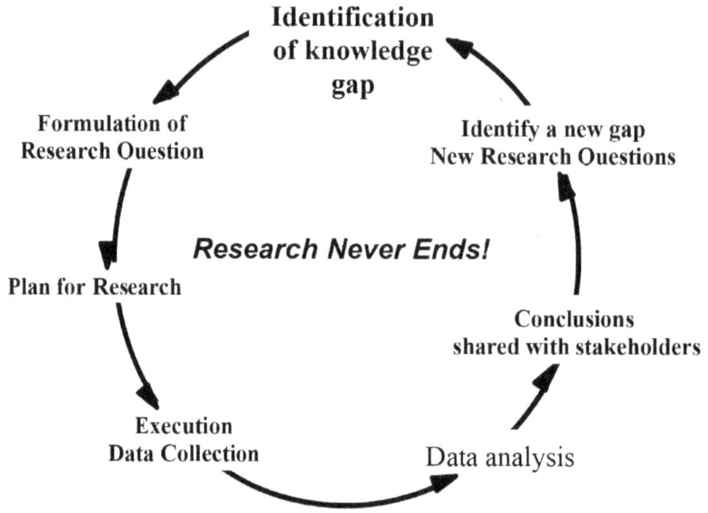
Identification of knowledge gap
Formulation of Research Question
Identify a new gap New Research Questions
Research Never Ends!
Plan for Research
Conclusions shared with stakeholders
Execution Data Collection
Data analysis

Figure 2.1: Research Life

Research Question

The research question reflects the investigator's proposed approach to resolve an identified uncertainty by making measurements in the study population. There are six steps involved while conceiving a research question (Figure 2.2):

(a) Review of the state-of-art information from literature by the researcher
(b) Identification of a research need and a question
(c) Assess if it is worth investigating through a peer review
(d) Define measurable exposures and outcomes
(e) Sharpen the initial question based on the above
(f) Refine the question by specifying details based on the above steps.

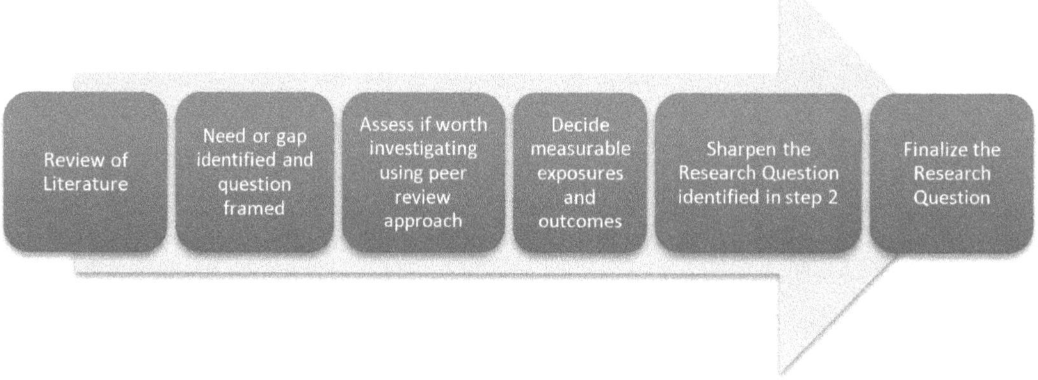

Figure 2.2: Six steps in finalizing a Research Question

While translating uncertainty or a perceived knowledge gap into a research question it is important to frame the problem in specific terms. In health research, it could be in the domains of laboratory-based, clinic-based, field-based or data-based research questions written in simple language. After framing a research question, it must be evaluated for the FINER criteria [3] [Figure 2.3]. Feasibility refers to the practical possibility of completing the research within available resources. The project should not only be interesting but novel as well because it will facilitate funding support, collaboration opportunities and eventually peer acceptance. Studies which have either ethical challenges or no logical relevance in the context of the country where it is going to be conducted or for people who would be participating, it would face difficulties in getting the necessary approvals to initiate such studies.

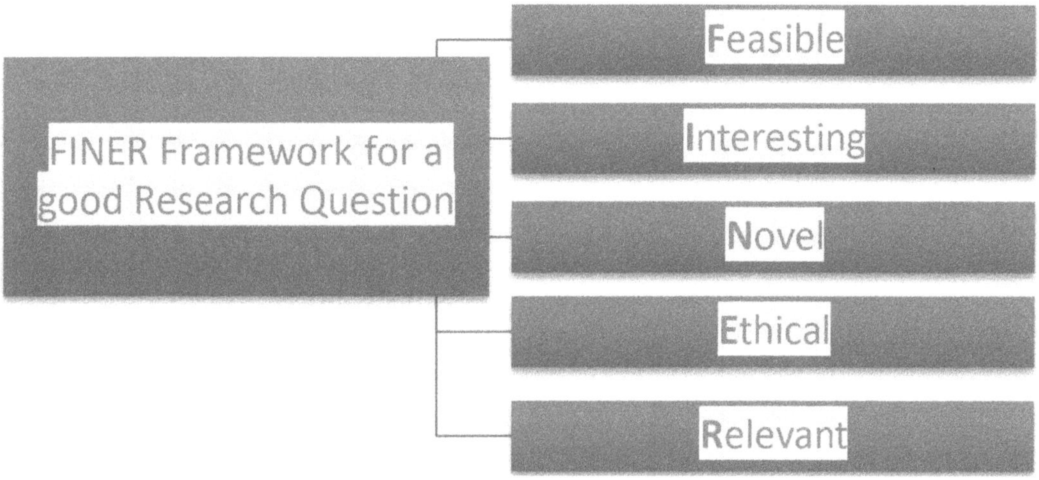

Figure 2.3: Five key characteristics of a good research question

The research question could be descriptive or analytical. The descriptive questions measure the person-specific characteristics [age, height, weight, BMI, gender, socio-economic status, family background, income, race and ethnicity, diet, etc.] or place-specific characteristics [urban or rural, low or high altitude, cities-villages-jungles, etc.] or time dimensions [season of the year, frequency of occurrence] against the disease or events related occurrences. In such type of research, there are no comparison groups or interventions for the research participants. In contrast, an analytical question involves comparison group/s or intervention to test a specific hypothesis. Therefore, while framing the research questions, researchers need to find out that the question will fall into which of these two categories. This has implications for framing objectives and choosing study designs [Figure 2.4].

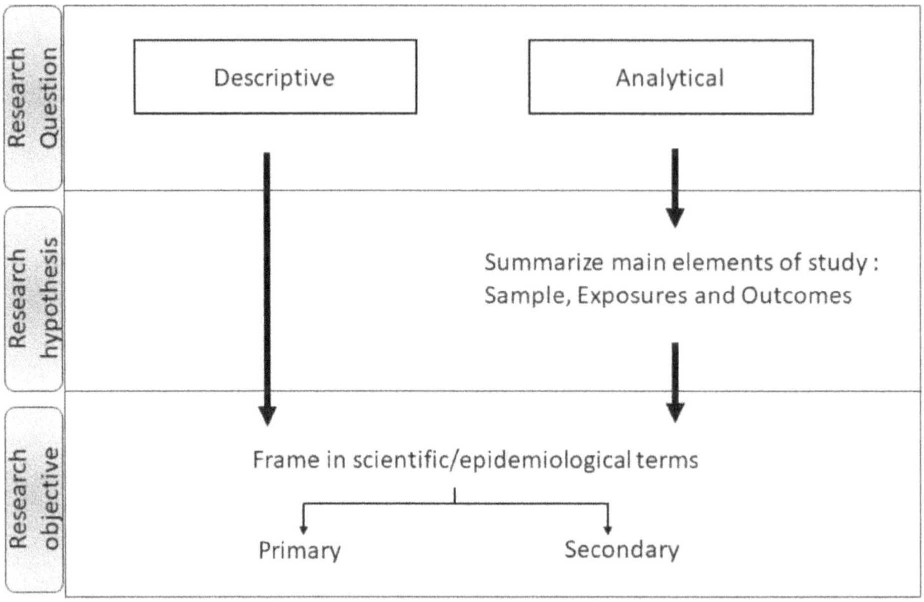

Figure 2.4: Categories of the research question, hypothesis and research objectives

Research hypothesis

A research hypothesis is an explanatory specific version of the research question that summarizes the main elements of the proposed research and provides basis for statistical analysis. A hypothesis is stated only for analytical questions involving comparison groups. The analytical questions usually contain terms such as factors, causes, relationship or association with, comparison to, likelihood, etc. Purely descriptive questions do not require a statement of hypothesis. [3]

Research objectives

The finalized research question must be translated into meaningful statement/s of objectives in scientific and epidemiological language. If there are multiple objectives, it is ideal to sort them as primary and secondary objective/s.

The primary objective must reflect the main focus of the proposed research. It is critically important that the sample size calculated for a research study must be able to find an answer to the stated primary objective. Sometimes, more than one primary objective is stated for a research study. In such circumstances it is important to determine the sample size for each primary objective and use the largest sample size for the study. As the name suggests, secondary objectives are of lesser importance but they often get framed because the researchers perceive a possibility of creating additional evidence while exploring the primary objectives. It is possible that the sample size determined based on the primary objectives might not have adequate power to provide a satisfactory and scientifically robust answer to the secondary objectives. Still, based on the evidence generated, additional larger studies can be planned, if necessary [4]

The statement of objectives should differentiate between descriptive questions and analytical or experimental questions.

Some examples of descriptive objectives are:

1. To describe the host characteristics of people affected in an outbreak of food poisoning in a village after a large function.
2. To estimate the age and gender-specific incidence of COVID-19 disease in people aged 18 and above in Pune district of India.

Some examples of analytical objectives are:

1. To identify which food item served during a party could have resulted in food poisoning among those who attended the party.
2. To measure the association between the presence of co-morbidity, age, high CRP values, and high CT scores with fatal outcomes in COVID-19 patients admitted to intensive care units.

4. Types of Epidemiological Study Designs

Study designs can be broadly divided into observational and intervention studies [Figure 2.5].

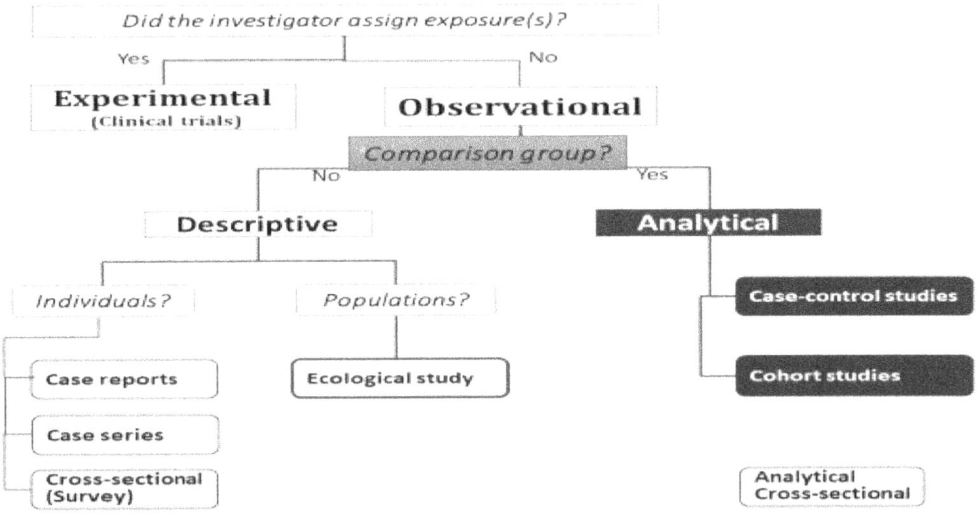

Figure 2.5: Overview of epidemiological/clinical research study designs

In observational studies, the investigator simply observes what happens as a result of the natural course of events and records and analyses the relationship between exposure status [exposed and not exposed] and the outcome [those who had and did not have the outcome of interest]. In contrast, in intervention studies, which are also called experimental studies or Clinical Trials, the investigator allocates research participants to specified intervention(s) and then follows different groups of individuals exposed to different intervention(s) to observe the outcome(s) of interest. For example, the occurrence of a disease in a vaccine trial or cure/recovery from a disease in a therapeutic trial.

Table 2.3: Description of epidemiological/clinical research designs

Type of Study	Description
Cross-sectional Study	Snap-shot
Case-control Study	Thinking backwards
Cohort Study	Looking forward in time
Randomized Controlled Trial	Testing Intervention (s) with Comparison Group (s)

4a Descriptive Studies

Case Report/Case Series:

Case report is the most basic type of descriptive individual case narrative. It provides a detailed report or account of the case by one or more clinicians. Generally, the 'atypical' or 'other than normal' type of clinical presentation is published as initial case report. Multiple individual case reports of similar nature result in a case series which describes the characteristics of a given disease among several patients. Inferences based on such studies are not considered applicable to the general population [5]. ([Figure 2.6]

Such observations made by an astute clinician may unveil so far unknown features associated with a condition or disease and may also lead to the formulation of a new hypothesis that can be tested in larger observational or analytical studies. Thus, case reports and case series represent a vital interface between clinical medicine and epidemiology as well as public health practice.

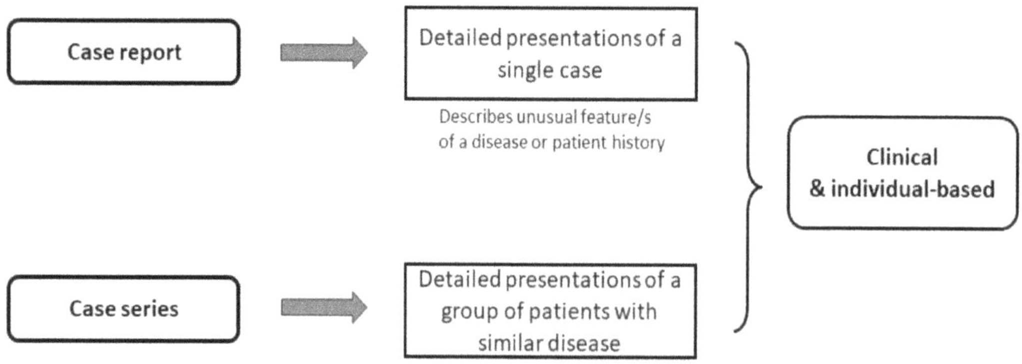

Figure 2.6: Describing Case-Control vs Case Series

Cross-sectional Study

Cross-sectional or prevalence studies are descriptive studies which are carried out in well-defined populations to simultaneously assess the exposure and outcome or disease status among individuals participating in the survey. They can be considered as "snapshots" of the population of interest at a given time. Based on the information obtained on the frequency and characteristics of the disease and related variables, the health administrators get valuable information on the disease burden, health status and health care needs of the surveyed population. Since the cross-sectional research design measures the exposure and the disease or outcome status simultaneously, they cannot conclude whether the exposure preceded the development of the disease or whether the presence of the disease affected the individual's level of exposure. This type of dilemma or limitation to establish temporal association is common to virtually all data generated by cross-sectional studies.

Further, cross-sectional studies do not have the ability to distinguish old [prevalent] and new [incident] cases. The data obtained reflects determinants of survival as well as aetiology. However, a cross-sectional study of factors that remain unaltered for life (such as gender, race, and blood group) can provide evidence of a causal association and thus, may be useful to test hypotheses. However, such instances are rare. In general, cross-sectional studies provide preliminary information to formulate a hypothesis and plan analytical studies to test the association or establish causality [6].

Links to some publications that have employed cross-sectional study design

6. Prevalence of psoriasis and associated risk factors in China: protocol of a nationwide, population-based, cross-sectional study. Li J, Yu M, Wang YW, Zhang JA, Ju M, Chen K, Jiang Y, Li M, Chen XS.BMJ Open. 2019 Jul 24;9(7):e027685. doi: 10.1136/bmjopen-2018-027685.PMID: 31345966

7. Predictors of health-related quality of life among patients with diabetes on follow-up at Nekemte specialised Hospital, Western Ethiopia: a cross-sectional study. Feyisa BR, Yilma MT, Tolessa BE.BMJ Open. 2020 Jul 28;10(7):e036106. doi: 10.1136/bmjopen-2019-036106.PMID: 32723738

8. Rotavirus gastroenteritis in Indian children < 5 years hospitalized for diarrhoea, 2012 to 2016. Giri S, Nair NP, Mathew A, Manohar B, Simon A, Singh T, Suresh Kumar S, Mathew MA, Babji S, Arora R, Girish Kumar CP, Venkatasubramanian S, Mehendale S, Gupte MD, Kang G.BMC Public Health. 2019 Jan 15;19(1):69. doi: 10.1186/s12889-019-6406-0.PMID: 30646867

Ecological study

In ecological studies, measures that represent the characteristics of the entire population or population of a very large administrative unit, such as age, calendar time, utilization of health services or consumption of food, medication, or other products are correlated to the presence and absence of disease or outcome(s) of interest. Ecological studies frequently provide initial clues on a possible exposure-disease relationship in a population. The main strengths of ecological studies are that they can be done quickly, are inexpensive and often use already available information. However, they have certain limitations as well. They include the inability to link the exposure with a disease in a particular individual, control other factors that might affect the study outcome and depend on average population-based exposure levels rather than actual individual-level values [7].

Links to some publications that have employed ecological study design

1. Ecological studies on influenza infection and the effect of vaccination: their advantages and limitations. Masakazu Washio 1, Asae Oura, Mitsuru Mori. Vaccine. 2008 Nov 25;26(50):6470-2. doi: 10.1016/j.vaccine.2008.06.037. Epub 2008 Jun 23. PMID: 18573289.

2. Air pollution exposure and bladder, kidney and urinary tract cancer risk: A systematic review. Zare Sakhvidi MJ, Lequy E, Goldberg M, Jacquemin B.Environ Pollut. 2020 Dec;267:115328. doi: 10.1016/j.envpol.2020.115328. Epub 2020 Aug 20.PMID: 32871482

3. A pilot study using ecological momentary assessment via smartphone application to identify adolescent problematic internet use. Gansner M, Nisenson M, Carson N, Torous J.Psychiatry Res. 2020 Nov;293:113428. doi: 10.1016/j.psychres.2020.113428. Epub 2020 Aug 23.PMID: 32889344

Analytical epidemiology

Evidence generated by descriptive studies is weak and has limited inferential significance in cause-and-effect relationships. The analytical epidemiology approach tests hypotheses based on descriptive studies and provides stronger evidence on determinants of a disease, thereby helping in designing and employing dependable strategies for prevention and control. In analytical study, the comparison between exposure [cause] and disease [effect] is explicit, and the investigators assemble a group of individuals for the specific purpose of systematically determining whether or not the frequency of occurrence of a particular event or disease is differential for the individuals exposed or not exposed to a specific exposure of interest. The presence of an appropriate comparison group is the strength of analytical studies that allow the testing of hypotheses. It is possible to test a hypothesis using any of the two basic types of analytical studies - case-control or cohort studies [Figure 2.7]. Each of these designs has certain unique advantages and disadvantages.

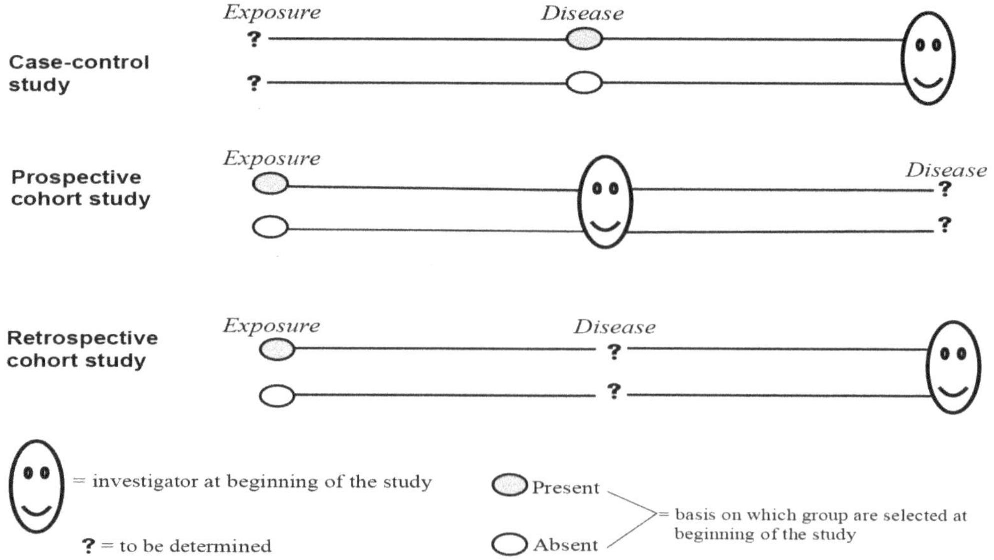

Case-control Studies

Figure 2.7: Designs of Case-control, Prospective and Cohort Studies

Case-control Study

In terms of exposure [cause] and outcome [effect], the directionality of the case-control study design is retrospective that is from outcomes [events or cases of interest] to exposures [causes/factors/variables of interest]. Case-control studies are relatively quick and cheap to carry out and have been used in many studies. They can be used to investigate multiple exposures, risk factors or aetiologies in the case of rare diseases [6].

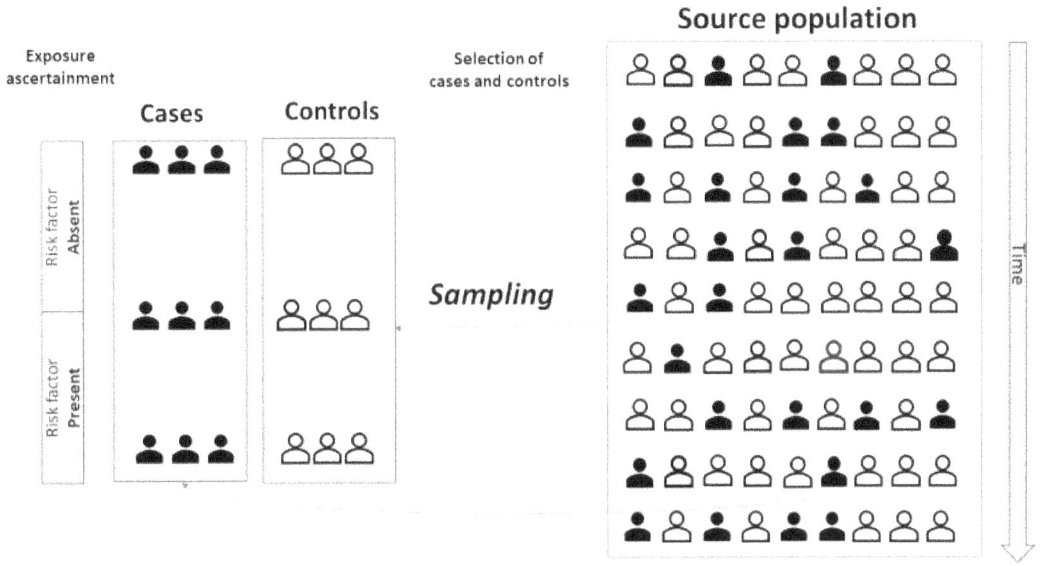

Figure 2.8: Design of the Case-control Study

In a case-control study, a group or series of patients with disease/cases (or outcome of interest) and a control or a comparison group of individuals (without the disease or outcome of interest) are selected from the source population (Figure 2.8). The cases and controls should be selected from the same population to ensure a similar representation of exposure among both groups. In practice, controls are usually selected from the general population (population-based case-control study) or the same hospital as the cases (hospital-based case-control study). It is important to select the cases and controls appropriately for reliable and meaningful conclusions. Matching ensures similarity between cases and controls in certain characteristics such as age, sex, race, occupation, socio-economic status, etc. Matching enables the identification of risk factors or exposures that are not due to differences between the cases and controls. To assess and ascertain the exposure status of cases and controls, they are interviewed or past medical records/laboratory files are examined. Then, the frequency of exposure of interest in each of the groups is compared.

Links to some publications that have employed case-control study design

1. Case-control studies of sporadic enteric infections: a review and discussion of studies conducted internationally from 1990 to 2009. Fullerton KE, Scallan E, Kirk MD, Mahon BE, Angulo FJ, de Valk H, van Pelt W, Gauci C, Hauri AM, Majowicz S, O'Brien SJ; International Collaboration Working Group. Foodborne Pathog Dis. 2012 Apr;9(4):281-92. doi: 10.1089/fpd.2011.1065.PMID: 22443481.

2. Assessment and comparison of the antioxidant defense system in patients with type 2 diabetes, diabetic nephropathy and healthy people: A case-control study. Lotfi A, Shapourabadi MA, Kachuei A, Saneei P, Alavi Naeini A.Clin Nutr ESPEN. 2020 Jun;37:173-177. doi: 10.1016/j.clnesp.2020.02.018. Epub 2020 Mar 14.PMID: 32359740.

3. Night-Shift Work and Risk of Prostate Cancer: Results From a Canadian Case-Control Study, the Prostate Cancer and Environment Study. Barul C, Richard H, Parent ME.Am J Epidemiol. 2019 Oct 1;188(10):1801-1811. doi: 10.1093/aje/kwz167.PMID: 31360990.

Because the information about the exposure would have happened sometime in the past in a case-control study, recall bias can be a problem since cases may remember and report exposures differently from controls. This problem is less serious when the exposure can be objectively assessed (e.g. height), accurately recalled (e.g. age), or verified (e.g. treatment received based on prescriptions or hospital case records). Such studies can suggest a causal relationship but cannot prove the same. There is also potential for selection bias particularly in the selection of controls. Case-control studies can suffer because of these limitations but are designed and executed thoughtfully. They can provide the same information as cohort studies but in a shorter time and at a lower cost.

Cohort Studies

In terms of exposure [cause] and outcome [effect], the directionality of cohort study design is generally prospective, that is, from exposures [causes/factors/variables of interest] to outcomes [events/cases of interest] [Figure 2.9]. However, cohort studies may be classified as either prospective or retrospective cohort studies. For both these study designs, the starting point is essentially the categorization of the study participants based on the presence or absence of exposure. In a retrospective cohort study, all relevant events [both exposure(s) and outcome(s)] have already occurred. Although the investigator initiates the study subsequently the directionality is always kept from exposure to outcome. However in the case of a prospective study, the exposed and unexposed study populations are followed systematically to record outcomes as they keep happening. The strengths of the cohort study design include the ability to measure the incidence of disease (rate of occurrence of new cases), more accurate and dependable exposure assessment and the ability to measure several outcomes in one study. Cohort studies are commonly employed or preferred when the suspected exposure is known and rare, but the anticipated incidence of disease/outcome of interest in the exposure group is expected to be high. Cohort studies provide strong evidence of a causal relationship but may not prove the same [6].

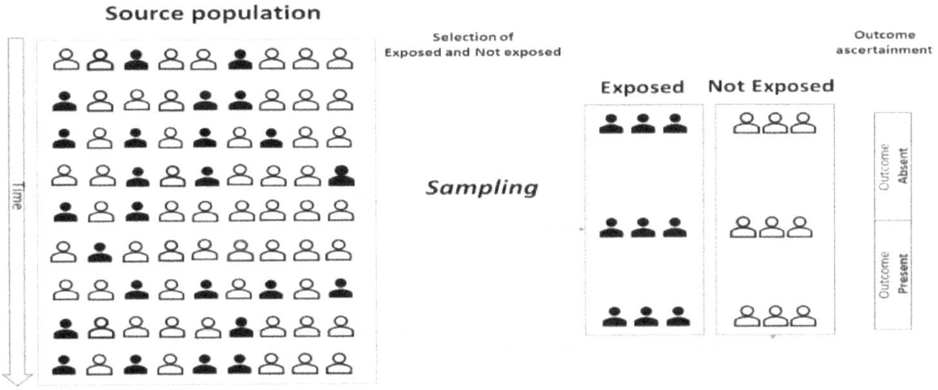

Figure 2.9: Design of Cohort Studies

A cohort study begins by identifying a study population that is free from the disease or outcome of interest, which can be characterized as "exposed" or "unexposed", depending upon exposure or lack of exposure to a particular exposure variable/factor/cause. Most often cohort study designs are used to study outcome(s) from a single exposure or risk factor. The most important characteristic feature of a cohort study is that individuals in these groups are evaluated in real-time as per a pre-determined follow-up schedule. The 'new' (incident) cases of the disease are captured in both the exposed and unexposed individuals.

The main drawbacks of cohort studies include the requirement of a large sample size to observe comparatively rare outcomes and the need for long and consistent follow-up to accumulate enough study endpoints or outcomes [to achieve sufficient power to make meaningful inferences]; moreover, they are expensive and time-consuming. Biases observed in the case of cohort studies include selection bias and information bias. Some individuals who have exposure may refuse to participate in the study or may not regularly report for follow-up. In such instances, interpreting the association between exposure and outcome is difficult. Also, if the information obtained from the past records is inadequate and inconsistent [retrospective cohort study], the inferences are non-dependable. In such instances the exposure status cannot be correctly ascertained and the measurement of association between the exposure and outcome becomes difficult to interpret.

Links to some publications that have employed case-control study design

1. Case-control studies of sporadic enteric infections: a review and discussion of studies conducted internationally from 1990 to 2009. Fullerton KE, Scallan E, Kirk MD, Mahon BE, Angulo FJ, de Valk H, van Pelt W, Gauci C, Hauri AM, Majowicz S, O'Brien SJ; International Collaboration Working Group. Foodborne Pathog Dis. 2012 Apr;9(4):281-92. doi: 10.1089/fpd.2011.1065.PMID: 22443481.

2. Assessment and comparison of the antioxidant defense system in patients with type 2 diabetes, diabetic nephropathy and healthy people: A case-control study. Lotfi A, Shapourabadi MA, Kachuei A, Saneei P, Alavi Naeini A.Clin Nutr ESPEN. 2020 Jun;37:173-177. doi: 10.1016/j.clnesp.2020.02.018. Epub 2020 Mar 14.PMID: 32359740.

3. Night-Shift Work and Risk of Prostate Cancer: Results From a Canadian Case-Control Study, the Prostate Cancer and Environment Study. Barul C, Richard H, Parent ME.Am J Epidemiol. 2019 Oct 1;188(10):1801-1811. doi: 10.1093/aje/kwz167.PMID: 31360990.

4b Experimental Studies/Intervention Studies/Clinical Trials

Randomized Controlled Clinical Trials:

Intervention studies (also referred to as experimental studies or clinical trials) are a type of prospective cohort study. However, exposure to intervention is decided by the investigator [Vaccine versus placebo or treatment A versus treatment B, etc.], and the study groups are followed to determine the occurrence of disease or cure from the disease [Figure 2.10]

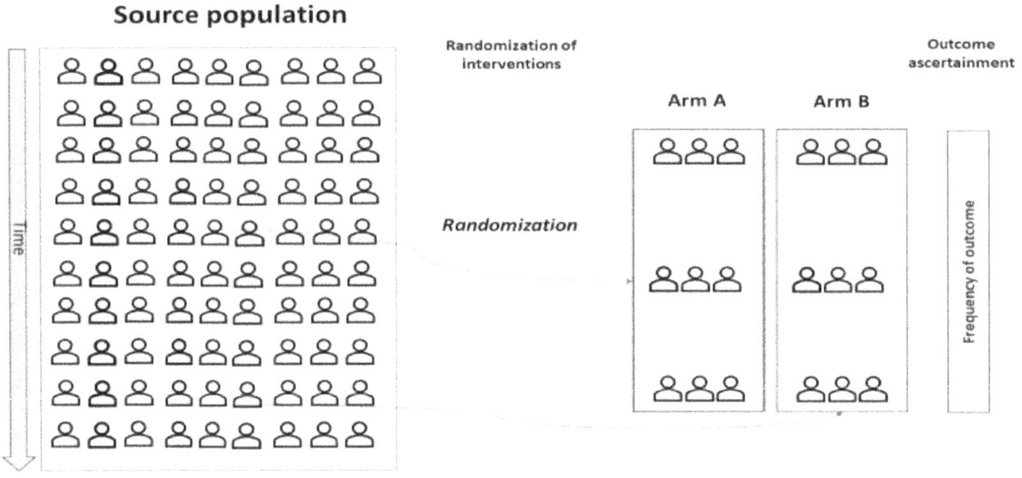

Figure 2.10: Design of Randomized Controlled Clinical Trials

Characteristic design features of randomized controlled clinical trials [RCTs] include:

1. Multiple arms such as test and control treatment arms. The results are compared between intervention and control arms to prove that the outcome resulted from the intervention and not due to chance.
2. Randomization procedure that provides an equal chance for any participant to be placed in any of the study arms
3. Blinding or masking of the trial participants, investigators and trial data analysts (as decided by the design of single, double or triple blinded study) to minimize information and diagnostic bias
4. Selection of outcome indicators which can be clinical, laboratory, images, etc. An ideal endpoint is a purely clinical outcome, for example, cure, survival or death in case of drug trials or occurrence or freedom from disease in case of prevention vaccine trials.

But due to this, the clinical trials are likely to become very long and expensive. In certain circumstances, surrogate endpoints are used that are biologically related to the ideal clinical endpoints. Surrogate endpoints must be reproducible, easily measurable and demonstrable much earlier than the clinical outcome. A Randomized Clinical Trial (RCT) can compare old versus new drugs, two different types of vaccines or different types of behavioural or nutritional interventions [8].

Intervention studies are considered high in hierarchy among various research study designs. This is primarily due to the unique strength of randomization which provides an equal chance of getting allocated to intervention or control arms. Moreover, random allocation helps in averaging the distribution of other known and unknown factors that might also affect the study outcome independently, controlling all other factors that may affect disease risk.

Ethical dilemmas related to intervention studies include exposing participants in one arm to a more superior or inferior treatment or potential adverse reactions of a new drug or unknown and possibly dangerous side effects of a new vaccine. One critical requirement to address such concerns is to provide complete information about the study and potential risks and benefits of interventions to all the study participants in a most transparent way and obtain their informed cConsent. Even though the trial participants may agree and consent to participate, they might not truly represent the population from which they are taken. Hence, another criticism of a clinical trial is about the generalisation or external validity of its results. Therefore, while designing a clinical trial, steps may be taken to ensure that the selected population is representative of the general population.

Non-randomized Clinical Trial

In non-randomized clinical trials controls are selected without randomization. Some kind of approach is used for the selection of two arms (test vs control treatment arms) either on specific dates or days of the week or certain sectors of a locality. This makes the study operationally easy, quick to complete and cheaper but allows some level of selection bias due to typical participant selection which may affect the validity of the study findings. One such example is of studies using historical controls (8) [controls used from past data like medical case records, insurance records, etc].

Cross-over Clinical Trials:

In the cross-over clinical trial study design, the same group of individuals act as their controls, for example, in the case of a drug trial involving two-drug regimens. Arm 1 starts with Treatment A and Arm 2 with Treatment B, and the pre-defined outcome parameters are measured. After a specified time period, both regimens are stopped for a period of washout to allow the blood levels of both Treatment regimens A and B to go down. After the residual effect of the previous regimens is over, the regimens are switched. Thus, in the next phase, Arm 1 receives Treatment B and Arm 2 receives Treatment A. The pre-defined outcome parameters are measured during this phase also. This study design allows the researcher to observe the possible differential effect of the two drug regimens in the same set of individuals. Such type of study design can be employed only if the study outcomes are reversible after the stoppage of intervention [like in the case of drug treatments for chronic diseases], and this design is not possible in the case of surgical interventions or radiotherapy [8].

Links to some publications that have employed Clinical trials designs

1. International open trial of uniform multidrug therapy regimen for leprosy patients: Findings & implications for national leprosy programmes. Manickam P, Mehendale SM, Nagaraju B, Katoch K, Jamesh A, Kutaiyan R, Jianping S, Mugudalabetta S, Jadhav V, Rajkumar P, Padma J, Kaliaperumal K, Pannikar V, Krishnamurthy P, Gupte MD.Indian J Med Res. 2016 Oct;144(4):525-535. doi: 10.4103/0971-5916.200888.PMID: 28256460.

2. Safety & immunogenicity of tgAAC09, a recombinant adeno-associated virus type 2 HIV-1 subtype C vaccine in India. Mehendale S, Sahay S, Thakar M, Sahasrabuddhe S, Kakade M, Shete A, Shrotri A, Spentzou A, Tarragona T, Stevens G, Kochhar S, Excler JL, Fast P, Paranjape R.Indian J Med Res. 2010 Aug;132:168-75.PMID: 20716817.

3. Safety and Efficacy of the BNT162b2 mRNA Covid-19 Vaccine. Polack FP, Thomas SJ, Kitchin N, Absalon J, Gurtman A, Lockhart S, Perez JL, Pérez Marc G, Moreira ED, Zerbini C, Bailey R, Swanson KA, Roychoudhury S, Koury K, Li P, Kalina WV, Cooper D, Frenck RW Jr, Hammitt LL, Türeci Ö, Nell H, Schaefer A, Ünal S, Tresnan DB, Mather S, Dormitzer PR, Şahin U, Jansen KU, Gruber WC; C4591001 Clinical Trial Group.N Engl J Med. 2020 Dec 31;383(27):2603-2615. doi: 10.1056/NEJMoa2034577. Epub 2020 Dec 10. PMID: 33301246.

Community trials

Community trials are also called cluster-randomized trials or community field trials. They involve assigning groups of individuals with and without the disease to different interventions. Some examples include:

(a) Village-based assignment for use of iodized salt versus non-iodized salt to study its impact on goitre prevention;
(b) School-based anthelmintic program involving yearly treatment of children in specific schools versus treatment of children and their siblings in other schools to evaluate better control over soil-transmitted helminthic infections in children
(c) Use of anti-COVID-19 vaccine A versus Vaccine B in two adjacent districts or states. The results of such studies are always on a larger scale and it is not possible to tease out variability at an individual level [8].

5. Critical considerations in relation to design, implementation and interpretation of various research studies

Internal and External Validity:

The objective of any clinical or epidemiological study is to obtain an accurate, dependable, reproducible and consistent result. The study is conducted on a specific population sample, and the study results must match the truth as it exists in the sample [Figure 2.11]. This reflects the study's internal validity and depends on the validity of the methods for collecting individual socio-demographic, laboratory and clinical data. Sometimes despite optimum data collection methods, internal validity is lost because of incorrect and inappropriate statistical methods. These are undoubtedly preventable and hence data must be handled by competent and experienced statisticians along with the study investigators for meaningful inference [9].

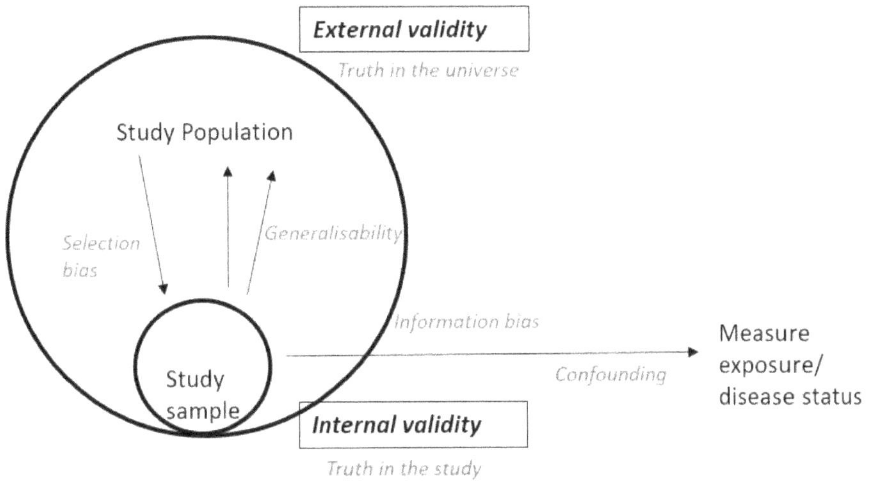

Figure 2.11: Internal vs External Validity

The goal of a research study is to ensure that the results and conclusions that have been drawn based on the sample can also be generalized to the relevant target populations from which the sample was drawn. This aim of external validity is challenging. Therefore, it is critical to ensure that both quantitative [adequate sample size] and qualitative [representation of the sample to the targeted population] dimensions should be carefully considered. High external validity permits the extrapolation of results to the relevant target population.

Accuracy of measurements

The accuracy of an estimate is described in terms of its precision and validity. The aim should be to achieve high precision and high validity [hitting a Bull's eye correctly and consistently]. If either validity or precision is poor, mechanistic improvement in measurements and laboratory methods and training of the staff can be helpful for improvement [Figure 2.12].

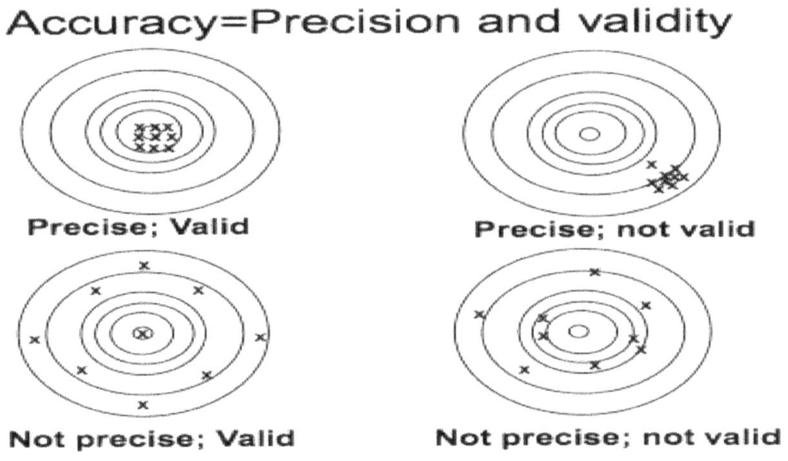

Figure 2.12: Illustration of precision and validity

Random and Systematic Errors

Random errors and systematic errors are likely to happen. It is desirable to be aware of the possibility of their occurrence and take steps to minimize or eliminate them. Random Errors happen due to chance, primarily due to variability between study participants due to unknown or uncontrollable reasons. They can be minimized by taking a sufficiently large sample and following uniform study procedures and protocols.

Systematic errors or biases are problematic and serious because they can affect the validity of any epidemiological study. Three kinds of biases are likely to occur in epidemiological studies and are called as (a) selection bias, (b) information bias, and (c) confounding.

Selection Bias

The method of selection of study participants may result in selection bias because of serious differences in the basic characteristics of the groups being compared. In a surveillance program screening and diagnosis may happen more systematically among the exposed individuals [as against non-exposed] leading to selection bias. Prior knowledge of exposure history can artificially create biases. Another common way in which selection bias occurs is when we select live cases and their exposure status might actually be the determinant of survival among people with that disease. Thus, the selection of surviving patients can actually lead to selection bias. In cohort studies, selection bias can result from instances of study participants getting lost to follow-up because this might be related to their exposure status. Losses to follow-up in either of the comparison groups can result in bias and erroneous interpretation of the cause and effect relationship [9].

Selection bias needs to be anticipated and dealt with at the design stage of a study. One way to achieve that is to recruit incident cases and avoid prevalent cases because prevalent cases can have survival bias. To avoid selection bias in case-control studies, population-based or community-based esign should be preferred over hospital-based design. The use of proper and uniform selection criteria while selecting cases and controls is likely to make sure that the study does not favour any particular exposure among the cases and controls. Both cases and controls should undergo the same diagnostic procedures, preferably in a blinded manner and with the same intensity of surveillance, before recruiting them in the study to avoid selection bias. All possible efforts should be taken to minimize non-response, non-participation, and losses to follow-up in prospective studies.

At the analysis stage, a comparison of the baseline characteristics [age, gender and others as deemed necessary] between the lost-to-follow-up and those who remain in the study might identify if the two populations are different and hence, likely to introduce selection bias. If selection bias is suspected then based on assumptions of the extent and direction of bias, Sensitivity Analysis can help to examine the influence of selection bias on study results.

Information Bias

Information bias results from errors and inconsistencies in the measurement of exposure variables and outcomes among the study participants. Other variables can also influence the exposures and the outcome/s relationship under exploration in any study. These are called confounders or modifiers. Their presence is inevitable and it is critical to measure and analyze them during the interpretation of the results.

In case-control studies, information bias results from getting exposure details by the recall of events/s that have happened in the past. These are likely to lean towards getting more reliable exposure information from one group than the other group. When cases and controls recall their past history of exposures, it is likely that those who were affected with a disease/health event may recall certain exposures more accurately than the unaffected or the control group.

In cohort studies, information bias results from gathering more detailed information in the exposed group for a specific outcome. It can happen due to a more rigorous follow-up of the exposed population than the unexposed population. Information bias can be introduced in a study by the investigators or the study participants. It is possible that the investigators may consciously or unconsciously collect exposure information among cases [case control study] or assess disease outcome among exposed [cohort study] to favour the expected conclusions.

Falsification of information by participants can also introduce information bias. The primary measure to minimize information bias is the use of precise definitions of all operational variables that are proposed to be measured along with strict adherence to previously decided measurement protocol for each variable. Additional measures include repeated measurements of key variables, initial and periodic training and certification of all the investigators and strict adherence to the study protocol. Data audits, well-defined oversight mechanisms and monitoring during the entire study can help reduce information bias 9].

Confounding

"Confounding" in French means confusion of effects. In an epidemiological study, the objective is either to establish an association between exposure and an outcome or to measure the extent of the relationship. However, it is commonly seen that a third-extraneous variable can affect such a relationship as it can have an influence both on the outcome and the exposure. This is called a Confounder and the study of its distorting effect on the relationship is called Confounding [Figure 2.13].

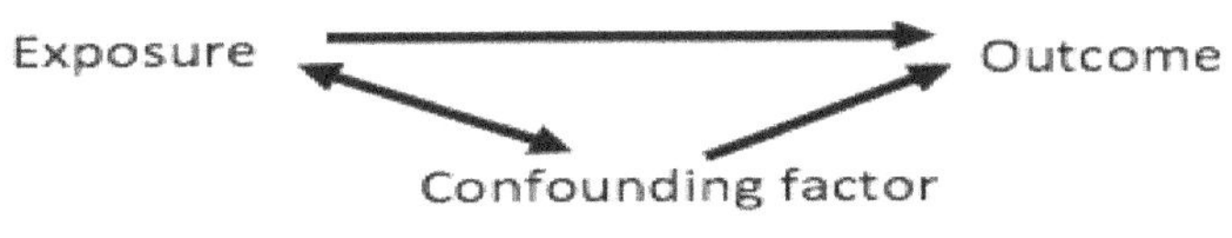

Figure 2.13: Illustration of a Confounding fact

Confounding can be an important threat to the validity of a study if its effect is not analyzed because it can suggest an association even if such an association does not exist. Confounding may result in hiding an existing association and may actually increase or decrease the strength of the association. More critically, confounding can reverse the directionality of the anticipated outcome.

Confounding can be dealt with both at the study design and also at the analysis stages. It is preferable to deal with confounders at the design stage than at the analysis stage. At the design stage, one strategy could be restriction of study participation to those not having any potential confounders that could vitiate the association between an exposure and an outcome. The other strategy of matching should ensure the presence of confounders in both the study groups to be in equal proportions. This procedure can negate the effect of the confounders on the relationship between the exposure and outcomes.

In experimental studies, the use of randomization automatically takes care of the confounders. It makes sure that the study groups are similar in terms of measured and unmeasured variables, including potential confounding variables. At the analysis stage, the presence and effect of confounding or confounding variables can be examined by stratified analysis, multivariate analysis and regression analysis such as logistic, linear or other advanced regression methods.

6. Developing Clinical Research Protocols

PR Researchers are encouraged to use existing guidelines to develop clinical research protocols, particularly in the earlier part of their career. Each research design has unique methodological considerations and challenges that must be addressed adequately in the protocol development phase. The EQUATOR Network [10] lists reporting and writing guidelines for several types of studies [11].

Table 2.4: Reporting Guidelines for main study types according to EOUATOR network {equator-network org}

Study Type	Network	
Randomised Trials	CONSORT	Extensions
Observational studies	STROBE	Extensions
Systematic reviews	PRISMA	Extensions
Study protocols	SPIRIT	PRISMA-P
Diagnostic/prognostic studies	STARD	TRIPOD
Case report	CARE	Extensions
Clinical practice guidelines	AGREE	Right
Qualitative research	SRQR	COREQ
Animal pre-clinical studies	ARRIVE	
Quality improvement studies	SQUIRE	Extensions
Economic evaluation	CHEERS	

7. Summing up

We encourage young medical researchers to adopt appreciative and suitable epidemiological study designs while designing clinical research proposals. They need to identify and address methodological challenges and considerations while developing such clinical research protocols. The protocols should adhere to the GCP and current regulatory requirements. We recommend making use of well-articulated and widely used guidelines while designing studies and writing protocols.

Acknowledgement

We thank Dr Nuzrath Jahan for helping with the illustrations and updating the references.

References

1. Park JJH, Grais RF, Taljaard M, Nakimuli-Mpungu E, Jehan F, Nachega JB, et al. Urgently seeking efficiency and sustainability of clinical trials in global health. The Lancet Global Health. 2021 May 1;9(5):e681–90.
2. Good Clinical Practice Guideline-India [Internet]. [cited 2021 Oct 16]. Available from: https://rgcb.res.in/documents/Good-Clinical-Practice-Guideline.pdf
3. Hulley SB. Designing Clinical Research. Lippincott Williams & Wilkins; 2007. 388 p.
4. Research Fundamentals: II. Choosing and Defining a Research Question - Kwiatkowski - 1998 - Academic Emergency Medicine - Wiley Online Library [Internet]. [cited 2021 Oct 16]. Available from: https://onlinelibrary.wiley.com/doi/abs/10.1111/j.1553-2712.1998.tb02673.x
5. Remenyi D. Case Study Research: The Quick Guide Series: 2nd Edition. Academic Conferences Limited; 2013. 219 p.
6. Celentano, David D,, M. Szklo, and Leon Gordis. 2019. Gordis Epidemiology. 6th ed. Philadelphia, PA: Elsevier,
7. Ahlbom A. Modern Epidemiology, 4th edition. TL Lash, TJ VanderWeele, S Haneuse, KJ Rothman. Wolters Kluwer, 2021. Eur J Epidemiol. 2021 Aug 1;36(8):767–8.
8. World Health Organization. Regional Office for the Western Pacific. Health research methodology: a guide for training in research methods. 2nd ed. [Internet]. WHO Regional Office for the Western Pacific; 2001 [cited 2021 Oct 16]. ix, 237 p. Available from: https://apps.who.int/iris/handle/10665/206929
9. Delgado-Rodríguez M, Llorca J. Bias. Journal of Epidemiology & Community Health. 2004 Aug 1;58(8):635–41.
10. The EQUATOR Network | Enhancing the QUAlity and Transparency Of Health Research [Internet]. [cited 2021 Oct 17]. Available from: https://www.equator-network.org/
11. Hoffmann T, Glasziou P, Boutron I, et.al., Better reporting of interventions: template for intervention description and replication (TIDieR) checklist and guide. *BMJ.* 2014;348:g1687.

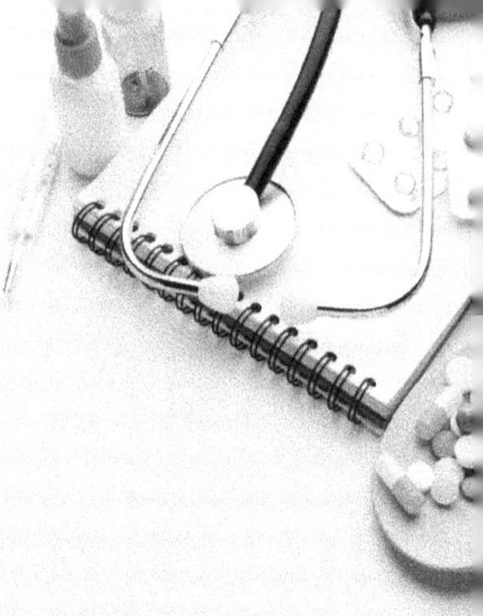

CHAPTER 3

Data Management and Biostatistics

Nikhil Gupte

1. Data Management

Biomedical researchers collect data under the assumption that a computer will perform its analysis. There are at least two essential steps between collecting data and its computer-supported analysis using statistical or biostatistical methods. Step 1 is to curate and clean the data for entry using appropriate data entry software like MS (Microsoft) Access. Once the data is entered correctly and quality check has been done, step 2 determines the statistical properties of the variables collected or entered in the database.

In this section, we will briefly discuss the issues related to the preparation of data for analysis using a statistical program. Any statistical software can be used like STATA, SPSS or SAS (Statistical Analytical Software), to name a few. There are two components to this process. The first one is the coding of data in a manner that permits analysis, and the second is the process of entering data or data entry. Data is typically entered in a spreadsheet or a database management program. One needs to remember that not all statistical programs can access data files created with a wide variety of software. Hence, investigate the data management capabilities of the statistical software before beginning data entry.

Measurement is defined as the process of assigning numbers to characteristics of persons, places, events, or things that can be observed. In the process of observing and measuring, each person, place or thing may be considered a primary unit of analysis and measured on a variety of characteristics. In an epidemiological experiment that measures time to death of HIV treatment, each patient represents a case.

Each case has a variety of characteristics. Each of these characteristics is known as a variable. The variable itself may take two or multiple values. The values can be defined as categories that constitute a variable. For example, the BMI of an individual can be expressed as actual value in kg/m^2, or expressed as underweight, normal, overweight or obese.

As stated above, measurement is defined as the process of assigning numbers to the characteristics of objects that we observe. In preparing data for analysis, we assign numbers to the categories of variables that do not normally take numerical values. This process of assigning numbers to each variable's value is called coding. For example, BMI could be coded as 1 = underweight, 2 = normal, 3 = overweight and 4 = obese. The choice of what codes to use is up to the researcher. Dichotomous variables are usually coded as 0 and 1. For example, 0 = Males and 1 = Females. A variable cannot have both numerical and text codes since most statistical softwares don't allow this. All variables collected on the cases must be coded if categorical and a codebook should be created for reference during analysis.

2. Types of Variables

While conducting a research study several variables are collected. Each variable consists of information that will be used in the statistical analysis. The type of statistical method used for analysis depends on the distribution of variables.

Variables can broadly be classified into two types:

i. Continuous and
ii. Discrete

Examples of continuous variables are height, weight, BMI, blood glucose level etc.

A discrete variable can be further classified into three types:

i. Binary
ii. Nominal
iii. Ordinal

Examples of binary variables are gender (Male/Female), HIV infection (seropositive/seronegative), etc. Nominal categorical variables are usually the socio-demographic characteristics of a case. For example, religion, education, occupation, income, etc. Ordinal categorical variables are measured on a Likert scale. For example: degree of pain (none/low/moderate/severe). Once the data is collected, it's important to note the type of variable since they will be treated differently for analysis.

3. Measures of Data Summary

Data collected must be summarised so that comparisons and interpretations can be made. Continuous data is summarized using mean and median. Mean is a sum of all the observations divided by the total number of observations, (Illustration 1). The mean blood pressure in this example is 99 mmHg. Mean is the simplest measure of summarizing data and has good statistical properties. However, it is sensitive to extreme observations.

Illustration 1

Five systolic blood pressures (mmHg) measurements (n=5)
120, 80, 90, 110, 95

Can be represented with math type notation:

x_1= 120, x_2=80,.....x_5=95

The sample mean is easily computed by adding up the five values and dividing by 5: in stat notation the sample mean is frequently represented by a letter with a line over it: for example (pronounced 'x bar')

$$\bar{x} = \frac{120 + 80 + 90 + 110 + 95}{5} = 99mmHg$$

12

Median is the central value of the data. To calculate the median, arrange the data in ascending order and select the value in the centre. In our blood pressure example (Illustration 1), the median is 95 mmHg.

In addition to mean and median, we also need to study the variation in the data. In simple terms, variation is the difference or the deviance of each observation from the mean (Illustration 2). This is called variance. The mean and the variance are key quantities used to describe properties of a variable.

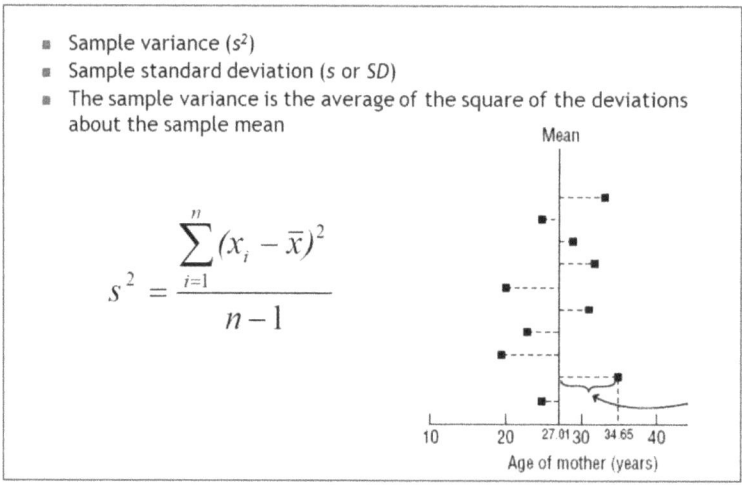

- Sample variance (s^2)
- Sample standard deviation (s or SD)
- The sample variance is the average of the square of the deviations about the sample mean

$$s^2 = \frac{\sum_{i=1}^{n}(x_i - \bar{x})^2}{n-1}$$

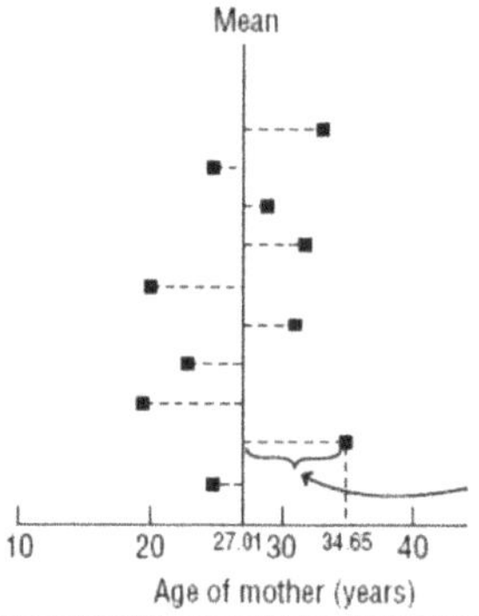

4. Exploratory Analysis

Researchers are tempted to immediately perform testing of hypothesis by using univariable and multivariable techniques and are often unaware of the starting point. In this section we will attempt to answer the question "where to start?" Many feel that data collection is the hard part and when it's done the computer will simply crunch the numbers and produce an analysis report. But this is not so. In fact, one needs to get a feel of the collected data and become comfortable with it before jumping into full-scale hypothesis testing procedures.

Examination of the characteristics of the data is a visual activity. A thorough inspection of data also makes use of tabular and mathematical calculations. Once the properties of data are understood completely, many questions regarding the ability of the data to meet the assumptions of sophisticated statistical analyses can be answered. We start by suggesting strategies for examining the distribution of a single variable, particularly the ability of that variable to approximate normality. This process is likely to indicate issues concerning the data that require some transformations before performing the analysis.

The initial step in exploring a data set is to examine the distribution of each variable that was collected during the study. The starting point of this process is to examine the frequency distribution of the variables irrespective of their type, categorical or continuous. This process helps in identifying skewness in the data. The term skew generally refers to the distribution's deviation from a preferably symmetrical shape. The data can be positively or negatively skewed. The type of skewness decides the methods for analysis. We will discuss more about this in subsequent sections.

Histogram

Refer to Figure 1, which is the age distribution of participants in an online HIV knowledge survey. This figure is called a histogram which has a superimposed normal distribution. The histogram clearly shows that the right tail of the distribution exceeds that of the superimposed normal curve and that the distribution is more peaked. This is an example of a positively skewed distribution. Depending on the type of variable, the histogram has different shapes (Illustration 3).

Illustration 3: Common shapes of the histogram (Distribution)

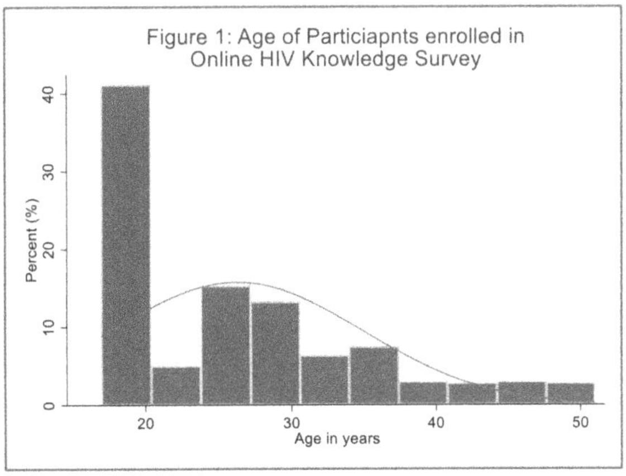

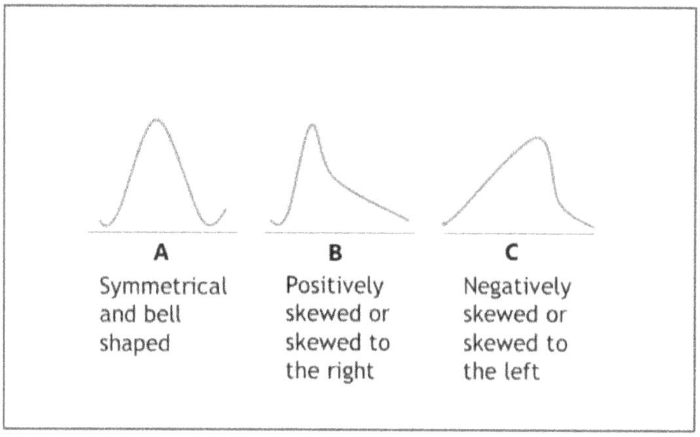

Box and Whisker Plot

This type of display is more informative than a histogram. The plot, Figure 3.2, consists of a box whose boundaries represent the upper and lower quartiles of the distribution. This means the middle, 50% of the cases, are contained within the box and the upper and lower 25% are excluded. The horizontal line within the box represents the median. The height of the box can be interpreted as the distance between the first and the third quartiles. The lines extending from the top and the bottom of the box are called the Whiskers. They represent the largest and smallest values, respectively.

When visualizing the data for trends and analytics, the box plot can also be stratified by other variables in the data set. For example, in Figure 3.3, the box plot is by gender of the study participants. From the plot, it can be concluded that the male study participants are marginally older than the females (the Median for males is bigger than that of females). Secondly, since the box for males is wider, the variance of males is bigger than that of females.

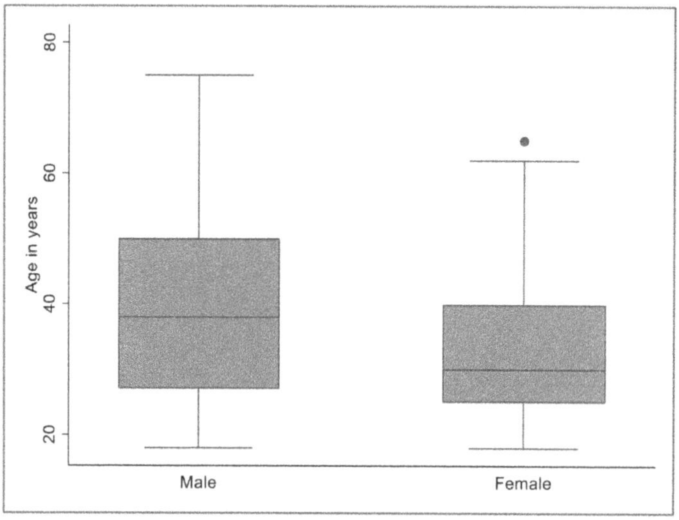

Figure 3.2: Box Plot of age of enrolled participants in a TB Cohort Study

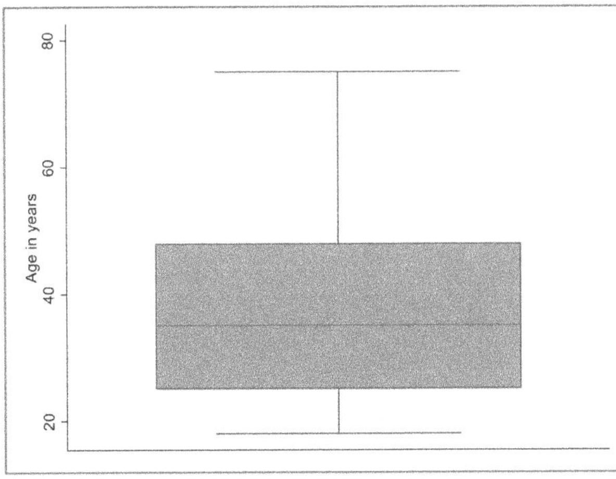

Figure 3.3: Box plot of the enrolled participants by gender

5. Normal Distribution

The term "Normal Distribution" appears several times in many statistical books and discussions. The distribution is a theoretical probability distribution and is a special case of a symmetrical bell-shaped curve. It is perfectly symmetrical around the mean, and for a theoretical normal distribution the mean and the median are the same. Normal distribution is also called a Gaussian distribution in honour of its inventor Carl Friedrich Gauss. Normal distribution is uniquely identified by the mean and standard deviation (square root of the variance). Based on the choice of mean and standard deviation, there are several normal distributions (Illustration 4). The normal distribution is most important to statisticians because of its unique properties. For any normal distribution, the mean ± 1 SD will contain 68% of the data, mean ± 2 SD will contain 95% of the data and mean ± 3 SD will contain 99% of the data.

Illustration 4

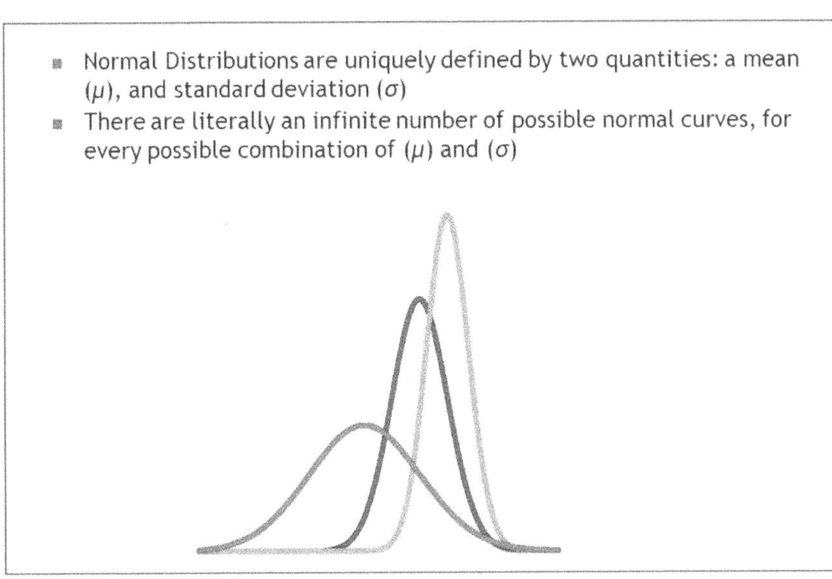

6. Population and Sample

Statistical analysis is viewed with two primary foci - the description of sample information or descriptive statistics, and the generalization of information obtained from the sample to the population or statistical inference. The goal of descriptive statistics is to organize and describe data obtained from a sample of observations. This involves the presentation of data obtained from the samples as tables and graphs.

Descriptive statistics that are used to describe samples such as percentages or measures of central tendency, for example, mean, measures of variability and the standard deviation, the measure of the strength of relationship, for example, the correlation of coefficient may be considered estimates of the value of the same measure in the population from which the sample was drawn. Thus, the sample mean can be considered an estimate of the population mean and the sample standard deviation is an estimate of the population standard deviation and so on.

Assuming that the sample has been selected using an appropriate sampling design, one may be able to use the information calculated from the sample to make inferences regarding the unknown characteristics of the population. This process of making such inferences is known as statistical inference.

The basic idea that serves as the foundation of statistical inference is generalization. We wish to generalise from the measures calculated from a sample to the population from which the sample is drawn. To be convincing, generalizations must have two features; first, they should be accurate and second, they should be precise.

A sample is defined as that which has been drawn in such a manner that each and every object in the population has an equal chance of being selected. A random sample ensures that random sampling error is minimized. However much one tries, there is still a minimum level of random sampling error in the sample that is drawn from the population. There are ways to measure a random sampling error through a special distribution called the sampling distribution. This is the distribution of a sample statistic that would be obtained if all possible samples of the same size are drawn from a given population.

7. Central Limit Theorem

A central limit theorem is a powerful mathematical tool that statisticians developed several years ago. Irrespective of any type of data, the sampling distribution of the sample statistic is always normal. Formally,

the central limit theorem can be stated as, if a variable X has a distribution with a mean (μ) and standard deviation (α) then the sampling distribution of mean based on random samples of size N will have a mean equal to μ and standard deviation equal to $^{\alpha}/_{\sqrt{N}}$ this will tend to be normal when sample size N increases.

8. Testing of Hypothesis

In addition to estimation, hypothesis testing makes inferences about the population. Hypothesis testing allows us to determine whether enough statistical evidence exists to conclude that a **belief** (i.e. ***hypothesis***) about a population parameter is supported by the data or not.

There are typically two types of hypotheses -the first is called the null hypothesis, and the second is the alternative hypothesis or the research hypothesis. The null hypothesis is usually the hypothesis of no effect. The alternative hypothesis is our hypothesis of interest. The hypotheses testing procedure starts by assuming that the null hypothesis is true. We now collect evidence (data) from the sample to prove otherwise. Rejecting the null hypothesis would conclude that the research hypothesis is true. During this two types of errors can occur: (i) the type I error and (ii) the type II error.

Type I error falsely rejects the null hypothesis, and type II error falsely accepts the null hypothesis. Type I error is also referred to as the level of significance. In a hypothesis testing procedure, one can never reduce or nullify both the errors. For any statistical testing procedure, statisticians have termed it reasonable to assume the type I error at 5% and type II error at 20% or 10%. Type II error is also referred to as the power of the test. P-value is another important measure in any testing of hypothesis procedures. P-value is a probability of obtaining a result as/or more extreme than you did by chance alone, assuming the null hypothesis (H_0) is true. If the level of significance is 5%, then the p-value is 0.05. One would reject the null hypothesis if the $p\text{-value} < 0.05$.

9. Common Statistical Tests

In this section, we will describe several common statistical tests that are used in public health or clinical research.

(NOTE: In the interest of space and context, only tests and scenarios are described. The focus is on interpretation of data. Any standard statistical software such as SPSS or STATA can be used to perform these tests.)

Paired t-test

A paired t-test is used in a scenario where data is collected before and after a certain intervention. For example, if you are assessing the effect of a training program, study participants are assessed before and after the training program. Other situations of paired data are data on twins, data on pair of eyes and matched study designs. Pairing is done to control extraneous noise where each observation acts as its control and it's a good way to obtain preliminary data.

Example: Ten non-pregnant, pre-menopausal women aged 16-49 years old who were beginning a regimen of oral contraceptive (OC), had their blood pressures measured prior to starting OC and then three months after OC use. The goal of this small study was to see what, if any, changes in average blood pressure were associated with OC use in such women. Data is shown in Exhibit 1.

The null hypothesis in this scenario is that there is no difference in the mean blood pressure before and after use of OC pills. We will reject the null hypothesis if $p < 0.05$. Using STATA the p-value for comparing the before and after mean blood pressure is 0.01. Since the p-value is < 0.05 we will reject the null hypothesis.

Interpretation: Statistically, the blood pressure measurements after oral contraceptive use were significantly higher than before oral contraceptive use since $p < 0.05$.

Blood Pressure and Oral Contraceptive Use

	BP Before OC	BP After OC	After-Before
1.	115	128	13
2.	112	115	3
3.	107	106	-1
4.	119	128	9
5.	115	122	7
6.	138	145	7
7.	126	132	6
8.	105	109	4
9.	104	102	-2
10.	115	117	2
	$\bar{x}_{before} = 115.6$	$\bar{x}_{after} = 120.4$	$\bar{x}_{diff} = 4.8$

Exhibit 3.1: Example of Paired t-test

Unpaired t-test

An unpaired t-test is used in situations where one wishes to compare two populations. Mean difference in the quantity of interest is compared across two independent populations. For example, comparing mean exam scores by gender.

Example: Effectiveness of low carbohydrate versus a low-fat diet in weight loss among severely obese people. In this study 132 severely obese males and females were randomized to either the low-fat diet or a low carbohydrate diet. All individuals were followed for six months. Data summaries are given in Exhibit 2. The null hypothesis in this example was that the mean weight change was the same in both groups. Statistical software was used to calculate the p-value, 0.0013.

Interpretation: Subjects on low-carbohydrate diet lost more weight than those on a low-fat diet.

	Diet Group	
	Low-Carb	Low-Fat
Number of subjects (n)	64	68
Mean weight change (kg) Post-diet less pre-diet	-5.7	-1.8
Standard Deviation of weight change (kg)	8.6	3.9

Exhibit 3.2: Summary of data in the randomized trial comparing low fat versus low carbohydrate diet.

One Way Analysis of Variance (ANOVA)

Often, it is of interest to compare more than two populations. In such scenarios, two sample unpaired t-tests cannot be performed. One can argue that multiple unpaired tests can be done. For example, if there are three groups, one would need to carry out three unpaired tests. However, if the number of populations to be compared is for example, 6, the researcher will need to carry out 15 comparisons. In the ANOVA testing procedure, multiple populations are compared using a single test.

Suppose the researcher is interested in the relationship between smoking and mid-expiratory flow (FEF), a measure of pulmonary health. He recruits study subjects and classifies them into one of six smoking categories: Non-smokers (NS), Passive smokers (PS), non-inhaling smokers (NI), light smokers (LS), moderate smokers (MS) and Heavy smokers (HS). The outcome variable here is forced mid-expiratory flow (FEF) in litres per second. The null hypothesis is that the mean FEF does not differ across the different smoking groups. The alternative hypothesis here is mean FEF which differs in at least two smoking exposure groups. Data is given in Exhibit 3.

The variation in the sample between groups is compared to the variation within a group. If the between-group variation is a lot bigger than the within-group variation, it suggests that there are some differences among the populations. Using statistical software p-value was calculated as 0.001.

Interpretation: Analysis of variance showed statistically significant ($p < .001$) differences in FEF between the six groups of smokers. Non-smokers had the highest mean FEF value, 3.78 L/s, and this was statistically significantly larger than the five other smoking-classification groups.

Group	Mean FEF	SD FEF	
	(L/s)	(L/s)	n
NS	3.78	0.79	200
PS	3.30	0.77	200
NI	3.32	0.86	50
LS	3.23	0.78	200
MS	2.73	0.81	200
HS	2.59	0.82	200

Exhibit 3.3: Summary data of Mean FEF by smoking exposure

Comparison of Proportions using a Fisher's Exact Test

Categorical data is summarized using proportions. Often it is warranted to compare proportions of outcomes across two or more groups. A Fisher's exact test can be used for making such comparisons and estimating p-values.

Example: Randomised double-blinded, placebo-controlled trial was conducted to measure efficacy and safety of zidovudine (AZT) in reducing the risk of maternal-infant HIV transmission. A total of 363 HIV infected pregnant women were randomized to AZT or the placebo group. Of the 180 women randomized to AZT group, 13 gave birth to children who tested positive for HIV within 18 months of birth. Of the 183 women randomized to the placebo group, 40 gave birth to children who tested positive for HIV within 18 months of birth. Data is summarized in Exhibit 4.

	AZT	**Placebo**	**Total**
HIV Positive	**13**	**40**	**53**
HIV Negative	**167**	**143**	**310**
Total	**180**	**183**	**363**

Exhibit 3.4: Observed data of the randomized clinical trial on prevention of HIV transmission from mother to child

The proportion of infants who tested positive for HIV within 18 months of birth was 7% in the AZT group and 22% in the placebo group. The study results estimate absolute decrease in the proportion of HIV-positive infants born to HIV-positive mothers associated with AZT to be as low as 8% and as high as 22%. The null hypothesis is that there is no difference in the proportion of HIV-positive infants born to HIV-infected mothers in the AZT and placebo groups. The p-value from a Fisher's exact test is < 0.001.

Interpretation: The proportion of infants diagnosed as HIV positive within 18 months of birth was compared between the AZT and placebo groups using a Fisher's exact test. The proportion of infants who tested positive for HIV within 18 months of birth was 7% in the AZT group and 22% in the placebo group. This difference is statistically significant ($p < 0.001$).

CHAPTER

4

Ethics in Biomedical & Health Research

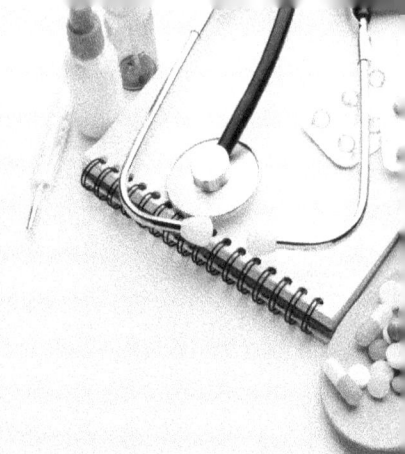

Roli Mathur

1. Introduction

Rapid advances in the last few decades have added complexities to the understanding of ethical issues surrounding medical research. There is a need to raise awareness for better understanding. Biomedical and Health research needs to be done on priority. However, we need to ensure that research is conducted in a manner that safeguards and protects the research participants, builds their trust and overall it is responsive to the nation's needs. There should be no compromises on the scientific aspects to maintain the quality of research outputs. As biomedical research evolves, it also brings forward novel challenges with advancements and newer technologies impacting the need to revisit research ethic requirements.

Studies involving human participants are necessary to improve scientific knowledge and developments in health care. The primary objective of researching humans is to create new knowledge in disease prevention, diagnostics, therapeutics and larger public health goals. As new knowledge becomes available, we need to continually check the safety, efficiency, effectiveness and accessibility of existing regimens or interventions. The social and scientific value of biomedical and health research has to be central. When the need and expected benefits outweigh the risks and burdens of the study then research involving human participants becomes meaningful. The researcher must have adequate knowledge of the ethical, legal and regulatory norms of conducting research involving human participants. Every biomedical and Health research must be suitably aligned with the core ethical principles as per the ICMR National Ethical Guidelines [1].

2. Historical Perspective

Ethics, morality and values are the essential virtues that form the basis of biomedical health research ethics. Historically, one of the earliest mentions of the principles of ethics has been made in Charaka-Samhita as well as Sushrut-Samhita. These ancient Indian scriptures have discussed the moral obligations of medical professionals towards society, the need to have moral standards and to be a humanist [2]. In Western literature, a key concept of the Hippocratic Oath is primarily to 'do no harm' [3]. Unfortunately, the world witnessed numerous inhumane crimes against humanity in the name of human welfare, such as around World War II when unethical and brutal experiments were carried out in many countries such as Germany, Japan and China on the prisoners of war without obtaining their consent.

Further exploitative research studies were conducted for over four decades such as the Tuskegee Syphilis study in which unaware persons were given false promises and not informed about the disease and its available treatment since they were being followed up to understand the course of the disease. They were denied the rightful treatment even after it became available. Following these unethical experiments, a series of guidelines, documents and codes of conduct were prepared and released from time to time by various international agencies and bodies. A few of these codes are the Nuremberg Code, Belmont Report and Declaration of Helsinki by the World Medical Association [4, 5, 6]. Further to this, other international agencies such as the World Health Organisation (WHO), Council of International Organisations of Medical Sciences (CIOMS), United Nations Educational, Scientific and Cultural Organisation (UNESCO), Nuffield Council and others have brought out guidelines for research in specific areas which provide direction on how the research should be undertaken. The International Council of Harmonization - Good Clinical Practice Guidelines (ICH-GCP) provide detailed harmonized standards for ethics committees, investigators and sponsors to conduct clinical trials involving drugs or devices in different countries [7].

These numerous documents, policies and guidelines have discussed the importance of having a framework for the ethical conduct of research to protect human rights, welfare and safety of the participants. They suggest the need for a prior review by an ethics committee comprised of independent members to undertake an unbiased ethics review before any research is conducted. These have further highlighted the need for obtaining informed consent to ensure that the participation is not coerced or forced but is completely voluntary, and the consent is provided by the participants after ensuring comprehension. Even though the fundamental principles remain the same, the ethical guidelines have evolved over the years as and when newer issues come to the fore with emerging technologies and their applications.

3. International and National Guidelines

Every nation should formulate its own ethics guidelines or regulatory framework based on its need and requirements and for the protection of its people. They may adopt the existing International guidance documents or develop their own National Guidelines according to their specific requirements. In India, the Indian Council of Medical Research (ICMR) has been at the forefront in setting up ethical standards needed for biomedical research. In 1980, ICMR prepared the first ethical Guidelines called the Policy Statement on Ethical Considerations involved in Research on Human Subjects. The ICMR has set up a Central Ethics Committee on Human Research (ICMR-CECHR), which functions as the National Ethics Committee to guide its research and develop a National policy and guidelines around emerging ethical issues. Over a period of time, the ICMR ethical guidelines were thoroughly revised to include more details and were published in the year 2000 and 2006. The latest guidelines, the ICMR National Ethical Guidelines for Biomedical and Health Research Involving Human Participants, were prepared and released in 2017. During the Covid-19 pandemic the ICMR came up with additional guidelines for the ethics committees to review research [1, 8]. It prepared a handbook on the National Ethical Guidelines, which is a useful brief guidance relevant to students and Researchers. Further, the Standard Operating Procedures (SOPs) for Emergency reviews by the Ethics Committees, which are not only useful but facilitated research reviews during the pandemic, were prepared. In addition, ICMR has come up with a number of other guidelines and policies, such as Research Integrity and Publication Ethics which discusses in more detail Responsible Conduct of research [9]. The ICMR has also prepared other reports such as Definitions pertaining to End of Life Care and Do Not Attempt Resuscitation Consensus Guidelines, which gives insight into the end-of-life care issues [10]. It has also developed templates for Common Forms to make submissions to ethics committees which are useful in harmonizing the submission to EC and ensuring their completeness [11]. The ICMR is working closely with the Department of Health Research (DHR) to set up a National Ethics Committee Registry for Biomedical and Health Research on the Naitik Portal [12]. After years of efforts, The New Drugs and Clinical Trial Rules, 2019, have made it mandatory for all to follow the ICMR National Ethical Guidelines for any biomedical and health research in India and to register every Ethics Committee with the DHR [13].

4. General Principles

No where in the world can research be conducted on humans, their data or biological material without obtaining ethical clearance. Both national and international guidelines have highlighted the importance of the principles that need to be followed to ensure ethical standards. These are Autonomy, Beneficence & Non-Maleficence and Justice. They are discussed below:

i. **Autonomy** translates into 'Respect' for participants who become part of the research. They must be provided adequate information about the research and given ample time to think and decide about participation. Their decisions should be respected and their participation must always be voluntary and never forced. Special protection has to be given to vulnerable persons who are unable to safeguard their rights.

ii. **Beneficence and Non-Maleficence:** Research has to always be beneficial and never harmful. All human research should follow the principle 'maximize benefits and minimize risk'. Research must have a favourable benefit-risk ratio to be ethically acceptable and steps to minimise the risks should be planned.

iii. **Justice:** This principle deals with the concept of fairness. The researcher designing the research should consider what is just in terms of recruitment of participants and choice of location to conduct the study. There should be no selection bias, stigma or discrimination towards any participant or community. Results or outcomes of research should be shared with the participants.

Autonomy:

Research needs to protect the rights of individuals and respect their preferences. Furthermore, one of the fundamental principles of research ethics is protection of individual autonomy. In order to impart due respect, the ICMR Guidelines no longer refer to persons who join the study as 'Subjects' but have switched to using the term 'Participants', indicating how patients or persons who join the research are equal partners and deserve due respect [1]. The principle of autonomy further necessitates the need for informed consent to respect the individual's rights and facilitate autonomous decision making without any coercion or influence. All research on humans should reflect the respect and concerns given for human rights and welfare of individual participants. The responsibility of protecting research participants rests with all stakeholders involved in the research enterprise, such as researchers, EC members, sponsors and other regulatory bodies. It encourages autonomous decision-making.

Informed Consent

The informed consent process facilitates autonomous decision-making thereby protecting the autonomy of the individual participant. It further requires provisions to be in place to ensure that the research study participants have been provided with relevant information about the nature of research, procedures, outcomes, possible adverse events, etc., and that they have comprehended the same. The purpose of the informed consent form is to disclose and discuss relevant details of the research with the participants. The informed consent process is not only about disclosing relevant information but also about comprehension and understanding of the participants. The researcher must make a meaningful effort to assess the participants' understanding of the research process and appropriately communicate their role as participants.

The informed consent document is signed and obtained from potential research participants by explaining all the relevant information regarding the study. It has to be obtained without any kind of influence or pressure to allow individuals to make informed decisions. It is the responsibility of all stakeholders to ensure that there is voluntariness in the consenting process. When a potential research participant gives consent, he/she acknowledges their participation in a designated role in the study. The informed consent document should especially emphasize that the participation is completely voluntary and that the participants are authorized to withdraw from the study without any negative effects or consequences.

In some situations, the potential participants may not be able to give fully informed consent as in the case of minors or persons with some types of disabilities limiting their decision making. In certain scenarios, researchers may be required to take consent from the Legally Authorized/Acceptable Representatives and prior approval from EC is required for the same. In the case of children, it is important to respect their autonomy and seek assent while the consent may be obtained from the parents or LAR before enrolment. In situations where the potential participant cannot give signatures or thump impression in the informed consent form, the researcher can obtain verbal or oral consent in the presence of an impartial witness with prior permission from the EC [1].

An Informed Consent Form must be prepared in a simple language and manner that a person can easily understand the same. It should have basic elements such as to state that it is a research, mention briefly the purpose of study, explain the methods and procedures involved, inform about the risks and benefits, how confidentiality would be maintained, contact information, provisions for compensation, the voluntary nature of research and possibility to withdraw at any time. It is also important to understand that informed consent process is not a one-time activity of signing a sheet of paper, but a process that is initiated before the research begins and it continues while the research is ongoing and then after the study is completed. There is an ethical responsibility to communicate the outcomes and findings and share the benefits with the participants as far as possible.

Privacy and Confidentiality

Research has to be conducted with sensitivity respecting the private and confidential information of the participants and their family members. An individual's health information is sensitive data and it has to be kept confidential. It is the responsibility of the researchers to safeguard the information from any unauthorized access, disclosure, loss or theft. There should be clarity on how the information will be collected, stored and shared. There should be safeguards to protect the information and ways to protect from any unauthorized access. The participant has a right to determine the extent of their personal information obtained through the study and control the use and manipulation of their sensitive information.

The confidentiality clauses may protect the participant from harm and this responsibility is vested with the researcher/sponsors/research team and all other relevant stakeholders involved in the study. The limitation to ensure fail-proof confidentiality must be explained and also who would be able to access their information or how it will be published must be informed. Research on sensitive topics needs care since any breach may lead to stigmatization or discrimination thereby harming the participants.

Similarly, any identifiable data from a participant cannot be published without prior informed consent from the participant. Biological samples and clinical records should be collected and stored with care. Institutions involved in bio-banking or storing the records and data must have adequate infrastructure to protect against a breach. They should also have defined policies regarding who can access the data/information and how. Research participants' data may be coded or anonymized to maintain privacy and confidentiality. Further, if any identifying information is collected which is required to be shared or published or if leftover samples are stored for future research purposes or sent to bio-banks then specific informed consent would be required [1, 8].

BENEFICENCE & NON-MALEFICENCE

The term Beneficence highlights the need and importance of doing good. In terms of research, it translates to qualities of kindness, helpfulness and humanity, and in general, refers to promoting the good of others to further their important and legitimate interests, often by preventing or removing possible harm. Beneficence is closely aligned with the principle of Non-maleficence, which stipulates the obligation of "first of all, do no harm". The principle of beneficence requires the researchers to use scientific knowledge and protect the participants from harm. On the other hand, the term Non-maleficence is also an inseparable pillar of ethics reflecting upon the duty to not allow any harm to the research participants due to neglect or oversight. Researchers must try to do good and refrain from providing ineffective treatments or acting with malice towards the participants [1].

BENEFIT-RISK ASSESSMENT

Before recruiting participants, a favourable benefit-risk assessment should be ascertained to understand the risks, benefits and the social and scientific value of the research. Primarily every research must have a social and scientific value. The benefits, which could be direct or indirect, must justify the risks, inconveniences, discomforts or harms that may be caused due to participation in the study. These benefits need to be identified and could be direct health benefits such as psychosocial support, counseling or indirect benefits such as care of allied diseases, referrals and others. Any monetary payments or reimbursements are not taken in terms of benefits. On the other hand, the risks or harm could not only be physical related to intervention but also social or psychological, monetary or others. Every study would have inherent risks and efforts must be made to see how these risks or discomforts can be minimized or reduced. Risks can be categorized into less than minimal, minimal, low or high. This categorization is important as it helps to understand the category of risk and if the benefits are enough to cover these risks [1].

The ethical justification for exposing people to risk is the potential individual and community benefits derived from the study. It also helps in adding new knowledge to the field of medicine for the protection and promotion of people's health. The risk-benefit ratio is not a mathematical entity that can be expressed in numbers or as a formula. Rather, it is a conscious judgment and careful assessment of the risks involved and expected benefits based on the available evidence. The researcher has to provide a credible interpretation of available evidence to support their judgment that the study has a positive risk-benefit ratio before submitting the study to the Ethics Committee for approval. The Ethics Committee members further evaluate the benefit-risk ratio and ensure that the risk involved is balanced by the individual benefit from the study. The measures for minimizing the risk for the participants must be balanced with the competing interest of public benefit, scientific value and fair selection. There should be due provisions for addressing the health needs of the participants during the period of research. The risk-benefit assessment is also not a one-time activity but needs to continue when the research is ongoing as there may be altered risks as the study progresses or as new information becomes available or in light of participant's concerns or media reports. All relevant stakeholders including the researchers, sponsors, EC members must rigorously scrutinize the research protocol and look for ways and opportunities to minimize the risk for the participants.

Payments for Participation and Compensation for Research related injury

Payments for participation refer to the reimbursements or other payments in cash or kind to cover the additional research-related costs incurred by the research participants. Offering large monetary rewards or big incentives may pressurise prospective participants to agree to be part of the study. These are called undue inducements or coercion. On the one hand, there should be some provision to cover the costs related to reimbursements wherein these amounts should be reasonable and justifiable and preferably be in kind rather than in cash. Accordingly, researchers must make needful provisions for paying participants for their losses in wages or the cost incurred for transportation or other expenses incurred due to participation in the study or provide them with food during the time spent at the research facility. Any kind of extra payments in cash or kind or as gifts or incentives has to be declared to the Ethics Committees, which would review the same in line with the risk and inconvenience and cost of participation involved to ascertain if these would be ethically appropriate or not. The Ethics Committee needs to further ensure that the study has appropriate budgets and that the amounts to be paid for reimbursement of expenses are reasonable and will not become an undue inducement for participation [1].

Payment of Compensation for any research-related injury is another area which is not well understood or implemented. The ethical requirements for all types of research requires that the research participants be duly protected and institutions involved in the research must build corpus funds or plan insurance schemes to cover the costs related to medical management as well as payment for compensation of research-related injury. The research study must also plan to have dedicated budgets or insurance policies to pay for any medical management that needs to be provided to a research participant if he/she suffers from an injury. Compensation must be paid once the causality is determined and it is found that the injury is related to research. Often it is seen that only pharma-sponsored clinical trials have built-in provisions to pay for medical management and compensation whereas other academic studies, student thesis and investigator-initiated research studies do not have any provisions to pay compensation. Details of provisions made in the study for payment for participation, medical management and compensation for research-related injury have to be submitted to the Ethics Committee for review and approval before the initiation of the study [1, 13].

Conflict of Interest

Conflict of Interest (COI) is said to arise when a secondary judgment unduly influences a primary professional judgment. The primary interest should be research objectives; however, various secondary interests exist such as the need for promotions, fame, awards, publications, monetary incentives, friendships, relationships, power relationships, hierarchy and others that may unduly influence decisions. An independent observer may reasonably believe that the professional judgement is biased in the presence of Conflict of Interest. This COI can be at any level such as a researcher, member of the Ethics Committee or an institutional authority which may pressurize approvals. The existence of COI damages the trust invested in the relationship and affects the research's integrity.

Conflicts of Interest are very common and therefore having a COI does not imply that there is wrong-doing or improper motivation, but it is always imperative to identify the COI, declare it and manage it accordingly. Disclosure is the golden rule and the researcher must disclose their COI that may affect the research, to the EC in a timely manner. The Ethics Committee would deliberate and suggest useful steps to overcome the same. If the COI exists within the EC, the member must leave the room and not be part of decision making, and due recording of this has to be in the minutes. Institutions and organizations must focus on improving awareness about COI by promoting training and education for the students and Researchers. Institutions engaged in research should have a policy on managing COI and this policy must be shared with all the relevant stakeholders.

COLLABORATION

Research is a multidisciplinary enterprise and often requires collaboration at departmental, institutional, regional, National or International levels. This collaboration should be built on the principles of equal partnership, fair agreements and transparent processes to ensure that the fruits of research can be harvested well. Collaborations can have an exploitative potential if the partnerships are on unequal platforms and can cause unnecessary suffering to participants, violate their rights and cause agony among researchers. Collaborative research involving samples or data, sharing, analysis and publications must follow transparent procedures outlined in the research protocols and all stakeholders need to be responsible for the outcomes.

Whenever there is sharing of information of participants, samples, clinical data, genomic samples or epidemiological data, there should be clarity on the ownership and custodianship as well as long-term storage. Appropriate Memorandum of Understanding (MoU) or Material Transfer Agreements (MTA), need to be signed. All involved stakeholders need to be accountable and register the research on a public platform such as the Clinical Trial Registry of India (CTRI) [14]. Studies conducted in international collaboration must ensure that the rules of all partnering countries are applicable, respected and followed.

JUSTICE

Equitable Distribution

Justice implies that the burdens and benefits of the research are fairly distributed, and there is equitable distribution ensuring that there is no exploitation of participants at any point of the study. The researchers should not disproportionately focus only on the health needs of a limited class of people, but instead they should strive to address the diverse health care needs of the people across different social and cultural classes or groups. No particular person or group should be stigmatised, targeted or discriminated against. There should be fair processes to ensure that the right people receive the required care and share of benefits.

Protection of the Vulnerable

Special care must be given to ensure that the socially disadvantaged and marginalized populations are not over-represented due to ease of recruitment or by offering them undue inducements. Vulnerable persons need special care, support or protection because of age, disability or risk of abuse or neglect. They are often not in a position to protect their rights and interests and therefore, the Researchers must take due care and protect them from discrimination. It is unjust to selectively recruit those who may be easy targets or who may not have access to research benefits. In the past, groups considered vulnerable were excluded from the studies to protect their rights. As a consequence, the information on diagnosis, prevention and treatment of diseases which affect the particular group was limited. This created serious injustice to the disadvantaged population. The ICMR National Ethical Guidelines state that it is important to recruit persons who are vulnerable if the study would answer their health needs and if there are additional safeguards in place to protect their safety and well-being [1].

New knowledge and information about the disease would benefit society as a whole. It is unfair to intentionally deprive a specific group from the burden and benefit of the Research. Often it is not easy to identify who can be vulnerable. Certain groups of people such as children or pregnant women or tribals or refugees etc can be easily classified. However, certain others are socially or economically deprived or those who are made vulnerable due to the situation or hierarchy such as being a student or subordinate cannot be classified. It is important to adequately protect them when they are made part of the research and the researchers have the responsibility to identify these vulnerabilities and take care to avoid any suffering or hardship.

The Ethics Committee reviews a study and ensures that if the study involves any person or group of people who may be vulnerable, the protocol has built-in provisions to take care of their rights and safety. They may make suggestions for safety measures and the appropriate documentation of informed consent is important. Informed consent in such cases also needs more care and may be done in the presence of the legally authorised/ acceptable representative or the EC may suggest the need for an impartial witness depending on the type of research and the participant group involved.

Community Engagement

Often while planning research, the investigator's main concerns are related to their research objectives and not much focus is given on how to engage with communities that will be involved in the research or how the research should be planned in the best interest of the communities that would be involved. For meaningful research, it is important to keep the interest of the involved participants or the communities on board and tailor the research as per the needs and requirements. There should be plans for good communication to understand the needs and requirements and build relations and trust with the communities involved.

The research should cater to the needs of the groups who participate and the benefits of the research should be translated back to them. For this to happen, meaningful community engagement is crucial. Researchers and the study teams must plan methods to understand the needs and engage with the communities to improve the study design, plan its conduct and implementation. A useful suggestion is to make a community representative a part of the study team if the nature of the research permits so. Similarly, when the Ethics Committees conducts their ethics review, they can invite community representatives as special invitees to better understand their perspectives. This would help in ensuring that the study takes care of the ethical and societal aspects and will be better tailored to find answers to the group's health needs. For certain types of research studies, the Ethics Committee may suggest the formation of Community Advisory Boards which can strengthen the understanding of the community perspective and help in better engagement for meaningful research outcomes [1].

Benefit Sharing & Return of Research Results

All stakeholders involved in a research enterprise have a moral responsibility to ensure that the benefits of the research finally reach the participants. Normally researchers feel that the research ends with a publication. Unfortunately this is not true. The outcomes must go back to the people or there must be channels to ensure public health benefits. In both, clinical trials as well as biomedical and health research, efforts have to be made to have provisions for post-research access of products/benefits to the participants. This requires equal partnerships, ways of encouraging participation and fair distribution of the burden and benefit of the biomedical research.

The research protocol must be designed with careful consideration given to the protection of disadvantaged populations who cannot protect the patient's rights. Upon completion of the research, it is the moral responsibility to ensure its translation to health benefits of the persons or their communities who participated. Researchers must have a priori agreements and plans to provide access to products developed in the research. Similarly, where studies lead to knowledge generation, efforts must be made to communicate the research findings so that the participants are not left in a lurch and unknowing of what happened to the sample or data collected from them. In the event of commercialization of research products or patents or royalties that may be received, it is important to share the same with the people who have contributed their samples or data for the research. These benefits may go to actual individuals who were part of the research or also to the communities or population groups who were involved. Often these benefits may not be direct or monetary but could also be in terms of building infrastructure or providing counseling or better medical care or health care facilities or advocacy and education about health practices, and so on. The idea is to provide benefit in any form to those who have contributed to the research [1].

5. Ethics Committees

An Ethics Committee is an independent group of people with multidisciplinary backgrounds who are responsible for undertaking an ethics review of biomedical and health research before it is initiated to safeguard the rights, safety and well-being of participants involved in the research. They must be competent and trained to review the research and must be independent in their decision-making to ensure robust ethical review processes [1].

Composition

The Ethics Committee is composed of a multidisciplinary group of experts with the primary objective of protecting the dignity, rights, safety and well-being of the participants. The members are drawn from a variety of fields to have a wider perspective that will help protect the interests of the research participants. There are clinicians, basic medical scientists, legal experts, social scientists, ethicists, theologians, philosophers and laypersons from the community whose role is critical as they represent the interest of society. The committee can further co-opt or invite special invitees such as subject experts, community representatives, patient representatives and others who can provide firsthand information to tailor the protocol and informed consent process to suit the best interest of people at large.

Functions

Every research study has to be submitted to an Ethics Committee before it is initiated. The committee reviews the research protocols and ensures that the study is conducted in a manner that it safeguards the rights, safety and well-being of research participants. The Ethics Committee must consider feasible methods of risk reduction, maximize benefits and protect vulnerable persons such as children, pregnant women, the elderly etc., who may be recruited into the study. The Ethics Committee reviews both science and ethics since a study with bad science can never be ethical. Depending on the risk involved, the Ethics Committee decides on the type of review required for the study. The introduction of innovative methods of informed consent, data collection, participant recruitment, etc., is under the purview of the Ethics Committee and prior approval is necessary before its implementation.

The approval of the Ethics Committee is not a one-time process it is also required to monitor the research to ensure that it is being conducted in compliance with the approved protocols. The EC may monitor site visits whenever required to ensure that the research team is carrying out the research as per plan and that the participants are duly safeguarded. Ethics Committee reviews possible modalities for reducing study-related risks and their management. It ensures that there is provision for the management of research-related injuries and measures are taken for risk reduction. It also ensures that the rights, dignity and well-being of the participants are protected throughout the study.

Ethics Committee Considerations

The Ethics Committee looks at all aspects of the research study. They look at its science and social value and how it will be implemented on the ground. They review the selection of participants at the site, facilities, study team qualifications and infrastructure available to support the research. They also look at study related risks to the participants and the possible benefits. The Ethics Committee reviews all the measures taken to protect participant confidentiality, privacy of individuals and safety and security of the stored research data. Inappropriate disclosures or use of data may bring unnecessary hardships to participants. All stakeholders of the study have a moral obligation to uphold the privacy of each participant. In case of any breach or loss of data, the researcher has to inform the Ethics Committee which decides the further course of action depending on the sensitivity of data and potential implications due to the breach.

The Ethics Committee reviews how data is being stored, how it will be used in future and who can access it. Research needs to be conducted by duly qualified people with necessary training and expertise. Ethics Committee requires a declaration of conflicts of interest by researchers and EC members whether financial, academic or personal, and suggest suitable mechanisms for managing the same. Ethics Committee members have also to declare their conflict of interest. They also look at the payments involved in the study and if adequate arrangements are in place to pay compensation in case of research-related injury. The Ethics Committee reviews the process of taking informed consent and ensures the voluntariness of participants. They are also involved in monitoring the implementation of the study on the ground and are wary of any societal concerns, if any. All these functions of the committee need to be supported by an EC secretariat appointed by the institution with adequate staff and infrastructure.

Ethics Committee Registration and Quality Assurance

Ethics Committees have to be competent and timely in the process of review. They must be abreast with national and international guidelines as well as developments that relate to biomedical and health research. Recently, it has become mandatory for the Ethics Committees to be registered with central agencies. Ethics Committees reviewing biomedical and health research must register on the Naitik Portal with the Department of Health Research, Ministry of Health and Family Welfare, and the Ethics Committees reviewing clinical trials need to be registered on the SUGAM portal with the Central Drugs Standards and Control Organisation, under Department of Health, Ministry of Health and Family Welfare. This structure has been created to ensure the Ethics Committees' accountability and to make sure that they have appropriate composition and are functioning as per the national guidelines and regulations. This also helps to ensure that they undertake monitoring of research and thereby safeguard the rights, safety and well-being of research participants. Further to the mandatory registration, provisions are available for participation in Quality Assurance Programs such as by the National Accreditation Board of Hospitals (NABH) to receive accreditation [15]. National and international agencies benchmark the Ethics Committees' performance against set standards to grant them accreditation. This helps to improve quality and be recognised to follow the best ethical practices.

6. Conclusion

Ethical considerations have to be central in the conduct of any biomedical or health research. There is a need to ensure that research is sensitive, more meaningful and tailored to answer the needs of the people and is carried out in a manner that respects their rights and safety. The research needs to work towards uplifting the health and prosperity of the participant as well as the community at large. These considerations help protect the participant's rights and well-being and protect them from unnecessary hardships. For every research, there has to be a mechanism for time-to-time monitoring of the participants' safety and well-being, especially those who are most vulnerable.

Institutions that engage in biomedical research need to make facilitatory provisions to support the ethical aspects of research. Ethical safeguards are required from inception to conduct of research, its actual implementation in the field and also in the follow-up and reporting of Research results, publications and finally in translating the findings for the public good. The participants and care for their perspectives and rights need to be safeguarded at every step. Research ethics is an ever-evolving vibrant and dynamic subject and requires time-to-time updating of guidelines brought out by various agencies. Ethical guidelines help to provide a framework to preserve the integrity of science and safety of participants and must be followed in letter and spirit.

References

1. National Ethical Guidelines for Biomedical and Health Research Involving Human Participants. New Delhi: Indian Council of Medical Research. 12 October 2017. Available from: (http://ethics.ncdirindia.org//asset/pdf/ICMR_National_Ethical_Guidelines.pdf). (Last accessed on 6th January 2022)
2. Mehta, PM, The Caraka Saṃhita Expounded by the Worshipful Atreya Punarvasu, compiled by the Great Sage Agnivesa and Redacted by Caraka & Dṛḍhabala. 1949. Available from: https://archive.org/details/in.ernet.dli.2015.63710/page/n7/mode/2up. (Last accessed on 6th January 2022)
3. Hippocrates, Jones WHS. Aphorisms I in W.H.S. Jones (trans). Hippocrates with an English translation, Cambridge, MA: Harvard University Press; 1959.Vol I. Available from: https://archive.org/details/hippocrates01hippuoft/page/n31/mode/2up. (Last accessed on 6th January 2022)
4. The Nuremberg Code, 1947. In: Trials of War Criminals Before the Nuremberg Military Tribunals Under Control Council Law No. 10, Vol. 2. Washington, DC: US Government

Printing Office; 1949. pp. 181-2. Available from: https://www.loc.gov/rr/frd/Military_Law/pdf/NT_war-criminals_Vol-II.pdf. (Last accessed on 6th January 2022)

5. The National Commission for the Protection of Human Subjects of Biomedical and Behavioural Research (1979). The Belmont report: ethical principles and guidelines for the protection of human subjects of research. Washington (DC): Department of Health, Education and Welfare. Available from: https://www.hhs.gov/ohrp/regulations-and-policy/belmont-report/index.html(Last accessed on 6th January 2022)
6. Declaration of Helsinki: Declaration of Helsinki: ethical principles for medical research involving human subjects. Fortaleza: World Medical Association. 1964, 1975, 1983, 1989, 1996, 2000, 2004, 2008, 2013; Available from: https://www.wma.net/wp-content/uploads/2016/11/DoH-Oct2013-JAMA.pdf. (Last accessed on 6th January 2022)
7. International Council for Harmonisation of Technical Requirements for Pharmaceuticals for Human Use (2016). Integrated addendum to ICH E6(R1): guideline for good clinical practice E6(R2). Available from: https://database.ich.org/sites/default/files/E6_R2_Addendum.pdf. (Last accessed on 6th January 2022)
8. National Guidelines for Ethics Committees Reviewing Biomedical & Health Research During Covid-19 Pandemic; April 2020. Available at: https://ethics.ncdirindia.org//asset/pdf/EC_Guidance_COVID19.pdf. (Last accessed on 6th January 2022)
9. ICMR Policy on Research Integrity and Publication Ethics, 2019; 31 July 2019 Available at: https://ethics.ncdirindia.org//asset/pdf/ICMR_PRIPE2019.pdf. (Last accessed on 6th January 2022)
10. Mathur R. ICMR Consensus Guidelines on 'Do Not Attempt Resuscitation'. Indian J Med Res. 2020 Apr;151(4):303-310. doi: 10.4103/ijmr.IJMR_395_20. PMID: 32461393; PMCID: PMC7371064. Available from: https://www.ncbi.nlm.nih.gov/pmc/articles/PMC7371064/pdf/IJMR-151-303.pdf. (Last accessed on 6th January 2022)
11. ICMR Common Forms for Ethics Review. 7 December 2018. Available from: (http://ethics.ncdirindia.org/Common_forms_for_Ethics_Committee.aspx). (Last accessed on 6th January 2022)
12. Department of Health Research (DHR), MOHFW, Government of India, National Ethics Committee Registry for Biomedical and Health Research (NECRBHR). Available from https://naitik.gov.in/DHR/Homepage. (Last accessed on 6th January 2022)
13. Drugs and Cosmetics Act, 1940, and Rules, 1945, India. Available from: https://cdsco.gov.in/opencms/export/sites/CDSCO_WEB/Pdf-documents/acts_rules/2016DrugsandCosmeticsAct1940Rules1945.pdf (Last accessed on 6th January 2022)
14. Clinical Trials Registry-India. (CTRI) Available from: http://ctri.nic.in/Clinicaltrials/login.php. (Last accessed on 6th January 2022)
15. National Accreditation Board for Hospitals & Healthcare Providers. (NABH). Available from: https://nabh.co/EducationTraining.aspx. (Last accessed on 6th January 2022).

CHAPTER

5 Commonly used Laboratory Procedures

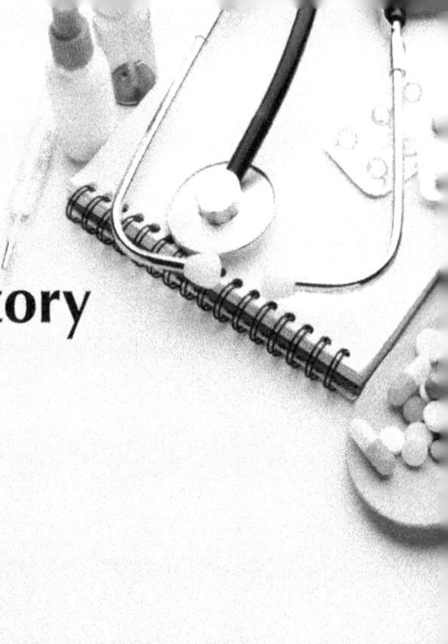

Rita Mulherkar

This chapter describes few of the basic procedures used in the laboratory to study Nucleic Acids (DNA/RNA) and Proteins.

1. Nucleic Acid Based Techniques

Principle

The nucleic acid techniques are based on the property of DNA or RNA to hybridize in a rapid, highly specific, reversible manner to a complementary strand. Double stranded DNA can be denatured at very high temperatures where the two strands separate and can anneal to complementary strands or primers at lower temperatures.

Commonly used laboratory techniques are Nucleic Acid isolation, Restriction digestion of DNA, Polymerase Chain Reaction (PCR), reverse transcriptase-PCR (RT-PCR).

DNA Extraction

Genomic DNA can be isolated from any frozen/fresh/formalin fixed, animal or plant tissue or cell line. A piece of the tissue or cell pellet is taken for DNA isolation. The tissue is initially homogenised and then freeze–thawed in PBS or normal saline to lyse the cells. The tissue can be digested with Proteinase K overnight at 56°C to break all proteins. Cell debris is discarded by centrifugation. The supernatant is added to phenol: Chloroform: Isoamyl alcohol, mixed vigorously, centrifuged and the aqueous phase collected. Phenol removes most of the proteins and chloroform removes lipids and fats. The DNA in the aqueous phase is precipitated with ice cold ethanol and the precipitate rinsed with 70% alcohol to remove residual salts.

For isolating DNA from blood, the following protocol can be followed:

Collect 1 ml blood (with anticoagulant) in a 15 ml centrifuge tube and spin at 10000 rpm (Rota4R) at 10°C for 10 min

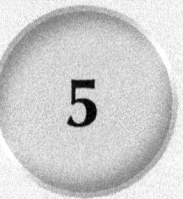

↓

Carefully remove the plasma and collect the buffy coat in a separate 15 ml centrifuge tube. (Some RBCs can be taken so that all white blood cells are collected)

↓

Add 3 volumes of RBC lysis buffer (0.83g NH_4Cl+0.1g $KHCO_3$+0.18ml 5% EDTA make up volume to 100 ml)

↓

Leave on ice for 10 min and mix by vortexing for 5 min

↓

Spin at 10000 rpm for 10 min at 10°C

↓

Discard supernatant and repeat above 3 steps 2x to completely remove any traces of haemoglobin

↓

Re-suspend pellet in 0.2 ml TMK1 Buffer (10mM Tris HCl pH 7.6, 10mM Magnesium Chloride, 10mM Potassium Chloride, 2mM EDTA and 10% Nonidet P-40). Incubate at RT for 5 min.

↓

Spin at 12000 rpm for 10 min at RT

↓

Re-suspend pellet in 200 µl TMK2 Buffer (10 mM Tris HCl pH 7.6, 10mM Magnesium Chloride, 10 mM Potassium Chloride, 2 mM EDTA, 0.4 M NaCl and 10% SDS) and vortex for 5 min

↓

Incubate the suspension at 55°C for 10 min

↓

Spin at 12000 rpm for 10 min at RT

↓

Collect supernatant which contains the nucleic acids and add 100 µl 3M Sodium Acetate. Incubate on ice for 5 min

↓

Add twice the volume of chilled absolute alcohol. Invert the tube few times. DNA strands will be visible. Leave at -20°C for 1 hour

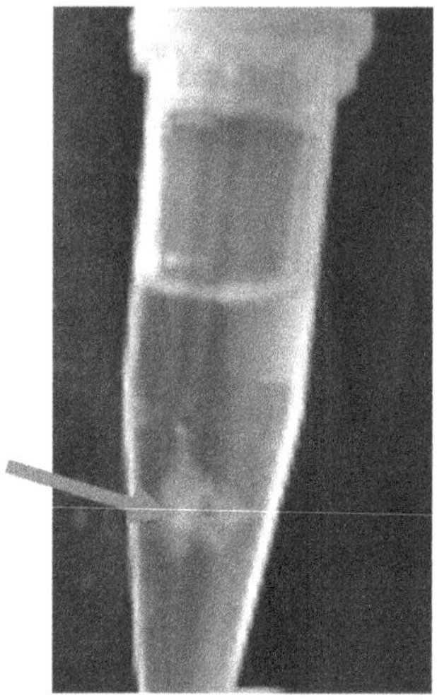

Arrow indicates DNA strands

↓

Centrifuge at 4°C for 20 min at 10,000 rpm. Discard supernatant and add 0.25 ml 70% alcohol and centrifuge at 10000 rpm for 10 min

↓

Carefully discard the supernatant and air dry the pellet. Re-suspend the pellet containing DNA in 50 µl TE (10mM Tris HCl+1mM EDTA). Store frozen until use.

Various DNA isolation kits comprising of spin columns and buffers are available which can be used.

Restriction Enzymes (RE)

RE are commonly used in all molecular biology techniques. They are enzymes found in bacteria which cut double stranded DNA at specific sites. The role of restriction enzyme systems in bacteria is to monitor the origin of incoming DNA and to destroy it if it is foreign. Restriction enzymes are called nucleases. The two types of nucleases are:

- **Exonucleases** which cut the DNA from one end of the molecule. Many of the REs cut specifically either 5' to 3' or in 3' to 5' direction, i.e. they remove nucleotides either from the 3' or from 5' end.
- **Endonucleases** cut DNA in the interior region, reducing them to smaller fragments. They cut within the DNA strand and are therefore called **Restriction Endonucleases.**

RE recognize and cut DNA strands specifically at a particular sequence of nucleotides. The bacterium *Hemophilus aegypticus* produces an RE called Hae III which cuts DNA between G and C (or C and G) wherever it encounters the DNA sequence.

Example of Lambda (λ) phage DNA cut with two RE - EcoR1 and Hind III and run on agarose gel

Place assay buffers and restriction enzymes on ice

↓

Keep the microfuge tube containing sample DNA on ice

↓

Prepare the reaction mixture using following constituents

Reaction 1 (EcoR I digestion)

Lambda (λ) DNA – 20 ul

2X Assay Buffer– 25 μl

EcoRI – 3.0 μl

↓

Reaction 2 (Hind III digestion)

Lambda (λ) DNA – 20 ul

2X Assay Buffer – 25 μl

Hind III – 3.0 μl

↓

Incubate the vial at 37°C for 1 hour

↓

Prepare 1.5 % Agarose gel for electrophoresis by weighing 1.5 gm agarose and making volume to 100 ml with TAE (40mM Tris base+20mM Acetic acid+1mM EDTA) buffer

↓

Melt agarose in a microwave oven, add *Ethidium Bromide (EtBr) to a concentration of 0.5 µg/ml to the gel and pour ~50 ml in a small gel electrophoresis tank. Place the comb in the gel

↓

Allow gel to set. Remove comb carefully and fill the tank with TAE containing *EtBr

↓

Electrophorese the restriction digested DNA sample and DNA molecular weight marker

(Add 5µl gel loading buffer to RE sample & Load 15-20 µl of mixture in well)

↓

Note down the sequence of the samples loaded

↓

Observe the gel under UV Trans-illuminator using protective glasses

*EtBr is a Carcinogen. Care should be taken while handling and discarding it.

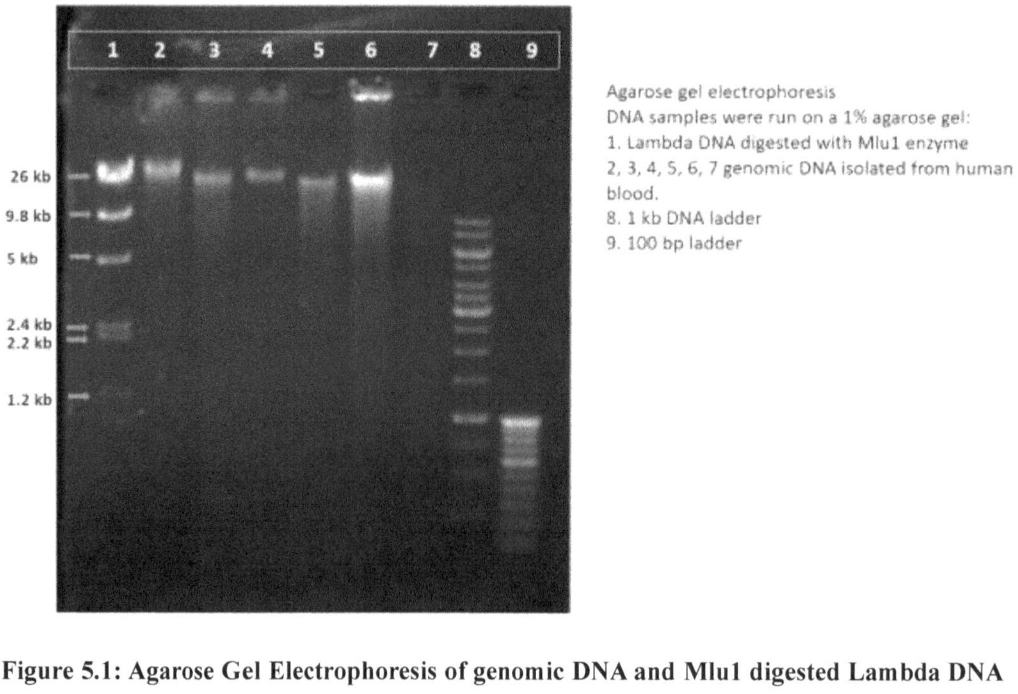

Figure 5.1: Agarose Gel Electrophoresis of genomic DNA and Mlu1 digested Lambda DNA

RNA Extraction:

Care has to be taken while working with RNA since it gets easily degraded due to the presence of RNA degrading enzyme – Ribonuclease which is present everywhere including on human skin surface and dust. Also, by its structure RNA is weaker than DNA. Utmost precautions have to be taken while working with RNA.

For extraction of RNA from tissue, the tissue is generally minced in Guanidium Isothiocynate (GITC) containing mediumvery quickly. GITC is a strong protein denaturing chemical and would inactivate all enzymes including nucleases. Commercially available reagents such as Trizol contain phenol as well as GITC which solubilizes biological material and denatures proteins. Chloroform is added to Trizol containing tissue or cell lysate and spun to give three phases. The aqueous phase containing RNA is carefully collected and precipitated in cold Isoamyl alcohol. Precipitate is then washed with 70% ethanol and dried.

To check the purity of RNA, the ratio of relative absorbance at 260nm/280nm is taken on a spectrophotometer. The ratio should be between 1.7 and 2.1. One unit of absorbance at 260nm is equivalent to 40 µg single stranded RNA per ml. To check the integrity of the RNA, it can be run on an Agarose gel and visualized by Ethidium Bromide staining which should give two prominent bands of 28S and 18S ribosomal RNA when viewed on a trans-illuminator under UV. Intensity of 28S band should be almost double that of 18S band. A smear would indicate degraded RNA.

RNA isolation kits are commercially available from Thermo Fisher, Ambion, Qiagen, etc.

Polymerase Chain Reaction (PCR)

PCR is a powerful tool used in research and diagnostics. By this method specific regions of DNA and RNA can be amplified in a test tube using a Thermal Cycler. One has to design Forward and Reverse primers which are 18-21 bases long oligonucleotides which flank the DNA segment that has to be amplified; deoxyribonucleotides (dNTPs), buffer and a heat resistant DNA polymerase such as Taq polymerase. All these are added to a micro centrifuge tube and the tube is placed in a Thermal cycler which is programmed to repeat cycles of Denaturation, Annealing and Extension at different temperatures. During the cycle of Denaturation, the temperature is set at around 95°C at which the two strands of the DNA template separate. The next step is Annealing where the Forward and Reverse primers anneal to the separated template DNA strands. This temperature is lowered to 50-70°C for the primers to anneal to the DNA. The last step is Extension where the DNA polymerase enzyme extends the primers by copying the template strand. The temperature is set around 72°C. These three steps comprise one cycle and each cycle is repeated 25-30 times so that many copies of the required DNA are made.

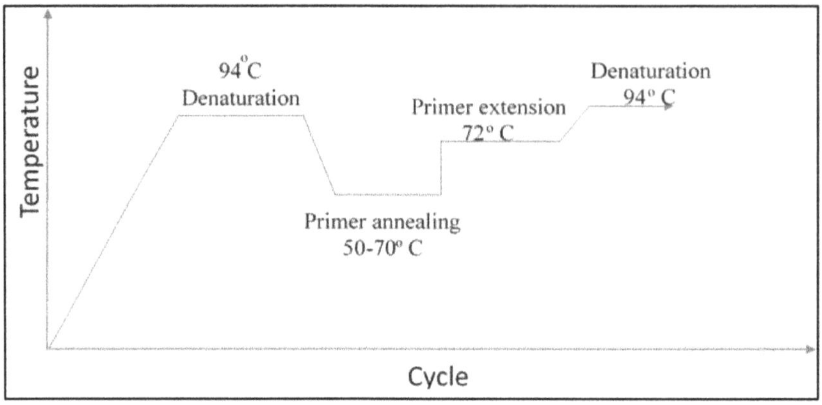

Figure 5.2: Typical Cycle Programme:

The amplified DNA called Amplicon, is run on an Agarose gel along with Ethidium Bromide and checked under ultraviolet light, on a transilluminator. The amplicon can be sequenced to detect mutations in the template DNA or cloned or used for detecting pathogens in a given sample.

Reverse Transcriptase Polymerase Chain Reaction (RT-PCR)

In this technique the RNA is reverse transcribed into complementary DNA (cDNA) using a Reverse Transcriptase enzyme. The cDNA is then amplified by PCR as described above. RT-PCR is useful for detecting RNA viruses as well as for studying eukaryotic gene expression where mRNA is converted into cDNA and further subjected to PCR amplification. RT-PCR is semi-quantitative. For quantitative RT-PCR the technique of real-time RT-PCR also known as qPCR is carried out. The amount of DNA after each cycle of replication is measured using a fluorescent probe such as an interacting dye or a hydrolysis-based probe.

SYBR Green based qPCR

SYBR Green binds to all newly synthesized double-stranded DNA complexes and fluoresces. The fluorescence accumulates after every PCR cycle and is measured at the end of each PCR cycle. The intensity of fluorescence generated by SYBR Green above background level (the Cq value or quantification cycle or Ct Cycle threshold) is measured and used to quantitate the amount of newly generated double-stranded DNA. After repeating the denaturation, annealing and extension cycles approximately 35-40 times, one can start the analysis. The Ct is defined as the number of cycles required to produce a constant emission of fluorescence. The constant fluorescent emission is recorded relative to a defined threshold setting and the cycle number at which the fluorescence generated crosses the threshold is the reaction Ct. The Ct value is used to calculate the initial DNA copy number, as the Ct value is inversely related to the starting amount of target. Ct or Cq values above 40 are generally not accepted.

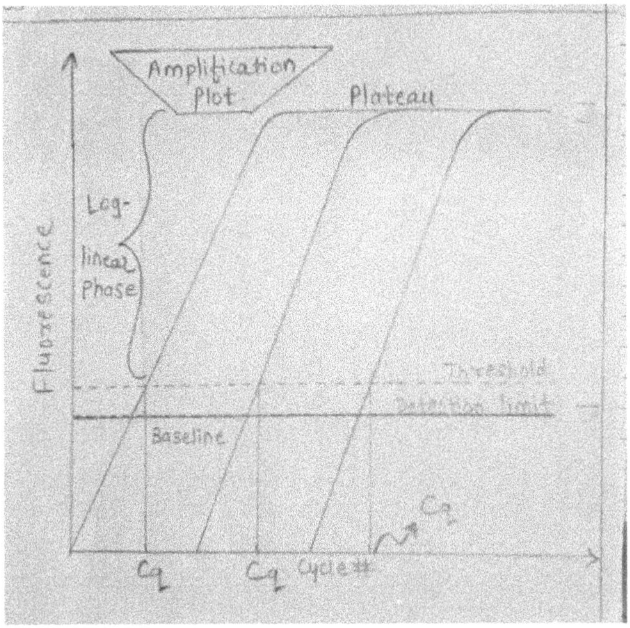

Figure 5.3: A typical Amplification Plot

Amplification plots are fluorescent signal (Y-axis) from each sample plotted against the cycle number (X-axis). Amplification plots represent the accumulation of product over the duration of real-time PCR experiment.

2. Basic Techniques for Studying Proteins

SDS-PolyAcrylamide Gel Electrophoresis

One of the commonest methods for separating small amounts of proteins on the basis of their molecular weight on a gel is by using SDS-PAGE. The gels are made up of polyacrylamide and bis-Acrylamide that results in a cross-linked gel matrix. The gel acts as a sieve through which the proteins move when an electric field is applied. The size of the pores can be regulated by changing the polyacrylamide percentage. High percent gels such as 15% SDS-PAGE gels are used for detecting low molecular weight proteins. Low percent gels such as 8% SDS-PAGE gels are used for detecting high molecular weight proteins. Gradient gels can be used if high and low molecular weight proteins are to be visualised.

Proteins contain an overall positive or negative charge which enables the movement of a protein molecule towards the Isoelectric point at which the molecule has no net charge. The proteins are denatured in the presence of SDS thereby giving them a uniform negative charge. Thus the proteins are separated based on the size as they migrate towards the positive electrode. High molecular weight proteins travel slowly compared to low molecular weight proteins. The protein bands are visualised by staining the gel with Coomassie Brilliant Blue.

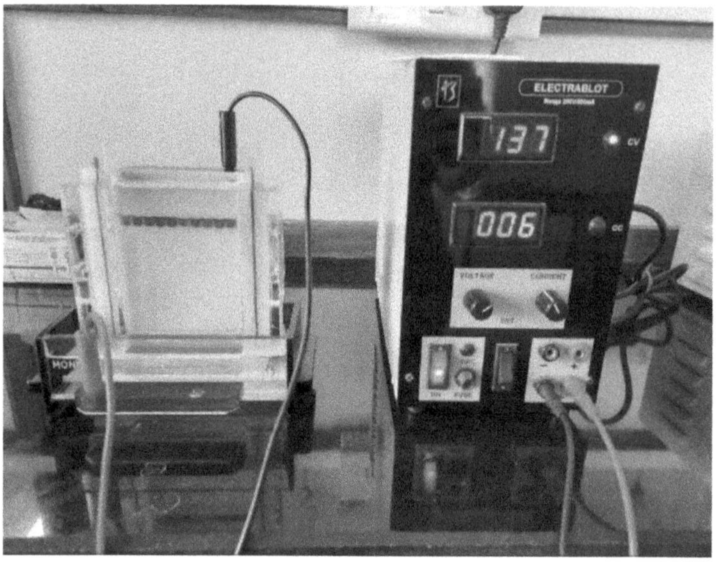

Figure 5.4: SDS-PAGE

Set-up for SDS-PAGE

On the left is the apparatus consisting of two glass plates separated by thin spacers between which the SDS-polyacrylamide gel is poured. After it polymerises, it is placed between two buffer tanks one at the top and one at the bottom. The protein samples are loaded in wells (seen in blue). A current is applied such that it flows from anode (black) to cathode (red) connected to a power supply on the right. After the blue dye reaches the bottom of the gel, the run is stopped, the gel is removed from between the two glass plates and fixed in methanol:acetic acid:water (5:1:4) and then stained with Coomassie Blue R-250.

Western Blotting:

In order to identify the proteins, specific antibodies can be used against the protein of interest and the protein developed by using a chromogen. The most common chromogen used for western blots is DAB (3, 3′ Diaminobenzidine Tetrahydrochloride. This is a carcinogen and should be used safely) which gives a brown colour when acted upon by the enzyme Horseradish peroxidase. The proteins run on SDS-PAGE are transferred to a Nitrocellulose paper and processed for staining with specific antibodies.

A brief protocol for western blotting is given below:

After the proteins are separated on a SDS-PAGE gel as described above, the gel is removed carefully with gloved hands

↓

The gel is briefly rinsed in distilled H2O and placed in Transfer Buffer (25mM TRIS, 190mM Glycine, 20% Methanol) for 30 min

↓

Prepare a sandwich to be placed in the Trans- blot apparatus by soaking 3MM filter papers and nitrocellulose membrane (all cut to the size of the gel) and the sponges in Transfer Buffer

↓

Assemble the sandwich carefully in the gel holder cassette by placing the sponge, followed by the filter paper, gel, nitrocellulose membrane, filter paper, sponge. Close the cassette and place it such that the membrane is on the cathode side and gel on the anode side.

↓

Place the cassette in the trans-blot apparatus. Fill the tank with transfer buffer and connect to a power pack

↓

Run overnight in a cold room at a constant current of 10mAmp

↓

Remove the cassette and carefully remove the membrane. Rinse it in water and stain in Ponceau S solution (0.2% Ponceau S in 5% Acetic acid). Photograph the blot

↓

Rinse the blot with tap water to de-stain and seal it in a plastic bag containing 3% BSA or milk powder in Tris-buffered saline with Tween 20 (TBST, 20mM Tris, pH 7.5, 150mM NaCl, 1% Tween20) to block protein binding sites on the blot. Keep on shaker for 1 hour at RT

↓

Incubate O/N at 4°C in antibody containing solution. Wash blot in TBST 3-5x

↓

Incubate in HRP conjugated secondary antibody for 1hour at RT. Rinse 3-5x

↓

Incubate with substrate DAB for a few minutes in dark. Stop the reaction as soon as the bands are visible by washing in TBS

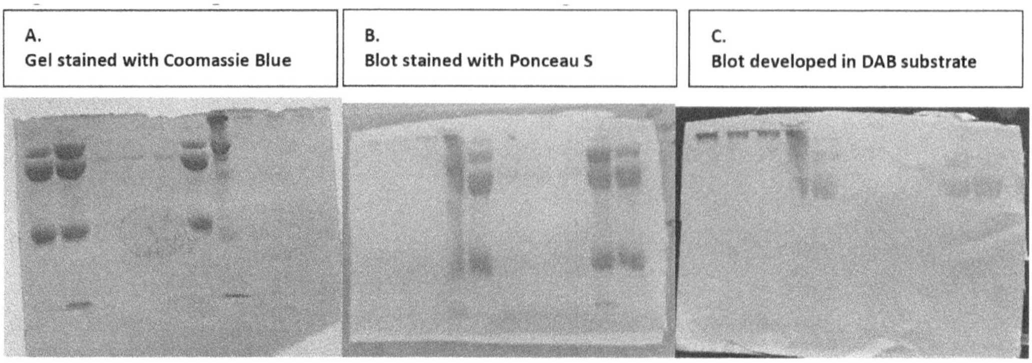

Figure 5.5: Proteins separated on 12% SDS-PAGE gel

A. Gel stained with Coomassie Blue;

B. Mirror image of the gel in A transferred to nitrocellulose membrane and stained with Ponceau S;

C. Blot developed with HRP-DAB.

Antibody against a specific protein was used. Brown bands indicate presence of the protein of interest.

Additional Reading

1. Green MR and Sambrook J. Molecular Cloning: A Laboratory Manual *(Fourth Edition). Cold Spring Harbor Protococ. 2018*
2. Shapiro A.L. et al. Molecular weight estimation of polypeptide chains by electrophoresis in SDS-polyacrylamide gels. *Biochem. Biophys. Res. Commun.* 1967; 28: 815-820.
3. Towbin H, Staehelin T, Gordon J. "Electrophoretic transfer of proteins from polyacrylamide gels to nitrocellulose sheets: procedure and some applications". *Proceedings of the National Academy of Sciences USA*. 1979; 76 (9): 4350–54.

CHAPTER

6 Immunodiagnosis – The Tools

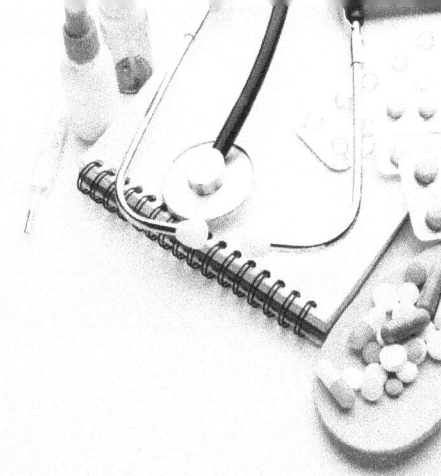

Madhuri Thakar

1. Introduction

Immunodiagnostic is a tool that uses the important and amazing characteristics of an antigen and the antibodies generated against that antigen. Antibodies are molecules produced by our immune cells against antigens (foreign bodies) and have the property of binding to the antigens in a specific manner. This characteristic is referred to as 'Specificity'. The immunodiagnostic tool can use either an antigen or antibodies to diagnose a particular disorder.

The concept of immunodiagnostics was introduced for the first time in 1960 when the antibody against insulin was used to detect insulin in serum samples. Soon after, in the 1970s a second test was developed to detect Thyroxine levels in human blood. Due to the specificity between antigen and antibody reactions coupled with technological advances, immunodiagnosis has become a sensitive, specific and time-saving technology that plays a vital role in understanding and diagnosing various diseases.

Immunodiagnostic tools have wider applications in the diagnosis of infectious, endocrine, and neoplastic diseases as well as measure blood drug concentrations and innumerate lymphocyte populations to diagnose various immunodeficiencies. Over time, immunodiagnostic tools have become simple, cost-efficient, highly sensitive, specific, acquired high throughput capability and have become easy to use in the field. The immunoassays use three factors, the antibodies and antigen-specific to each other and the signal generating system to detect the antigen and antibody complex.

This chapter provides a brief introduction to immunodiagnostic tests, including but not limited to Immunofluorescence Assays, ELISAs, Immunohistochemistry and Flow Cytometry for lymphocyte enumeration.

Table 6.1 details the uses of different immunodiagnostic assays in clinical settings.

Table 6.1: The Immunodiagnostic Tools used for Diagnosis and Measurement of various Biomarkers

Sr. No.	Biomarkers	Testing Principle	Examples
1	Antibodies	ELISA	HIV (Human Immunodeficiency Virus) antibody detection in serum
		Rapid detection using chromatography techniques and flow-through devices	Detection of antibodies in infectious diseases such as HIV, HBV (Hepatitis B Virus), HCV (Hepatitis C Virus) infections Mycotoxin detection
		Rapid detection using agglutination	Widal test for Typhoid fever, Blood Group Test
		Western Blot	Antibodies against different viral proteins for example, HIV infection
2	Antigen	Haemagglutination	HA antigen of Influenza virus
3	Hormones	RIA, ELISA	Luteinizing Hormone, Follicle Stimulating Hormone (FSH), Testosterone Markers for Thyroid function
4	Enzymes	ELISA	Liver Function Test: Serum Glutamic Oxaloacetic Transaminase (SGOT) & Serum Glutamic Pyruvic Transaminase (SGPT)
5	Absolute counts and percentages of Lymphocyte subsets	Flow Cytometry	Primary and secondary immunodeficiencies, Cancer
6	Biopsy Tissues	Immunohistochemistry (IHC)	Detection of malignant cells in cancers

2. Types of Immunodiagnostic Assays

Radioimmunoassay (RIA):

RIA was the earliest immunodiagnostic assay developed in the 1950s. These assays use radioisotopes of iodine, ^{125}I, ^{131}I, or Tritium (^{3}H) as labels to detect the antigen-antibody binding. These assays were one of the most sensitive methods. However, due to safety concerns in handling and disposal of the radioactive reagents, the use of RIAs in clinical laboratories has declined and has been replaced by non-radioactive techniques.

Agglutination

Agglutination is the cross-linking of insoluble antigen with the corresponding antibody which forms a visible lattice or clump. In these tests, the antigen is bound to a surface of particulate material such as red blood cells (RBCs) or latex beads. In the case of RBCs, the reaction is called hemagglutination while in the case of latex beads the reaction is called latex agglutination. In these tests, the antigen absorbed on the lattice must have two antigenic determinants so that it can bind to two antibodies and so on to form a lattice. The Latex Agglutination Test can be easily adapted as a rapid test which can be used in a field or in a facility with minimum equipment. For example, the Widal Test for typhoid and the Regain Test for syphilis.

Viral hemagglutination

In these types of assays, the property of some of the viruses to agglutinate the RBCs by binding to receptors on the RBCs is used to detect the antibodies against that virus. The test is commonly used in the case of Rubella or Influenza virus infections. The modified viral heamagglutination i.e. Viral Hemagglutination Inhibition Tests are used to detect the presence of antibodies in the patient's sample. In this reaction, the antibody inhibits the virus from agglutinating the red blood cells, and no haemagglutination indicates the presence of specific antibodies against the virus.

Enzyme-Linked Immuno-Sorbent Assay (ELISA)

ELISA uses the enzyme-substrate principle to detect either antigen or antibody of interest in the biological samples. In this assay, the antibodies are labelled with an enzyme and in the presence of this enzyme the substrate gets converted into a coloured product, the intensity of which can be measured colourimetrically. ELISA was first employed for the determination of levels of IgG in rabbit serum. In the same year, scientists were able to quantify Human Chorionic Gonadotropin (HCG) in urine by using the Horseradish Peroxidase enzyme. Since then, ELISA has become a routine laboratory research and diagnostic method worldwide. It is very sensitive and is used to detect and quantify substances including antibodies, antigens, proteins, glycoproteins and hormones, even in small amounts of a test sample. Hence ELISA is considered the gold standard of immunoassays. ELISA is a high throughput assay when adapted to the 96 well plate format in which so many samples can be tested at one time. Different uses of ELISA are given in Table 6.2.

Table 6.2: Applications of ELISA

Sr. No.	Application	Example
1	Infectious diseases diagnosis	Infectious diseases: For example, Human Immunodeficiency Virus (HIV), Hepatitis A, B, C
2	Autoantibodies	Antinuclear Antibodies (ANA), Anti-Desmoglein (anti-dsg) etc.
3	Tumour Markers	Prostate-Specific Antigen (PSA) & Carcinoembryonic Antigen (CEA)
4	Disease outbreaks	Cholera, Influenza
5	Past exposures	Lyme Disease, HIV
6	Screening donated blood	Hepatitis B Surface Antigen (HBsAg), Human Immunodeficiency Virus (Anti-HIV) & Hepatitis C Virus (Anti-HCV)
7	Detection of drugs in blood/urine samples	Methamphetamine, Cocaine etc.

Principle of ELISA

To detect the antibodies against a particular antigen (for example, anti-HIV antibodies in the serum samples), the antigens are coated on the bottom of each of the 96 well plates. After incubation, the unbound antigen is washed and the unbound sites are blocked with agents like Bovine serum Albumin or any other animal protein so that unrelated antibodies from the sample would not bind to the well. The sample is then added to the well and the plate is incubated at an ambient temperature of 37°C. If the antibodies against the antigen coated on the plate are present in the sample, those will bind to the antigen fixed at the bottom of the well. Washing the plate will remove all the unbound antibodies, leaving the complex of antigen-antibody in the well.

In the next step, the anti-IgG antibodies raised against the human IgG antibody are added to the well. This antibody is conjugated to the enzyme such as Horseradish Peroxidase (HRP) or Alkaline Phosphatase and is commonly called conjugate. Since these antibodies are specific to the human IgG attached to the antigen fixed to the well, these antibodies bind to the antigen–antibody complex in the well. After washing to remove the unbound conjugate, the substrate specific for the enzyme used in the conjugate is added. The presence of the enzyme converts the substrate into a coloured product, which the naked eye can see and the optical density of the color can be read at the suitable wavelength (usually at 450nm) on a colorimeter, ELISA reader. Figure 6.1 illustrates the principle of ELISA.

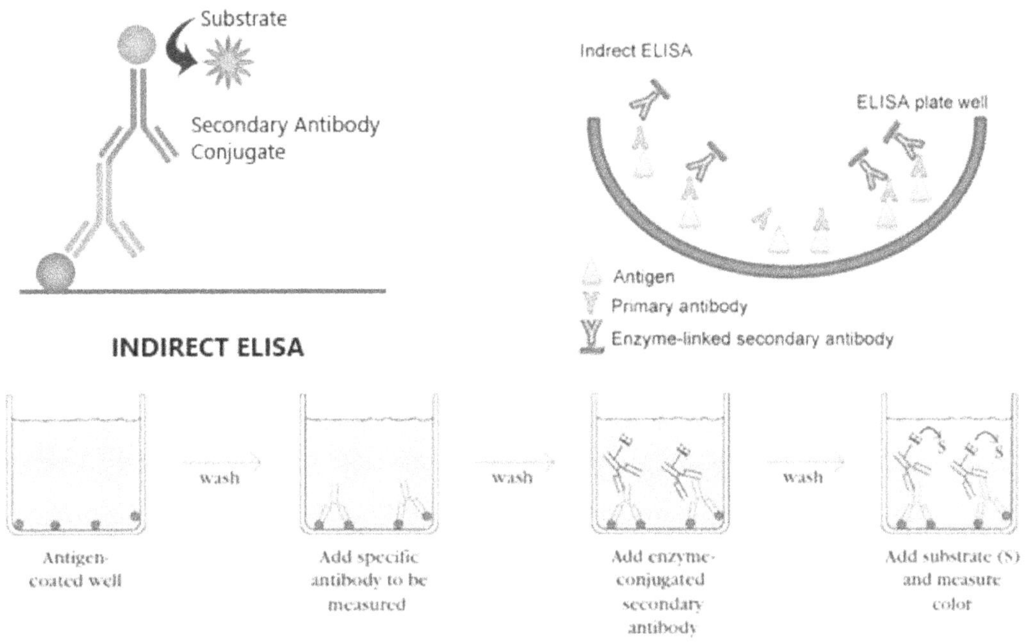

Figure 6.1: Principle of ELISA

Indirect ELISA - Introduction, Steps, Advantages and Protocol. May 22, 2021
https://microbenotes.com/indirect-elisa-introduction-steps-advantages-and-protocol/

This simple principle is modified further to develop different types of ELISAs.

There are four main types of ELISA: Direct ELISA, Indirect ELISA, Sandwich ELISA and Competitive ELISA. Each has unique advantages, disadvantages and suitability.

Figure 6.2: gives the illustrations of different types of ELISAs:

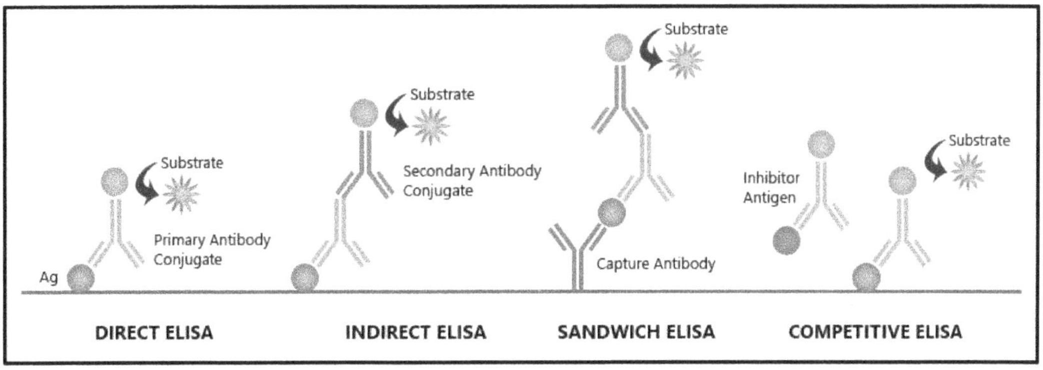

Figure 6.2: Types of ELISA

Source: https://www.bosterbio.com/newsletter-archive/20170728-which-elisa

Direct ELISA

In Direct ELISA, the antigen is immobilized to the surface of the multi-well plate and detected with an antibody specific for the antigen. The antibody is directly conjugated to the enzyme, such as HRP or any other detection molecule. The test can be used to detect both antigens and antibodies.

Indirect ELISA

Indirect ELISA requires two antibodies, a primary antibody (antibody under test) that binds to the immobilized antigen and a secondary enzyme-linked antibody complementary to the primary antibody. As compared to Direct ELISA, Indirect ELISA has a higher sensitivity.

Sandwich ELISA

Unlike Direct and Indirect ELISA, the antigen is immobilized by first using a specific antibody and then the steps of Indirect ELISA are followed. Thus, the antigen is sandwiched between two layers of antibodies (the captured antibody and the antibody to be detected) hence, the name Sandwich ELISA is used. This format is most commonly used in clinical diagnosis. As with other forms of ELISA, this can also be used to detect both antigens and antibodies. In the case of antigen detection, the captured antibody immobilizes the antigen from the biological sample, which is then detected by the conjugated antibody against the same antigen. In this case, both the antibodies should bind to different epitopes (part of the protein) of the antigen to be detected. For example, the ELISAs detect various cytokines from the sample. Sandwich ELISA has the highest sensitivity among all the ELISA types.

Competitive ELISA

As the name suggests, Competitive ELISA uses the competition between two different antibodies; one that might be present in the sample and the other known as specific antibody conjugated to an enzyme to bind to the immobilized antigen. In this ELISA, the higher the binding of the antibody present in the sample, the lower is the colour intensity. The absence of colour indicates a positive test and the presence of antibodies in the test sample. The test format can be modified to detect the antigen in the sample where two antigens, one from the test sample and the other known antigen compete to bind to the labelled specific antibody. Competitive ELISA has low specificity.

3. Nature of Results Obtained from Elisa

The results of ELISA can be quantitative, qualitative or semiquantitative. Quantitative results are obtained by plotting the optical density values against the concentrations of the serially diluted reagent with known concentrations. In contrast, qualitative results give information on whether a particular biomarker is present or absent in the sample. The semiquantitative results compare the relative antigen levels in a sample by measuring the intensity of the signals.

4. Immunofluorescence Test

Although the principle for the Immunofluorescence Test is the same as ELISA, the secondary antibody is conjugated to a fluorescent dye known as Fluorochromes, to detect either antigen or antibody. The intensity and the location of the fluorescence are then visualized using a Fluorescence Microscope. Both direct and indirect fluorescent antibody assays are in use. In the direct method, fluorochromes tagged antibody reacts with the antigen present in the tissue/cell enabling direct detection of antigen in the sample. In Indirect Immunofluorescence method, the known antigen (fixed to a surface: slide, Microspheres etc) is allowed to react with the antibody from the sample. This antigen-antibody complex is visualized with a secondary antibody conjugated to a fluorochrome. Fluorescein Isothiocyanate is the most commonly used fluorochrome in the Immunofluorescence Assay.

5. Lateral Flow Assay

The principle of ELISA is further modified to develop an antibody or antigen detection that can be used for field testing or the testing that can be done at the point of care facility. These tests use the lateral flow device in which the antigen is immobilized on a Nitrocellulose membrane of the sample under testing, followed by the conjugate and substrate which are added in a sequential manner. The results are usually obtained in the form of a coloured spot or a line indicating the presence of an antigen/antibody. Some of the examples are detection of HIV antibodies using a rapid test and pregnancy test. These tests can be used at point of care and require minimal training.

The sensitivity of an immunoassay is an important parameter and is under continuous improvement. The advanced signal generation systems such as Avidin-Biotin Amplification System or the use of Chemiluminescent Substrates have been shown to improve the sensitivity by many folds. These applications require different set-ups and thus become expensive and may reduce the portability of the assays.

6. Chemiluminescent Immunoassays (CLIAs)

In CLIA, the formation of antigen and antibody complexes is detected by the luminescent chemical molecule for eg: Isoluminol. The reaction triggers the emission of visible or near-visible ($\lambda = 300–800$ nm) radiation and the resultant potential energy in the atom gets released in the form of light. The intensity of light is measured on a spectrophotometer or a Luminometer and is directly proportional to the concentration of antibodies present in the sample. The assay can be automated, has high sensitivity, can be modified into multiplex testing (testing a number of biomarkers simultaneously) and can express the result in quantitative terms. Due to all these advantages, CLIAs are becoming popular in clinical diagnosis.

7. Limitations of Immunodiagnosis for antibody detection

Although the serological immunodiagnostic tests are commonly used to diagnose various disease conditions by detecting antibodies, the limitations of these assays should also be kept in mind while interpreting the test results. The first limitation is the presence of lag between the onset of infection and the development of antibodies. Another limitation is that Immunosuppressed patients may be unable to mount an antibody response. In both these situations, false results might be obtained. Also, the presence of IgG antibodies against the pathogen does not necessarily reflect the current infection, it may be a past infection.

8. Flow Cytometry as Immunodiagnostic tool

Flow Cytometry is a technique that uses the principle of immunodiagnostics for the identification of different immune cells i.e. the use of antigen (specific surface markers present on different immune cells) and the monoclonal antibodies raised against the specific surface marker coupled with fluorescent dye. The technique is being used not only to enumerate lymphocyte subsets but also to determine functional and differentiation abnormalities of different cells present in the blood and other tissues.

History

The first-ever Flow Cytometry was developed by Wallace Coulter in 1954. It could measure cell size and count the absolute number of cells. Immunologists started using this instrument with modifications to further identify and study the functions of immune cells. In the 1970s, the hybridoma technology for the development of monoclonal antibodies and the technology for coupling antibodies with fluorescent dyes became available. The use of these technologies along with the Flow Cytometer helped greatly in understanding the differentiation, function and phenotypes of human Lymphocyte subsets at the cellular level and started a new era of immune diagnostics and immunopathology research. This advancement came in handy in the early period of the HIV pandemic, when the appearance of opportunistic infections in previously healthy gay men was rapidly recognized as a cellular immune deficiency and the first human disease characterized by the selective loss of a specific T-cell subset namely, CD4+ T-helper/inducer cell. Flow Cytometry, a research tool until then, was thereafter used increasingly in diagnostic testing at clinical facilities.

Principle of Flow Cytometry

The Flow Cytometer typically includes four components- fluidics, optics, electronics, and computer interface. For analysis of different cells, it is necessary that the information on the surface protein specific to the cell is available. These proteins are known as Cluster of Differentiation or Cluster of Designation (CD). Monoclonal antibodies that identify different CD markers are used to differentiate and analyze different cell types in Flow Cytometry assays of peripheral blood or mucosal samples for clinical diagnosis of various immune disorders.

Table 6.3 gives information on the common CD markers useful in the Flow Cytometry analysis.

Table 6.3: Common Immune cells and their specific CD markers used in Flow Cytometry

Sr. No.	Immune Cells	CD Markers	Disease Diagnosis
1	CD4+ T-Cell (T_H Cell)	CD3+, CD4+	HIV Infection (AIDS)
2	CD8+ T-Cell (T_C Cell)	CD3+, CD8+	Immunodeficiencies like Severe Combined Immunodeficiency (SCID)
3	T_{reg} Cell	CD4+, CD25+, FOXP3+	Immune Dysregulation, Polyendocrinopathy, Enteropathy, X-linked (IPEX) Syndrome
4	Memory T-cells	CD45, CCR7	Common Variable Immunodeficiency (CVID)
5	B-cell	CD3-, CD19+	Primary antibody deficiency
6	Memory B-Cells	CD20+, CD27+	CVID
7	Natural Killer Cell	CD16, CD56	Familial Hemophagocytic Lymphohistiocytosis (FHL-2)
8	Monocyte	CD3-, CD14+	X-linked Agammaglobulinemia
9	Dendritic Cell	CD1c+, CD11c+	GATA2 deficiency
10	Macrophage	CD11b+, CD14+	Crohn's Disease

Figure 6.3 gives a schematic representation of the working of a Flow Cytometer. The cell suspension from the sample (blood, tissue or CSF) is labelled with monoclonal antibodies specific to the CD markers of the cell of interest. These antibodies are tagged with fluorescent dye. The labelled cells are suspended in a stream of fluid known as sheath fluid. This fluid moves through a flow cell in which a beam of light (usually a laser) is focused. As the cells pass through the laser beam (one cell at a time) they scatter the light so that Forward Scatter (FSC) and Side Scatter (SSC) light is captured. The FSC helps to determine the size of the cells whereas, the SSC gives information about the granularity of the cells. Using these two properties, three cell populations of the peripheral blood, viz; lymphocytes, monocytes and granulocytes, can be identified (Figure 6.3).

Additionally, the labelled cells emit light at a wavelength which is detected by fluorescent detectors; photomultiplier tubes (PMTs) convert the detected photons into electronic signals. These signals are captured by the computer interface having analysis software that can analyze the samples for size, granularity and antigen profile of the target cell population. The fluorescent dyes emitting light of different wavelengths can be coupled with antibodies against different CD markers and the combination can be used to perform multi-parametric analysis. One such example of simultaneous detection of CD4 and CD8 + T-cell percentages is shown in Figure 6.3. The Flow Cytometers in clinical use at present can analyze at least four fluorochromes simultaneously in addition to FSC and SSC.

Figure 6.3: Schematic representation of Flow Cytometer process

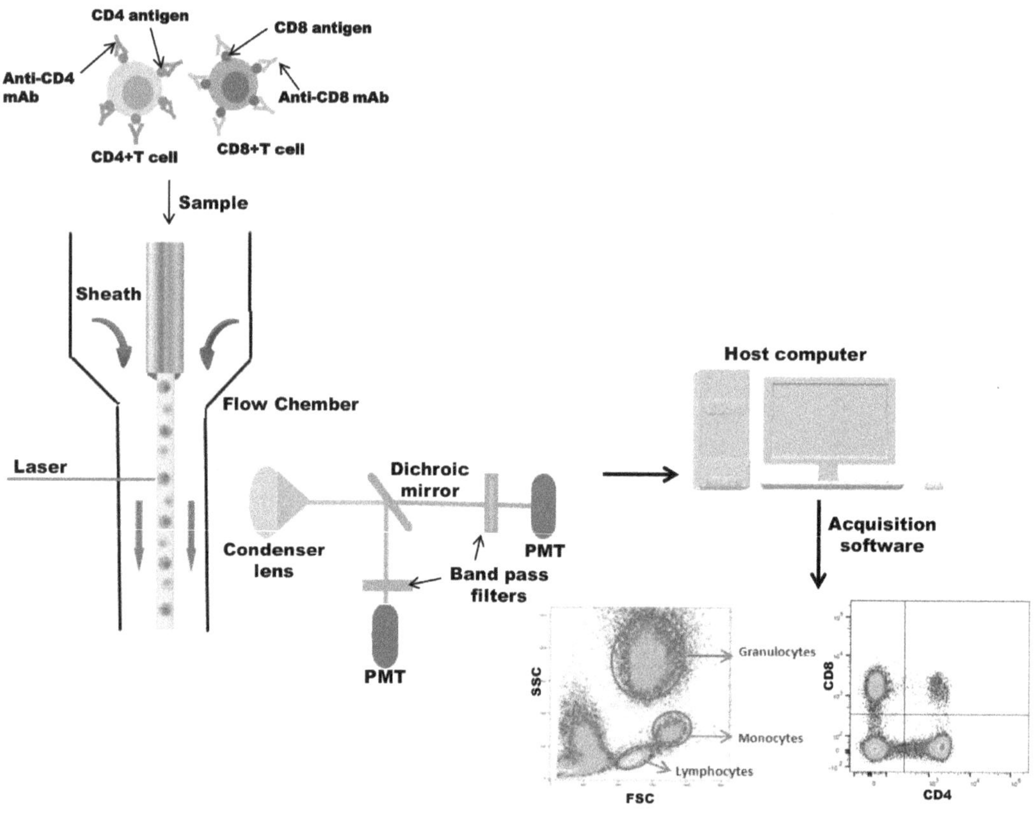

Figure 6.3: is modified from source:

https://adamasuniversity.ac.in/immunodiagnostics-an-emerging-opportunity-in-biotechnology/

Applications of Flow Cytometry

A Flow Cytometry analysis can be performed on peripheral blood, bone marrow aspirate, or cerebrospinal fluid samples. It is important that the single-cell suspension should be prepared for the Flow Cytometry analysis without any visible or invisible micro clots. It should also be kept in mind that only viable cells can be analyzed through this method. The choice of Flow Cytometry diagnostic parameters will depend on the clinical presentation of the patient and the results of basic laboratory tests. For instance, if a defect of adaptive immunity is suspected, then usually a basic lymphocyte phenotyping will be performed followed by some more specific testing (e.g. extended phenotype of B-cells in patients with antibody deficiency). The phenotypic assays investigating the numbers and proportions of immune cells and functional analysis of cellular processes (e.g. proliferation, cytokine secretion, cytotoxicity) can also be performed as per the need of the information based on clinical presentation.

The most frequent use of Flow Cytometer has been to estimate the CD4+ T-cell count in HIV infection for clinical staging of the infection and to determine the efficacy of the anti-retroviral treatment. The technique can be used in primary and secondary immunodeficiencies to assess the qualitative and quantitativeabnormalities in the immune cells of the patients. Flow Cytometry analysis is widely used in the field of cancer to differentiate between the healthy and malignant cells based on various properties. Flow Cytometry is also widely used for basophil testing in allergies in the Basophil Activation Test (BAT). The test measures the presence of activation markers on the basolphils as an indication of allergic response governed by the activated basophils.

Diagnosis of Paroxysmal Nocturnal Hemoglobinuria (PNH)

The diagnosis may be made based on a thorough clinical evaluation, a detailed patient history and Flow Cytometry to identify defective red blood cells showing the absence of GPI-anchored proteins.

Flow Cytometry is a powerful and versatile tool that provides a quantitative assessment of the physical and antigenic properties of platelets thereby, facilitating the diagnosis of inherited or Acquired Platelet Disorders.

Limitations of Flow Cytometry

Flow Cytometry is an expensive and technically demanding technique related to most of the applications. The advent of point of care Flow Cytometers is in use for CD4 count estimations. However, for other applications the standard Flow Cytometry still needs to be used. The protocols are not standardized. Thus, the results suffer in reproducibility and consistency. However, harmonization of protocols, use of commercially available standards for result comparison across laboratories such as calibrated beads, stabilized blood cells and following strict quality control in laboratories are measures that can make Flow Cytometry a more reliable and versatile tool.

The awareness and knowledge about the potential of Flow Cytometry

Clinicians and laboratory specialists should work together to devise a strategy to make the Flow Cytometry tool more useful for clinicians to decide on patient management. Furthermore, understanding the Flow Cytometry research involved in a disease or chronic condition and understanding the laboratory results will allow better patient assistance and education. By overcoming these limitations, the Flow Cytometry technique can provide an accurate estimation of the patients' immune status to the clinicians for better patient management and initiation of immunostimulating therapy.

9. Quality Control in Immunodiagnostics

The results of laboratory tests influence medical decisions and patient care. Therefore, it is very essential that clinical laboratories must ensure that right and accurate results are obtained at the right time and for the right patient. Hence, every clinical laboratory should adopt a Quality Assurance System which comprises of both Internal Quality Control (IQC) and External Quality Assessment (EQA). IQC includes pre-test, during the test and post-test measures to ensure accuracy and reproducibility of the test results. The pre-test parameters include collection of right kind of samples, proper labelling and transportation of the sample from the collection sites. At the laboratory, proper processing of samples as per requirements of the test advised, inclusion of positive and negative controls to assess the validity of the test, monitoring of quality in terms of variation in the values of controls in quantitative tests are important aspects of quality control. The post-test measures include reporting the results in a pre-decided format with all details of the testing.

The additional measures that a laboratory should take are proper maintenance of the equipment, training of staff in all required processes and monitoring the competency of the staff from time to time. The laboratory should also participate in External Quality Assurance (EQA) program provided by external agencies for a particular test. In EQA, the sample is provided by an external agency (usually a national laboratory) to a number of laboratories that process the sample and send the results back to the agency providing the sample. The performance of the participating laboratory is assessed by the EQA providing agency in comparison with the performance of other laboratories. Successful performance in EQA gives confidence to the laboratory and the clinicians.

10. Immunodiagnostics: Requirement of Collaboration from all arms of Healthcare

Immunodiagnostics is an integral part of medical care and scientific research and hence, cooperation and coordination of both the clinical and laboratory facilities is required for appropriate specimen collection, testing, interpretation, diagnosis and effective patient education and treatment planning. The immunodiagnostic assays are improving continuously and information on such tests will further improve the diagnosis and monitoring of infectious diseases in early detection, detection of picogram quantities of antigens and improvement of specificity of the same.

Additional Reading

1. Sheehan, Catherine. *Clinical Immunology: Principles and Laboratory Diagnosis, 2nd ed.*, Lippincott, 1997.
2. Alhajj M, Farhana A. Enzyme Linked Immunosorbent Assay. [Updated 2021 Feb 6]. In: StatPearls [Internet]. Treasure Island (FL): StatPearls Publishing; 2021 Jan-. Available from: https://www.ncbi.nlm.nih.gov/books/NBK555922/

3. Luigi Cinquanta, Desré Ethel Fontana and Nicola Bizzaro Chemiluminescent immunoassay technology: what does it change in autoantibody detection? Auto Immun Highlights. 2017 Dec; 8(1): 9. doi: 10.1007/s13317-017-0097-2.
4. Dawn M. Betters. Use of Flow Cytometry in Clinical Practice. J Adv Pract Oncol. 2015; Sep-Oct; 6: (5): 435–440.
5. Venet F., Lepape A. & Monneret G. Clinical review: flow cytometry perspectives in the ICU - from diagnosis of infection to monitoring of injury-induced immune dysfunctions. *Crit Care* 2011; 15: 231 https://doi.org/10.1186/cc10333.
6. Barnett D., Walker B., Landay A. *et al.* CD4 immunophenotyping in HIV infection. *Nat Rev Microbiol*2008; 6: S7–S15. https://doi.org/10.1038/nrmicro1998.

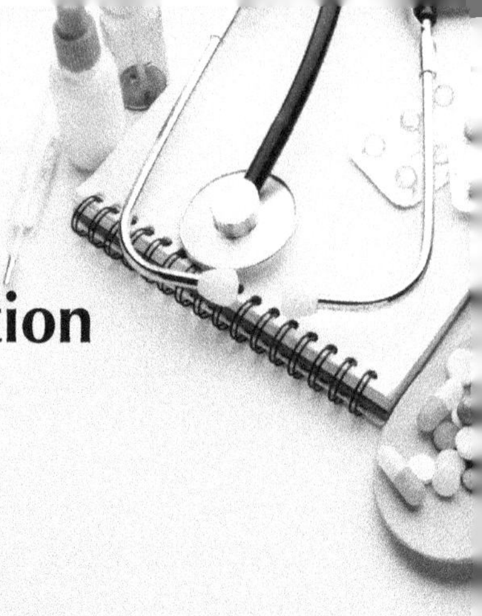

CHAPTER

7

Implications of Information Technology to Medical Research

Avinash Deo

1. Outline

Information technology has revolutionized the storage, access and analysis of information and changed medical research. The earliest impact was felt on the analysis of data through sophisticated statistical methods available on desktop computers. The potential of information technology goes beyond the statistical analysis of biomedical data. Information technology has the potential to affect all aspects of medical research. On one hand it can be used for insights into the structure and function of macromolecules, something that has an impact on drug discovery and preclinical development, and at the other end of the spectrum, it has the potential to improve efficiency of clinical trials making the process of drug development more efficient. An outline of this rapidly evolving field is presented here. Many concepts presented are still hypotheses, some have entered clinical trials, and a few have shown to have clinical implications.

2. Introduction to Information Technology

Data is central to research, wherein it is not only consumed but produces even more data. The amount of biomedical data produced has increased like no other data has, not only in the number of observations recorded but also in the expanse of the data recorded. The optimal use of this data is challenging. Technology has played a major role in the generation of biomedical data. The evolution of technology has made available a range of hardware and software resources that have aided data generation, collection and analysis. These include:

Increased computational power of mobile devices

The transistor count of a microchip doubles approximately every two and a half years. This is accompanied by a reduction in cost and increased power efficiency. These technological innovations have resulted in the development of powerful mobile computing devices that can perform operations that were performed only by large computers at the turn of the century.

Wearable sensor technology

There has been an explosion of wearable sensor technology driven by the wellness industry. Wearable sensor technology has opened up newer ways to collect patient data. Examples include Smartphones, Smartwatches, hearing aids, electronic/optical tattoos, head-mounted displays, subcutaneous sensors, electronic footwear and electronic textiles [1]. Data collection and analysis protocols of the devices need standardization before they can be used for clinical research. The paucity of patient monitoring options during the COVID-19 pandemic provided a push to the use of wearable device data for clinical research.

Availability of reliable high-speed communication

The availability of reliable high-speed communication has led to the evolution of Medical Internet of Things (MIoT). The Internet of Things is a group of objects embedded with sensors and processing ability that exchange data over the internet and other communication systems. MIoT has the potential to generate more data than anything that has ever been done in the past. The connectivity has also allowed the mobile computing device to connect with a powerful server and bring all its power to a mobile device. Operations that are demanding in terms of computing power, like many Artificial Intelligence tools, run on servers using data captured by the mobile device. This has implications on the quality and accuracy of the data collected.

Electronic health record (EHR) and personal health record (PHR)

EHR and PHR are sources of patient information. EHR is the health record entered by doctors. On the other hand, PHR can be generated by a diverse set of sources including physicians, patients, hospitals, pharmacies and others. The entries are controlled by the patient. Laws to encourage the adoption of EHR have been enacted by most countries. Over a period of time, the EHR is expected to become an important source of data for biomedical research.

Cloud computing

Cloud Computing is a term used for the delivery of a variety of services over the internet. The services can include data storage and programs to work with and analyze the data. Cloud storage is centralized storage and makes it easy to share data with multiple users and sites. Cloud Computing brings innovative and reliable services to consumers saving them the cost and burden of maintaining hardware and software.

Artificial Intelligence (AI) tools

Artificial Intelligence programs can be defined as those programs that perform tasks associated with human intelligence like natural language processing, pattern recognition and classification. There has been an explosion in artificial intelligence techniques and today they are used in almost all aspects of biomedical research. They have allowed insights into data that conventional data analytic methods could not.

Natural Language Processing (NLP)

Most medical data is in the form of notes. These notes are not computer-readable and cannot be used for computation. Natural language processing allows the conversion of unstructured medical notes to structured data that can be analysed by a computer. NLP has a potential application at every point where there is a free text record. NLP is a prerequisite to the application of AI tools to free-text data.

Internet and social media

The Internet and social media present unstructured and unconventional data sources in the form of news and patient experiences. If the challenge of harnessing this data can be overcome a lot of real-world experiences could be included in clinical trials. Social media monitoring has potential in Pharmacovigilance [2].

3. Information Technology in Modelling

Mathematical and statistical models play an important role in Medical research, be it clinical trials or predicting chemical structures or interactions between macromolecules. The complexity and usability of such models has increased manyfold by the widespread availability of powerful hardware and the development of Artificial Intelligence techniques for modelling and simulation. Computers allowed the creation of models that were too complex for non-computation methods. Two areas of medical research that have benefited from computer modelling include preclinical drug development and enhancing the power of clinical trials by the in-silico trials.

Preclinical drug development

Drug discovery is an expensive and time-consuming process. Preclinical drug development involves target identification, candidate molecule generation, efficacy, toxicity, and Absorption, Distribution, Metabolism and Excretion (ADME) screens and evaluation of *in vivo* efficacy. AI has a potential role in many aspects of drug discovery, including drug design and synthesis, drug repurposing, prediction of metabolism, drug interactions, off-target effects and adverse effects [3].

Target identification

Target identification relies on the development of models of macromolecular structure and interactions. Our ability to generate such models has been enhanced by Machine Learning. Models generated by Machine Learning are faster and appear to be accurate at least in preliminary studies. Some drugs developed by this method have entered early clinical trials.

Prediction of proteins folding

The 3D structure of proteins is the key to understanding protein function and a critical step in drug development. The traditional methods of determining the 3-dimensional structure were slow and labour intensive. Machine Learning has aided the prediction of 3D structure of proteins. Alphafold2, developed by Google AI DeepMind program, was at least as good as conventional methods at predicting protein folding. The prediction was possible with lower quality data and was faster. The performance was best in the category of "Free Models", where predictions are made for proteins with no related molecule known [4]. DeepMind and EMBL's European Bioinformatics Institute have partnered to create AlphaFold' freely accessible database (https://alphafold.ebi.ac.uk).

While AlphaFold can address the problem of protein folding, it cannot address other aspects of protein structure that have a bearing on protein functions like conformational change in proteins, addressing post-translational modifications and predication of structures as a part of multimeric complexes. Work on these aspects will contribute to the understanding of molecular biology.

In-silico trials

Statistical models can simulate the patient population participating in a clinical trial. These simulations can be used to run multiple virtual trials. Such trials are known as *In-Silico* trials. Randomized clinical trials are expensive, time consuming and often do not test the intervention on a population that is expected to be seen in clinical practice. *In-Silico* trials give an opportunity to test a set of different hypotheses on the clinical trial population. They extend clinical trials to patient sets that have not been adequately represented in a trial [5]. Multiple trials can be rapidly conducted on the same patient population. They are mainly hypothesis generating but can sometimes change practice. An example of this will be the emergence of a drug safety concern in a minority population where other options are available.

4. Information Technology in Data Management

Healthcare data is central to biomedical research. It ranges from clinical data recorded in electronic health records to laboratory data, imaging data, genomic data, insurance claims data and pharmacy prescription data. Wearable devices are a source of real-time data. Computers have increased the ease of data management and allowed the recording, storing and freely sharing of large amounts of data. Technology allows data to be gathered from various sources, but this has complicated data management and created new challenges in using this data for biomedical research. The challenges include capturing data, optimally using this data for conducting clinical trials, storing and sharing this data and evaluating real-world evidence for changing medical practice.

Biomedical data

Biomedical data is different from most other types of data. It is voluminous and complex, making capturing data at the point of care challanging. The process of data capturing comes at the expense of time spent on patient care, and the completeness of data is a casualty of the need to spend more time with the patient. Biomedical data, other than data captured from devices like machines used in the laboratory, is in the form of free text. There are no regulations about the format in which the data should be recorded, resulting in multiple storage formats that make the exchange of information difficult to even impossible at times. This unstructured data is unsuitable for computation and is an important limiting factor for the optimal use of computers in biomedical data analysis. Accessibility of biomedical data is another challenge arising on one hand from lack of central storage and on the other from Data Privacy Laws. Since Data Privacy Laws consider biomedical data sensitive they limit access by third parties. These laws are still being evolved.

Challenges of capturing unstructured data

Information technology can make the recording, storage and analysis of data efficient. Natural language processing has the capacity to generate structured data from free text. Data entry remains a challenge that can be overcome by speech to text engines. A computable phenotype is a clinical condition, characteristic or a set of clinical features that can be determined solely from data in EHRs and ancillary data sources. It does not require chart review or interpretation by a clinician. The term "EHR" broadly refers to data generated through healthcare delivery and reimbursement practices (https://rethinkingclinicaltrials.org/chapters/conduct/electronic-health-records-based-phenotyping/electronic-health-records-based-phenotyping-introduction/). Generation of computable phenotypes need conversion of unstructured data to structured data. Computational phenotypes have a range of application risk predictions, cohort identification and drug adverse effects prediction. It has also been used in predicting defaults in clinical trials.

Use of wearable devices to collect data

The use of wearable devices/sensors for collection of data is an attractive proposition because of its ability to collect real-time data at reduced cost. The use of commercially available wearable devices promoted by the wellness industry is widespread. Sensor technology as well as data collection and analysis protocols are proprietary and not standardized. While they have a potential for clinical trial monitoring and endpoint detection, these need to be validated in clinical trials. Wearable biometric devices are increasingly used to monitor clinical trials [6]. Mobile phones can be used for self-reporting of symptoms. Self-reporting has been used in clinical trials [7].

Real-world data

Real-world Data (RWD) is that data which has been collected from sources other than those used for a traditional clinical trial. These include EHR data generated during routine patient care, data generated by wearable devices and data from internet and social media. RWD is more diverse than clinical data posing challenges for recording, storing and interpretation. As it is generated as a part of routine patient care, no additional cost is incurred. It is available in real-time and does not suffer from collection bias. There are situations where clinical trials are not possible as in the case of rare diseases or drug repurposing, where clinical trial funding is difficult because of a lack of clear financial gains for the sponsor. Real-world data has the potential to generate evidence in such cases.

Real-world evidence is evidence generated by the use of RWD. Real-world evidence guided clinical practice before randomized clinical trials became the standard for evidence generation. These trials derive their power from the statistical model that allows a probabilistic interpretation of differences caused by intervention. Information technology has provided models for a similar interpretation of real-world data using Machine Learning [8, 9].

Acceptable uses of real-world data include post-marketing safety surveillance, hypothesis generation, feasibility assessment, performance improvement, guideline adherence, drug utilization, epidemiological studies (incidence/prevalence), a study of natural history and exploring new risk factors. Pharmacovigilance using real-world data has an advantage since it provides realistic rates of events. Conventional methods only capture what is reported [10].

5. InformationTtechnology in Clinical Research

Randomized clinical trials are the gold standard of evidence generation. Clinical trials are resource intensive and time-consuming. A successful trial needs matching the right patients to a clinical trial, recruiting as many of the eligible patients as possible and ensuring that the trial is completed without protocol violations. Information technology has made or has the potential to make each of these processes efficient.

Patient selection and retention in clinical trials

Recruiting patients for a clinical trial involves matching and incentivizing the patient to participate and complete the trial. The average dropout rate across trials is 30%. Eighty-five per cent of trials experience dropouts. Due to the exponential increase in the number of patients that dropout there is a need to recruit more patients to maintain statistical power. Eighty-six per cent of clinical trials do not meet the enrolment timeline, and about a third of the Phase III trials fail due to challenges of enrolment. The phase III trial accounts for 60% of the cost of developing a drug and efficient enrolment and retention will bring down the cost of drug development [11] and have an impact on access to new drugs.

Patient recruitment

Patient recruitment takes about one-third of the trial duration. A very small proportion of eligible patients are actually enrolled in a clinical trial. About 70% of adults in US were inclined to participate in trials. Over 95% of these patients do not because of unavailability of an appropriate trial. The inefficient recruitment process prolongs trials and also results in the termination of trials.

Recruitment needs to match a patient to a trial and has two components. Firstly, it involves identifying the right patient for the right trial. Computable Phenotypes described above can be used to identify groups of patients with required characteristics. Knowledge about the available trials may be obtained from clinical trial databases or by analysis of non-conventional sources like trial announcements and social medial monitoring. The effectiveness of AI-based clinical trial matching has been successfully demonstrated. [12, 13]

Participant retention, monitoring and protocol adherence

A patient excluded because of protocol violation or dropout not only increases the cost and time taken to complete the trial, but it can also diminish the value of the conclusion. The complexity of clinical trials makes adhering to protocols a challenge. Compliance requires patients to adhere to medication and keep detailed records, a process that can be overwhelming, particularly for those suffering from physically or mentally debilitating illnesses. On an average 40% patients become non-adherent after 150 days into a clinical trial. There are two approaches to use Artificial Intelligence for patient retention.
The first is to identify the participants who are at a high risk of non-compliance and intervene to ensure compliance. Examples of this include:

1. Incorporating an AI platform during the screening period to screen out potential poor compilers could be a valuable tool in mitigating the risks of suboptimal adherence during the treatment phase
2. AI platforms have been shown to increase adherence, rapidly detect non-adherence, and predict future non-adherence in patients with Schizophrenia [14] and anti-coagulation [15]
3. Drug-device combinations like a smart insulin pen, a smart pill or a smart inhaler can monitor compliance [16]
4. Manufacturers are building smartwatch capabilities to detect changes in tremors associated with Parkinson's disease [17]
5. Commercially available wearables have the potential to monitor patients as well as give reminders to take medication and give guidance on how to take it

properly. These applications also facilitate quick and easy access to site support, allowing patients and sites to interact in a way that alleviates questions and stress for the patients [18]

6. Real-time dose measurement can be utilized to dynamically predict medication adherence with high accuracy [19]

The second is to use AI to decrease participant study burden and improve participants' experiences. The approaches include passive data collection, use of NLP for clinical documentation and use of wearable devices.
Monitoring is intrusive and perceived invasion of privacy may be a barrier. The participants also need to be comfortable with technology.

End-point detection and safety signals

Machine Learning, by virtue of its classifying abilities, has the potential in endpoint identification and safety signals. The lack of standard definitions of outcomes makes this task challenging. The potential can only be realized if standard definitions of endpoints are evolved.

Artificial intelligence for missing data

Missing data is common in clinical research. Imputing missing data can use simple methods such as replacing the missing data with means or may use complex methods using Machine Learning [19]. However, the value of imputing missing data using complex methods needs to be determined [20)].

6. Information Technology in Information Management

Biomedical information is voluminous. The National Library of Medicine began publishing Index Medicus in 1879. The advent of computers saw this evolve into Medical Literature Analysis and Retrieval System (MEDLARS) in 1963, MEDLARS onLINE (MEDLINE) in 1971 and PubMed in 1997. The National Biotechnology Information Centre offers access to databases other than PubMed, including those for genes, proteins, associations between heritable DNA variation and human pathology and molecular pathways. There are other repositories of biomedical information.

Information is the key to the design and interpretation of experiments and clinical trials. Given the volume of information, timely access to complete information is a challenge. The traditional methods of dealing with biomedical literature includes reviews, guidelines, systemic reviews and consensus statements that are slow to develop and difficult to maintain.

Artificial Intelligence has been used in coping with medical literature. Some examples include:

Robot analyst

A web-based software system that combines text-mining and machine learning algorithms for organising references by their content and actively prioritising them, based on the relevancy classification model trained and updated throughout the process.

Rapid meta-analysis (RMA)

Meta-analysis and systematic literature review are useful techniques where clear answers do not emerge from clinical trials. These analyses require significant time and effort to produce and are difficult to update. RMA replaced as many manual meta-analysis steps as possible with Machine Intelligence, allowing a faster meta-analysis.

IRIS.AI

This is the search engine that was the first application to address the problem of screening vast amounts of scientific literature using AI.

Information technology has the potential to make research fast, cost-effective and extend the boundaries to areas that were untouched by traditional methods. As technology evolves newer aspects will be addressed. Information technology will have a role in every aspect of research sooner rather than later.

References

1. Yetisen AK, Martinez-Hurtado JL, Ünal B, Khademhosseini A, Butt H. Wearables in Medicine. *Adv. Mater.* 2018: **30**: 1706910.
2. Pappa D, Stergioulas LK. Harnessing social media data for pharmacovigilance: a review of current state of the art, challenges and future directions. *Int J Data Sci Anal* 2019; **8:** 113–135.
3. Paul D, Sanap G, Shenoy S, Kalyane D, Kalia K, Tekade RK. Artificial intelligence in drug discovery and development. *Drug Discov Today*.2021; **26**: 80-93.
4. Callaway E. 'It will change everything': DeepMind's AI makes gigantic leap in solving protein structures. *Nature*. 2020; **588:** 203-204.
5. Wedlund L, Kvedar J. Simulated trials: in silico approach adds depth and nuance to the RCT gold-standard. *NPJ Digit Med*.2021; **4:** 121.
6. Graña Possamai C, Ravaud P, Ghosn L, Tran VT. Use of wearable biometric monitoring devices to measure outcomes in randomized clinical trials: a methodological systematic review. *BMC Med*.2020; **18**: 310.
7. Osborn J, Ajakaiye A, Cooksley T, Subbe CP. Do mHealth applications improve clinical outcomes of patients with cancer? A critical appraisal of the peer-reviewed literature. *Support Care Cancer*. 2020; **28:** 1469-1479.
8. Visanji NP, Madan P, Lacoste AMB, Buleje I, Han Y, Spangler S, Kalia LV, Hensley Alford S, Marras C. Using artificial intelligence to identify anti-hypertensives as possible disease modifying agents in Parkinson's disease. *Pharmacoepidemiol Drug Saf*.2021: **30**: 201-209.

9. Kuang Z, Bao Y, Thomson J, Caldwell M, Peissig P, Stewart R, Willett R, Page D. A Machine-Learning-Based Drug Repurposing Approach Using Baseline Regularization. *Methods Mol Biol.* **1903**:255-267 (2019).
10. Cowie MR, Blomster JI, Curtis LH, et al. Electronic health records to facilitate clinical research. *Clin Res Cardiol.* 2017; **106**: 1-9.
11. Harrer S, Shah P, Antony B, Hu J. Artificial Intelligence for Clinical Trial Design. *Trends Pharmacol Sci.* 2019; **40**: 577-591.
12. Helgeson J, Rammage M, Urman, Roebuck CAM, Coverdill S, Pomerleau K, Dankwa-Mullan I, Liu LI, Sweetman RW, Chau Q, M. Paul Williamson, Michael Vinegra, Tufia C. Haddad, and Matthew P. Goetz. Clinical performance pilot using cognitive computing for clinical trial matching at Mayo Clinic. *Journal of Clinical Oncology* 2018;**36:15_suppl:** e18598-e18598.
13. Alexander M, Solomon B, Ball DL, Sheerin M, Dankwa-Mullan I, Preininger AM, Jackson GP, Herath DM. Evaluation of an artificial intelligence clinical trial matching system in Australian lung cancer patients. *JAMIA Open.* 2020; **3:** 209-215.
14. Bain EE, Shafner L, Walling DP, Othman AA, Chuang-Stein C, Hinkle J, Hanina A Use of a Novel Artificial Intelligence Platform on Mobile Devices to Assess Dosing Compliance in a Phase 2 Clinical Trial in Subjects With Schizophrenia *JMIR Mhealth Uhealth.*2017; **5**,: e18 (2017)
15. Labovitz DL, Shafner L, Reyes Gil M, Virmani D, Hanina A. Using Artificial Intelligence to Reduce the Risk of Nonadherence in Patients on Anticoagulation Therapy. *Stroke.* 2017; **48**:1416-1419.
16. Zijp TR, Mol PGM, Touw DJ, van Boven JFM. Smart Medication Adherence Monitoring in Clinical Drug Trials: A Prerequisite for Personalised Medicine?. *EClinicalMedicine.* 2019; **15**: 3-4.
17. Christie RH, Abbas A, Koesmahargyo V. Technology for Measuring and Monitoring Treatment Compliance Remotely. *J Parkinsons Dis.* 2021; **11**: S77-S81. doi:10.3233/JPD-212537
18. (Koesmahargyo V, Abbas A, Zhang L, Guan L, Feng S, Yadav V, Galatzer-Levy IR. Accuracy of machine learning-based prediction of medication adherence in clinical research. *Psychiatry Res.*2020.; **294**:113558.
19. (Weissler EH, Naumann T, Andersson T, et al. The role of machine learning in clinical research: transforming the future of evidence generation [published correction appears in Trials. 2021 Sep 6;22(1):593]. *Trials.* 2021; **22**: 537.
20. Guo CY, Yang YC, Chen YH. The Optimal Machine Learning-Based Missing Data Imputation for the Cox Proportional Hazard Model. *Front Public Health.* 2021; **9**: 680054.
21. Leurs R, Church MK, Taglialatela M. H_1-antihistamines: inverse agonism, anti-inflammatory actions and cardiac effects. Clin Exp Allergy. 2002 Apr;32(4):489–498.

CHAPTER

8 Preparing Research Proposal to Seek Funds from Public Sector Entities

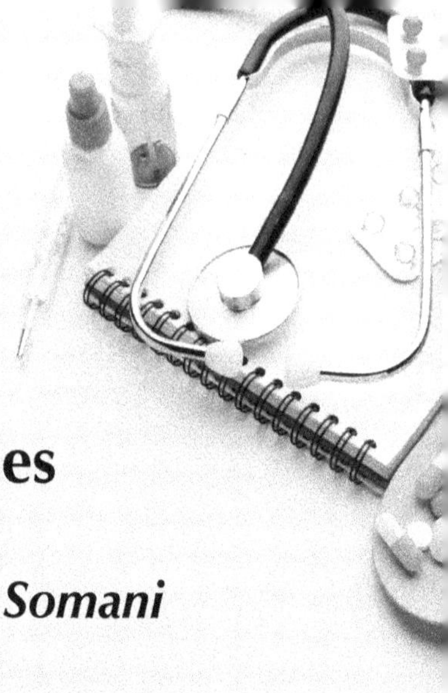

K Satyanarayana and Madhuri Somani

1. Background

It is well known that science and technology (S&T) can improve health, save lives, boost the economy and assure national security. Yet, in India S&T has not been able to match the growth of the economy. With a steady growth rate, India is the fastest-growing economy, poised to become the fifth largest in 2025 and third largest by 2030. Despite the healthy trend in global economic indicators, Indian contribution to global S&T continues to be rather modest. India averaged about 18.0% of total output of global papers (Scopus) during 2014-17 [1-2]. In 2018, it climbed to the fifth spot [1-2], well behind China which was at number 3 with about 28%. Significantly, Medicine was the second-largest contributor in publications from India. The same trend has been seen with the latest Covid-19 publications over the last two years [3]. India's share is a mere 6.7% as compared to 32.5% of the USA and 17.5% of China [3]. Data on new innovations from India are more depressing. The global PCT patent filing by India during 2020 is a mere 2314 (0.1%) as compared to 92032 (26.8%) by China [4].

What is more, India is at a lowly 51 in the Global Innovation Index [5].

However, in the recent past, there has been a new thrust and focus to boost S&T with new policy frameworks and increased funding. The Covid-19 pandemic saw a substantial increase in funding for biomedical research with a fair amount of positive returns. However, productive utilization of the increased funding needs high-quality institutional frame-work and overall ambience to promote innovative research both in the public and private sector entities manned by qualified and competent S&T personnel. Interestingly, unlike in India, globally much of the high-quality Research is done in the academic sector (Universities and Medical Schools) through extramural Research. The USA is an excellent example where a substantial portion of extramural funding is done by the National Institutes of Health, Bethesda primarily to the academic sector. In India due to various factors, including funding constraints, the pool of Researchers is still sub-critical, at least in the medical sector,. To address this critical issue of sub-optimal human resources in the medical/biomedical sector, the ***Moving Academy of Medicine and Biomedicine*** has been striving hard for several years, with fair amount of success. Clearly, more needs to be done both to attract and retain the best young doctors into research, and, more importantly retaining them. A major strategy is to ensure funding for carrying out research, in the formative years. This Chapter on writing a grant proposal aims to help young and middle-level Medical Researchers to seek funding from various publicly funded agencies in India.

The structure and format of the chapter are ICMR-centered for two reasons. Firstly, the ICMR (Indian Council for Medical Research) continues to be a major funder for Biomedical Research in India with a mission to promote Research in Medical Colleges. Secondly, the overall format and structure of the ICMR extramural funding, in our opinion, are quite comprehensive and include almost all major components of a grant application from other agencies. There could be a few agency-specific variations in certain sections. More information and expected commitments from the applicants can be found on the agencies' websites. Also, extensive grant writing guidance is available from various Research bodies [5-10] and others [11-14]).

2. Funding Opportunities in India

All Indian public funding agencies offer Extramural Research support to scientists from Medical Colleges, Universities and other institutions of higher learning in the all public sector and to a large number of private entities and voluntary agencies. The research priorities understandably vary with the agencies' objectives and priorities. Some may encourage projects with immediate relevance, utility and application, while others support any exciting research idea that enriches science irrespective of immediate application. Websites of these agencies can be consulted for more details. Major funding agencies for Extramural Research support in Biomedical Sciences are:

i. Indian Council of Medical Research (ICMR)/Department of Health Research (DHR);
ii. Department of Biotechnology (DBT); and
iii. Science and Engineering Research Board (SERB, DST), New Delhi.

Other agencies like the Council of Scientific & Industrial Research (CSIR), New Delhi, Defence Research & Development Organization (DRDO), New Delhi also offer extramural research support for biomedical research.

The ICMR, one of the oldest medical bodies in the world (Est 1911), offers Extramural Research support to short-term result-oriented projects that aim at filling critical gaps in the Biomedical field (https://main.icmr.nic.in/extramural-ad-hoc). There is also a unique scheme **"Short duration low cost proposals"** from ICMR that is worth a try by new researchers. This scheme has no age limit, focused towards Medical Colleges offering support up to Rs

10 lakh in about a year. This could be a good starter for doctors/ newinvestigators from Medical Colleges who tend to get into research rather late and with a limited publication-based track record.

The total funding by ICMR for a typical extramural project is restricted to Rs 1.5 crore for the complete duration of the project which is three years. The DHR also offers extramural support in some selected areas. Both the ICMR and DHR follow a two-tier web-based Extramural support system requiring the submission of Concept Proposals for review. Only approved concepts are eligible for submission as full-length proposals that are subjected to a peer review system for recommending for funding.

The DBT supports Research in all areas of Life Science with funding from Rs 5 lakh to up to Rs 5 crore, or more. riority areas for support, system of peer review *etc.* are given on its website (https://dbtindia.gov.in/). The SERB, DST encourages research projects in all areas of science and technology with no limit in funding. (http://serb.gov.in/emr.php).

All funding agencies also have periodic *Specific Call for Proposals* (SCP) on topics of relevance and urgency. The SCP is a good system to seek funding as:

i. There is committed funding;
ii. It is limited to a small focused area/priority/expertise; and
iii. Offers quick review with better chances of funding.

However, the SCP typically has a strict timeline for submission.

3. Planning the Proposal

There are a few important elements of any research proposal. These are:

i. The key Research Question;
ii. How it will be investigated (Research Plan or Methodology);
iii. What will be the likely outcome(s), and
iv. Potential impact in terms of new knowledge generated and broader impact/ utility/application for the society.

Project Review Committees (PRC) primarily look at these criteria for decision making with guidance from the funding agency in setting scoring criteria. Good preparatory work is essential before submission of a project. reviewers are flooded with dozens of applications and are often expected to take a call within a limited time frame. With a rather low success rate, it would greatly help the applicant to do a thorough groundwork to avoid getting knocked out in the 'heats'. Nothing can be more irritating for a busy reviewer if the message of why the grant is being sought is not available in one read. Importantly, the PRCs are normally advised to clear only a fraction of submitted proposals simply due to budgetary constraints. If the proposal is unclear in the first glance, chances of positive consideration are seriously diminished. A clear well-organized application with key elements clearly and lucidly articulated therefor is likely to clear the first hurdle with a better chance for support.

For starters, it is always a good practice to prepare a one pager for yourself about the project with the research question/ core research concept, plan of execution, proposed budget and expected outcome *etc.* Once the idea is put on paper, it will help to crystallize thoughts and expand the proposed research idea, set the boundaries and generally serve as a guide in the drafting of the complete grant application. As this 'extended summary' will be used to make the proposal, this write-up could be discussed with your Co-PI and mentor to seek inputs. The need for any collaboration from within or outside the Department and institution can also be decided. This extended summary can be finalized when everyone is on board. It will be good idea to not to share with any outsiders (even those from whom advice/guidance may be sought later) until the draft proposal is finalized). However, the final abstract/summary will be prepared only upon completion of the project preparation.

Where to send the proposal for support is another question that has to be decided at this stage as the objectives, focus, budget sought *etc.*, are agency-specific. For example, the ICMR expects uploading of concept proposals in the same format as the full proposal.

4. Project Format

It is important to know and understand the requirements of a funding agency in terms of format, structure., to plan and prepare according to their requirements. The main components of a proposal for the ICMR are:

i. Title;
ii. Summary/Abstract;
iii. Keywords and Abbreviations;
iv. Background/Introduction;
v. Literature Review;
vi. Novelty/Innovation;
vii. Study Objectives
viii. Methodology;
ix. Equipment & Supplies
x. Expected Outcomes;
xi. Limitations of the Study;
xii. Timelines;
xiii. Institutional Support;
xiv. Bio-data of Investigators
xv. Budget.

There could be minor variations in this format for other funding agencies.

Title

This is the first item read by any reader including the reviewer. It sets the first impression. The Title must be concise yet sufficiently descriptive, informative and catchy. The Title can include, depending upon the type of the project topic, study design viz., observational study, a case-control study or a randomized controlled trial *etc.* It should be descriptive, specific, appropriate and should reflect the importance of the proposal. A good title is usually a compromise between being brief and concise and explicit. If some important words are left out, they can always be included as Keywords.

Summary/Abstract

The purpose of the Abstract/Summary is to briefly describe every major aspect of the Proposed Project. It is read immediately after the title by everyone interested in the project to get the basic premise of the proposal. Typically, the abstract covers:

i. A brief background of the project;
ii. Specific aims, objectives, or hypotheses being tested;
iii. The methodology (action steps) to be used for achieving the objectives;
iv. The significance of the Proposed Research;
v. The unique features and innovation of the project;
vi. Expected results/outcomes; and
vii. How the results will impact other Research areas and/or relevance to public health/national policies.

As mentioned earlier, the Reviewers are chronically short of time (and patience). A well written abstract will catch and keep the attention of the Reviewer creating a positive image. The Abstract must convince the Reviewers that the proposed project is based on an innovative idea, will advance and complement the existing knowledge, be feasible and practical with a credible time-frame for achieving the objectives. The Abstract is typically stand-alone when read with the title. It should serve as a succinct and accurate description of the proposal.

Most agencies set a limit on the size of the Abstract. The ICMR expects a structured summary with sub-heads within 250 words. It is read by all the members of the PRC and grant managers some of whom may not be domain experts. The Abstract is also used in annual reports, presentations and put in public domain. Therefore, the language must be simple and easy to understand with less jargon. The time spent on writing a good Abstract is well worth, if the Proposal is accepted.

Keywords and Abbreviations

Keywords and important terms from the project are required mainly to facilitate search in the database for retrieval. Therefore, it is important that all the key terms that do not occur in the title are included. The ICMR limit for Keywords is six.

A list of Abbreviations must be provided. It is always better to use only standard abbreviations. Else, they must be spelt out at their first appearance. The ICMR limits the number of Abbreviations to a maximum of ten.

Introduction

In a project proposal, in common with a research paper, introduction sets the scene and puts the existing research idea/concept into perspective with the gaps clearly articulated and how this project proposes to fill those gaps. Introduction includes:

i. Rationale for the Research question, adequately supported by literature;
ii. What is already known?
iii. What and how much has been accomplished so far with Research gaps;
iv. How will this project help to fill that gap;
v. Justify why this is the best way and you are the best person
vi. Hypothesis/Novelty of the proposal;
vii. Will this project add new knowledge or push the frontiers of Science;
viii. Potential impact, practice and policy in this area

The Introduction must also convince the reviewers that the applicant(s) have a fair command and expertise over the current status/knowledge in this area and that they are the best people to execute this research. The ICMR limits the Introduction to about 500 words.

Review of Literature

The Literature Review must logically lead from what is known to the current status of the proposed Study. The available scientific evidence/data must be systematically navigated intelligently to help the reviewer to quickly grasp the key arguments related to the proposed study vis-a-vis published information/ data. It is important to convince the Reviewers that despite the plethora of earlier studies, the proposed research question is original and innovative and worthy of support. Literature cited must be very selective with critical appraisal to include only the important works highlighting critical details as relevant to the study proposed. The logical progression must be from the more general to the more focused. Often, historical progression is verbose- it must be summed briefly up with relevant (and recent) references. Review of Literature must be cohesive - not very comprehensive - to finally lead to the objectives and justifications. If there are any controversies they must be addressed in a balanced, objective and dispassionate manner, with relevant papers citing both the support and opposing the proposed hypothesis. Data available, even if preliminary or in pilot studies, relating directly to the Hypothesis could be given. It is important to recognize that the reviewers are chosen on their expertise and knowledge in the area.

It is a good practice to

i. Cite the most recent and relevant Literature;
ii. Papers quoted are balanced with both supporting and critical of the concept being proposed (it is likely that some of those cited could be Reviewers!);
iii. Include only papers from peer-reviewed journals;
iv. Double check for predatory open access journals;
v. Provide URL links and date of access for non-journal material, limited to the bare minimum;
vi. Limit self-citations to only those which are most relevant to the project.

There is usually a word limit and restriction on the number of References cited. The ICMR sets a limit of about 1000 words for a cohesive Literature Review with about 30 relevant publications to be given at the end in the Vancouver Style.

Novelty/Innovation

Every funding agency looks for novel idea(s) in a new project - the quality, currency and significance of the scientific/technical content. The first question that comes to a Reviewer's mind is: "So what is new"? It is therefore important to clearly and unambiguously articulate your research question with a clear plan, focusing on innovation or what is new in the proposal. Novelty sought in a project, just like in a research paper, is near universal. The reviewers could look for at least one or more of the following:

i. Are the proposed concepts, approaches or methodologies or interventions novel to this area alone?
ii. Do they have a refinement, improvement or new application of known theoretical concepts, approaches or methodologies, instrumentation;
iii. Are the interventions proposed known?
iv. Does it address an important problem or a critical knowledge barrier to progress in the field?
v. Will the project significantly advance scientific knowledge, technical capability and/or clinical practice be improved?

A clear justification must be provided to convince the Reviewers that there is something 'new' and 'novel' in your proposal and it is not just another me-too proposal. In other words, proposed Research idea must create some excitement and interest in their minds to coax them to read further.

Some guidance from funding agencies may provide further clarity. The ICMR stipulates that the Novelty/Innovation section must contain:

i. How the proposal challenges and seeks to shift the current Research/knowledge/ clinical practice paradigms etc. by utilizing novel theoretical concepts, approaches or methodologies, instrumentation, or interventions *etc.* indicating if there is a refinement, improvement, or new application of theoretical concepts, approaches or methodologies, instrumentation, or interventions in the proposed study.

To sum up, the project proposal must be innovative within the context of the subject/ discipline. The grant application should not appear to be used merely to enhance the skill-set of the investigators or upscale the infrastructure or merely reinforce a known idea/concept as a follow-up which could yield papers in high impact journals without adding any tangible benefit to the publicly funded research agency's objectives, or to the society.

As per ICMR guidelines, all this should be explained in a maximum of 250 words.

Study Objectives

This section essentially describes what is being tested and/or accomplished in the project. The ICMR expects the applicants to define the Objectives (primary and secondary) in clear and measurable terms. The Council (in fact all funding agencies) discourages projection of too many objectives. Most research projects typically focus on a central hypothesis that is testable, focused, clear and doable. Research questions may be used in place of hypotheses, especially if the proposed work is in the early stages. It is also possible that a working hypothesis is used in place of a central hypothesis. Whatever the concepts are, this section must focus on outcomes as opposed to processes. Some important points could be:

i. Write around each specific objective;
ii. For each specific objective state the expected outcomes, potential problems, if any; and
iii. Propose alternative strategies but if they impact timelines avoid proposing multiple strategies. Stick with the best preferred strategy with strong justification.

Some points may have already been made in the *Introduction/Background.* A brief recap will always help a tired reviewer. Don't propose more work than can be reasonably done during the proposed project period. The objectives proposed **must** match the methodology, expected outcome and budget. No page length is indicated underscoring the importance of the section in the project proposal.

Methodology/ Research Plan

This section describes the Execution Plan of the research question. This is a very important component of the project proposal. The Reviewers need to be convinced that it is the *best* plan to achieve the set objectives. The *Methodology* structure proposed by the ICMR is one of the most appropriate for biomedical/medical research proposals. It includes:

i. Study Design
ii. Sample Size
iii. Project Implementation Plan
iv. Ethics Review
v. Data Collection & Statistical Analysis Plan.

The relative importance/focus of each of the sections could vary with the kind of proposal *viz.*, clinical, epidemiological or basic science project.

Study Design

If well-known standard procedures are to be used, a mere reference should do. In case of deviation and/or for new methods detailed explanation may be provided as to why they are better than the existing methods. If a difficulty is envisaged about the success of the proposed methodology, it must be indicated as to how an alternative procedure can be undertaken to achieve the objectives with an appropriate modified timeline. The ICMR recommends that the proposed study design should be most appropriate/ideal to fulfill the objectives. Details of the study design whether descriptive, analytical, experimental, operational, or a combination of these or any other along with adequate description of the study population should be provided. It is essential to justify the selection of the research participants and controls (human) and whether the subjects will be chosen randomly, consecutively *etc.* For clinical trials, the criteria for inclusion and exclusion of study subjects, definitions of cases, controls and handling of subjects lost to follow up *etc.* must be given clearly. For interventional studies, a detailed description of Intervention (drug/device/behavioral) should be given. These issues have been well laid down in the ICMR Ethical Guidelines.

Whether it is a clinical or basic research project, it is important to clearly articulate the potential difficulties and limitations of the proposed methodology and indicate any measures to be taken to overcome these. Clear articulation of the limitations of the methodology by the investigators will give confidence to the reviewers on the ability of the team for successful and timely execution of the project.

Sample Size

Adequate sample size forms the veryfoundation for reliable conclusions/outcomes of the study. It is therefore essential to indicate in detail how the sample size and/or power calculations are done. If standard procedures are followed they could be mentioned with a reference. If data from earlier pilot/preliminary studies are being used for sample size calculation, necessary documentation/citation must be provided.

All operational definitions for key variables should be spelt out. Often these can be represented through a flow chart indicating the study design with the number of participants in each group etc. It will be good to seek the advice of a competent Biostatistician. In fact, an experienced Biostatistician should form an integral part of the team. It is also important to consult a biostatistician right from the conceptual stage of the project. It is important to recognize that projects rejected on faulty study design are unlikely to be reconsidered.

Project Implementation Plan

This section describes how the overall plan of work proposed will be implemented. In case using human subjects, how will they be enrolled [say from other Department(s)?] with details of the enrolment process within the system of referral. If follow-ups of enrolled participants is envisaged, details of how, when and where will they be followed up should be mentioned. collection, storage and testing of samples must be described along with details for ensuring data confidentiality, safety and security. In case of a collaborative study, it will be good to give detailed responsibilities of clinical collaborators. In case new tests are proposed, the process of standardization and quality assurance Procedures to reliably accomplish the Study Objectives must be provided. Often, based on the proposed time-lines for the execution of the projects, experienced reviewers assess the competence of the investigators for the timely execution of the project.

Ethics Review

It is imperative that the appropriate Ethical Guidelines are followed for the conduct of the project. For studies involving animals, the guidelines prescribed by the CPCSEA (Committee for the Purpose of Control and Supervision of Experiments on Animals) as revised from time to time must be given. In case of studies involving human subjects, it is imperative to follow the ICMR Ethical Guidelines. For human studies, it is essential to obtain and send a copy of the approval of the Institutional Ethics Committee. Details of how Informed Consent is obtained as also the system of documentation should be described along with risks and benefits to the participants [15]. Both the documents are mandatory national policy guidelines for studies involving animals and humans respectively to be clearly indicated in the project proposal to be submitted to any national agency in India.

For projects involving the utilization of genetically engineered organisms (GMOs), it is necessary to submit clearance from the Institutional Biosafety Committee and also commit that the appropriate Biosafety Guidelines of the DBT will be followed. Where field trials/experiments/exchange of specimens, *etc.* are envisaged in the project proposal, it is mandatory to not only follow the relevant rules of the Govt of India but also certify the same in the application. It is also necessary to obtain all other statutory approvals from appropriate authorities before submission of the project and the same must be clearly indicated in the application. [16]

For research using stem cells or use of radiation facilities *etc.* following appropriate regulatory guidelines is imperative and should be indicated in the proposal. Proposals with inadequate and/or incomplete information/compliance on regulatory compliance could well be summarily rejected.

Data Collection & Statistical Analysis Plan

For clinical studies, the plan and tools for collection, compilation and analysis methods as relevant to the project objectives and study design need to be given. Details of all key variables of the study, how will they be measured with units of measurement must be specified. Details of data entry, data storage (data safety), use of analytical platforms and analysis plan must be described comprehensively. The statistical methods to be used in order to answer/achieve the study objectives must be appropriate. Storage and safety of data are important as the ICMR has a Data deposition clause that mandates ".. .. submission (online) of all raw data (along with descriptions) generated from the project to the ICMR Data Repository within one month from the date of completion/termination of the project". For basic research studies, data collection and analysis plan, use of appropriate statistical method must be appropriate to the proposed project.

Equipment and Supplies

If there is a need for expensive chemical/biological equipment, detailed justification has to be given for the same. For chemicals and reagents to be procured, the source (supplier) must be indicated. For reagents that are not commercially available procedures for making them must be detailed. It is important to indicate a reasonable time-frame in case any of the chemicals, reagents, biologicals etc. have to be imported. Often, inexperienced and over-enthusiastic Investigators project impractical timelines which seasoned reviewers notice, causing avoidable embarrassment to the applicant. It will be good to seek appropriate advice from knowledgeable people while formulating this section.

To sum up, only such methods/experiments should be listed:

i. That are directly relevant to testing the Hypotheses
ii. In which demonstrated expertise is available for successful execution of the project
iii. Readily available with the Research Team and/will be procured under the project.

Limitations of techniques must be indicated. Many reviewers opine that the Methodology section truly reflects the depth of expertise and competence of the Investigator underscoring the need to pay attention. Not surprisingly, there is usually no word limit for this section. Methodology forms the heart of the study. A wrong/inappropriate study design/method could lead to unreliable outcome wasting resources and time. There are enough studies that have trashed research conducted over several decades (published in highly respected journals) as worthless due to inappropriate/incorrect study design/methodology.

Expected Outcomes/Potential Significance

Information on the impact of potential significance of the project is important for the funding agency to take a call if the project is not useful for the organization or the country. This short paragraph usually given at the end of the grant application is also obligatory and expected even though some of the information may have been given in the earlier sections as well. This statement provides another opportunity to showcase the scientific importance and (clinical) significance of the project. Some basic research Projects may have a broader impact at a later date which could be mentioned. In fact, funding agencies have clear policies about the potential impact of the proposed research. Some agencies like the DBT and SERB, unlike the ICMR, consider creation and advancement of new knowledge beyond the immediate field or even beyond the research per se as adequate. And significant for support. Writing about the broader impacts is not always easy. A balance has to be struck between being too modest ('proposal too tepid') to over emphatic ('impractical and over-ambitious'). So the lesson is not to overreach but to make a strong but modest pitch and hope the Reviewers are receptive to the idea. This is where mentors can play a role. The ICMR expects a quick wrap-up of the potential significance of the project in about **100** words.

Limitations of the Study

Many funding agencies like the ICMR expect the applicants to mention the Limitations of the study (about 100 words) describing potential difficulties and restrictions of the proposed study methodology and give alternative plans. In fact, it is a good place to honestly indicate the overall Study Limitations. Else, the reviewers can get the feeling that the Investigator is deliberately hiding the potential problems. Clear articulation of the possible weaknesses and/or ambiguities could well prevent potential criticisms by reviewers and may, in fact, "save" the proposal and enhance the credibility of the investigator.

Timelines

All projects are approved by funding agencies subject to the completion strictly within the approved timelines and sanctioned budget. Any delay could result in cost overrun which all funding agencies strongly discourage. It is therefore important to clearly plan at the very beginning. All funding agencies expect the applicants to clearly indicate achievable milestones with a set time-frame. These timelines must be carefully set taking into consideration the work climate in the host institute, approvals for hiring staff, delivery of chemicals and equipment *etc.* Where there are collaborators, they must be consulted to minimize avoidable delays. Bureaucratic lethargy is near universal and one should not fight shy to compute for such a likely procedural delay. Also, one should set aside some time for possible equipment failures, leaving personnel, import procedures *etc.* All funding agencies, being public funded, are very strict about timely submission of annual and final reports, audit statement of accounts *etc.* Investigators and Institutions have even been blacklisted for chronic undue procedural delays in the submission of details of fund utilization and audit statements.

Institutional Support

Here, details about support provided by the institute and collaborators have to be given along with necessary undertakings. For a single Department/Institute Study the Head of the Institute needs to certify providing all promised facilities for the smooth and timely conduct of the project. For projects with more than one Department, clarity on the system of co-ordination must be given with written commitment from all the Departmental Heads. In case where inter- institutional collaboration is proposed, details of coordination must be mentioned along with necessary written commitments. Responsibilities and leadership for execution of each component must be defined as also the governance and organizational structure. The funding agency must be in a position to fix accountability should something go wrong. Clarity is also needed on access to special facilities like computer/data management centers needed for the project. Institutional eligibility and written undertakings are closely examined with funds released only when the funding agency is satisfied.

One important and contentious issue not directly involving the funding agency is authorship of papers emerging from the project as almost all the projects have more than one investigator and more than own Department. If the grant has more than one PI/Co-PI (other than your team) a clear consensus on authorship of possible publications from the project (especially first and last authorship) should be defined before hand. If there is a potential for Intellectual Property (IPR) generation, a written agreement on the mode of IP (patents, copyright registrations *etc.*) ownership, cost sharing on their filing and maintenance, and distribution of the revenue generated *etc.* would greatly help the applicants and the institutions possible conflict at a later stage. The applicants can seek support for IP filing in the Budget section of the proposal.

Bio-data of the Investigators

While the research idea, methodology/plan of Execution, institutional facilities available are important, reviewers often look at the names of the Investigators. Simply put, will this PI (and his/her team) be able to deliver the committed outcome in the prescribed timeline? It could greatly help the not so 'well known' applicants, to give sufficient details about their qualifications to convince the PRC of their competence to successfully complete the study. This typically includes details of qualifications, research experience, record of earlier grants, if any *etc.* and these must be uploaded on the agency's database and an ID for the researcher should be generated. However, the format for seeking Bio-data varies as per the funding agency. The ICMR expects the applicants to upload their bio-data with a list of *all* their publications over a 10 year period. On the other hand, the DBT asks for a maximum of five recent publications relevant to the proposed area of work. The SERB seeks key publications on the theme over the last five years. Care must be exercised in the submission of bio-data as credentials and track record of PI/Co-PI/Collaborators are often critical in funding decisions It is very important to submit a crisp and uncluttered biodata.

For young scientists, submission of a grant application will be a good and useful starting point to build collaborations both within and outside the institute/area of interest. Complementary and integrated expertise is considered prized and will help serious researchers go a long way in ensuring not just successful funding but also in career building.

Budget

This section will give an estimate of the financial resources projected for the successful execution of the project in the given time period. Funding agencies state upfront the maximum amount that can be requested and under what heads. Funds are provided under two main heads - non-recurring and recurring costs. Non-recurring costs include funds for equipment and related infrastructure wherein the funds are typically released at the beginning of the project. Recurring costs include funds towards hiring manpower, travel, consumables (chemicals, disposables, contingencies, travel and outsourcing) *etc.* which are released as per a mutually agreed schedule.

It is important to get a clear idea very early in the writing of the application about the total funds requiredfor timely and successful execution of the project. Budget is best finalized once the grant proposal has been completely developed with consensus among the research team about the proposed budget.. Detailed justification of acquiring new equipment must be given with clear reasons why it cannot be shared, if available within the institute. Details of the consumables/contingencies item-wise and year-wise with some buffer for cost escalation must be given. About hiring personnel, funding agencies have clear guidelines about the type of people to be hired and their salary structure etc. Institutional commitment about their service conditions, continuation and liability after the project must be strictly as per the funding agency's policies. This 'justification' is very important as all funds given out are subject to Govt audit to ensure proper utilization of the tax payers' money. It will be good to seek inputs from the stores/ procurement section of the institute about the costing of chemicals and equipment as the taxation is sometimes complex. Advice from members of the PRC/mentors will be very handy as they will guide on what and how to project convincing demands for equipment and supplies.

Funds sought must be 'reasonable' and not inflated or padded. Funding decisions are typically taken by all members of Project Review Committee along with grant manager(s)..

Any ambiguity, discrepancy or incomplete/incorrect information may mean delay until the next meeting, which may be a year for major queries. It will be good not to ask for items that are not permitted by the funding agency as it exposes the ignorance of the applicants besides causing avoidable delay. Budget is a stand-alone item, independent of the rest of the application so it must be made accordingly. Internal consistency of the budget must be ensured. The numbers must match and be in agreement with what is proposed in the text. A good proposal will have the best match between objectives, timelines, outcome and projected resources (human, equipment, technical support *etc.*).

Budget decisions are always taken at the end once the 'quality' of the proposal has been agreed upon by the PRC. Almost always, budget is pruned in consultation with the grant managers, irrespective of the merit of the proposal as money is always in short supply. Also, almost always the PRC is asked to prune the budget to the bare essentials. Reviewers often have a fair idea of the budget required for projects. Any unreasonable and irrational demand will run the risk of the proposal being postponed to a later date and/or dumped.

For a beginner, it is wise to seek modest funding. Reviewers and grant managers are always impressed with good, simple proposals with reasonable budget.

5. Statutory Requirements/Codal Formalities/Declarations

All publicly funding agencies stipulate certain written, mandatory commitments and conditions to be fulfilled *before* money is released. This is to ensure that:

i. Money is utilized as certified in the project proposal by the Institute
ii. The PI/Institute keep their commitments to the project
iii. There is no liability on the funding agency should there be any violation of laws of India
iv. Research is done as per National/International statutory ethical/regulatory requirements
v. Statutory auditory provisions are ensured.

Details of mandatory declarations sought are available on the websites of funding agencies. Some agencies like the DBT also expect the Head of the University/Institute to declare that the:

i. Research work proposed in the Scheme/Project does not in any way duplicate the work already done or is being carried out elsewhere on the subject; and
ii. The same Project Proposal has not been submitted to any other agency for financial support.

However, the above two conditions are implicit for funding from the ICMR.

6. Writing Process

Clear and lucid applications are highly appreciated (and welcomed) by all readers including grant managers and reviewers. Clarity and brevity are also important as time-starved reviewers may simply ask for resubmission of the proposal with more clarity and brevity. A year could well be lost for an otherwise avoidable reason. In addition, verbose and unclear writing may well reflect muddled thinking. Unless it is an earth-shattering idea, poorly written projects get a poor ranking with likely rejection. therefore, makes tremendous sense to spend enough time to craft a clear, concise and a readable proposal. This is a case where time spent on multiple revisions is well worth. A well written proposal simply enhances the success rate besides leaving a very positive impression of the applicants

It is therefore a good idea to start early, very early, weeks in advance from the deadline. If possible, a good practice is to write every day at a set time stating all milestones till the completion of the project. In fact, most successful scientists keep a rigid, disciplined and organized schedule for writing papers, reviewing projects *etc.* Fortunately, like research papers, grant applications are also structured and therefore allow easy modifications. So, the writing process could be divided between routine portions like Methodology, collaborations, budget *etc,* leaving the tougher parts like objectives, justifications, expected outcomes *etc*., to when the mind is fresh. This will avoid the stress of last-minute rush to meet the deadline. The use of computers allows multiple changes and any number of drafts. It will be a good practice to save all versions, properly labeled as every revision could means deletion/addition of more material.

Sentences should be short, divided into neat paragraphs, logically arranged and always ensuring focus on the theme. Initially, one need not worry about the word limit putting everything on to paper. The second, third and subsequent revisions can help to ruthlessly cut the flab. Use of flow diagrams, figures and tables with appropriate legends of a size that are easily readable will not just improve clarity, reduce monotony and space as well As tables and graphics are stand-alone it must be ensured that the data matches with the text.

For longer projects there could be headings, sub-headings to help readers with easy navigation. It is a good practice to thoroughly check for the set sequence of sections and ensure there is no duplication, typographical errors, mis-spellings, grammatical mistakes or sloppy formatting. It will be a good practice to ask your-co-PI or a dependable colleague to give a critical reading.

It is very important to cite/acknowledge authors of *all* publications consulted and listed under References in the proposal. Besides being a very ethical practice, it minimizes the risk of potential plagiarism allegations. Use of quotations can be avoided: sentences could be suitably paraphrased. When absolutely essential, quotations could be minimally used with quotation marks.

A simple thumb rule for project writing could be: tell them what you are going to tell tell them and repeat what you told them, briefly within the word length set by the funding agency. Grant applications, like research papers, often offer enjoyable writing experience. Finally, if needed, there is no shame in seeking help in the writing, rewriting or editing of the proposal. Good Researchers may not necessarily be the best writers!

7. Responding to Revisions/How to handle Rejection

Three things can happen to a grant application submitted for support:

i. It can be funded as submitted
ii. It can be approved with minor/major changes
iii. It can be rejected with or without reason.

In fact, very few grant applications get approved in the way they are submitted. There are always minor or major revisions suggesting modifications, with pruning of budget being most common. If a major change is suggested which is not to your liking, it could result in anger in view of the time and effort that has gone into preparing the proposal. It is important not react immediately. Keep the letter of the grant manager aside for a day or more. If the comments are read again with a cool mind, you may appreciate that not all the criticisms/suggestions are unreasonable. It is better to take a little time to frame a point-wise response to all the reviewers' concerns. If there is a disagreement, most convincing reasons and explanations can be offered. Even if the comments are irrational and unacceptable, irrespective of the tone, tenor and reasonableness, it does not help to insult or question their wisdom of the PRC. One can always put across the message in a polite but firm way. Besides, bickering often does more harm than good. It is important to understand that the reviewing is anonymous and that the same persons could well be in other committees as well. For a young researcher it is important to develop a support-base rather than enemies. Often, reasoned arguments can help change the mind of even rigid reviewer(s), if put across politely.

Sometimes, there could be a long gap of a few months to a year or more before the final revised version is resubmitted to the funding agency. In case there are important developments that improve the quality and currency of the proposal during this period, these can be included provided it does not substantially alter the content with no change in the budget. This however, has to be clearly spelt out in the cover letter.

With intense competition, rejection of proposals is not uncommon. It is important to understand that 'rejection' is an integral and inevitable part of doing and publishing science. Even papers of Nobel Laureates have been rejected, funding discontinued and/ or denied. There is no reason to lose heart. Competition is fierce, funding is limited and most importantly, grant reviewing is done by our peers who can also err! If you do get a rejection letter, lock it up for a week. If seen again, you may better appreciate the reasons for rejection. It is possible that your project could not make the cut on *that* day.

The best way to handle rejection is to see whether there is scope for improving upon the earlier version in the light of criticisms for possible resubmission. While responding, one need not be overtly defensive: face the criticism head on and respond with facts and reasonable not emotional arguments. If there is no scope for resubmission, just move on and try elsewhere for support. Or just dump the project. Thick skin along with tenacity are essential to be successful. If you cannot swallow rejection easily, it is better not submit proposals, or research papers. It will be good to remember that reviewers often do a a largely thankless and underpaid or unpaid service to science. Good scientists are almost always overburdened, often working in less than/under less-than-ideal conditions – evenings, weekends, holidays, between clinical/ laboratory/teaching commitments *etc.* Learn to be a good loser.

Doing science, to my mind, should be a passion not a job. If there is no passion about the research project being proposed, it is very unlikely that the reviewers perceive the same feeling. Grant writing process should be a pleasure, a means to bounce new ideas to your peers, and demand attention and funds. They may have read your papers; but then papers cannot substitute a good grant application. Papers are after all what happened yesterday and may be work done with others. This grant is tomorrow – the future and *your* future. Grant writing will give an opportunity to char a new course for future. For young researchers it could often be frustrating – bias, delays, bureaucracy *et al.* Yes, me-too science and more worryingly, fashionable science, does get funded occasionally. But then, if you plan to spend a lifetime in science, this is but a passing moment. History tells us that good science *does* get funded, and funded well. And recognized! The only mantra is to keep going and never give up!

Acknowledgement

The authors have immensely benefited from the experience and wisdom of many scientists and grant managers who shared in their experience in the publications and reports included in the paper. We sincerely thank them.

References

1. India's global position rises both in innovations & publications. https://www.pib.gov.in/PressReleasePage.aspx?PRID=1691125 (Accessed on 28 September 2021).
2. S&T Indicators Tables Research & Development Statistics 2019-20. https://dst.gov.in/document/reports/st-indicators-tables-2019-20. (Accessed on September 26, 2012
3. Cai X. Fry CV Wagner CS. International collaboration during the COVID19 crisis: autumn 2020 development. *Scientometrics* 2021; 126:3683–3692.
4. *World Intellectual Property Indicators 2020.* World Intellectual Property Organization, Geneva. https://www.wipo.int/edocs/pubdocs/en/wipo_pub_941_2020.pdf (Accessed on September 26, 2021).
5. India at no. 5 in the world for science research, says new global report. https://theprint.in/science/india-is-now-a-leader-in-scientific-research-says-a-new-global-report/157204/. (Accessed on September 26, 2021).

5. Indian Council of Medical Research. *Guidelines for Extramural Research Programme.* https://main.icmr.nic.in/sites/default/files/extramural/Extramural_Projects_Guidelines.pdf (Accessed on September 6, 2021).
6. *Guidance for grant application.* National Institutes of Health, Bethesda, Maryland https://grants.nih.gov/grants/how-to-apply-application-guide/format-and-write/write-your-application.htm. (Accessed on September 6, 2021).
7. *NIH QUICK Guide For Grant Applications*, 2010. https://deainfo.nci.nih.gov/extra/extdocs/gntapp.pdf (Accessed on September 6, 2021)
8. *A Guide For Proposal Writing*, National Science Foundation Directorate For Education And Human Resources, 2004 National Science Foundation, Virginia, USA.: https://www.nsf.gov/pubs/2004/nsf04016/nsf04016.pdf (Accessed on September 6, 2021).
9. McInnes, R Andrews, B Rachubinski. R *Guidebook for New Principal Investigators: Advice on Applying for a Grant, Writing Papers, Setting up a Research Team and Managing Your Time. 2005.* Institute of Genetics (CIHR-IG), Canadian Institutes of Health Research, Ottawa, Canada.
10. *Guidebook For New Principal Investigators: Advice on Applying for a Grant, Writing Papers, Setting up a Research Team and Managing Your Time.* Canadian Institutes of Health Research, Ottawa, Canada. https://cihr-irsc.gc.ca/e/27491.html (Accessed on September 7, 2021).
11. *The Proposal Writer's Guide: Overview. Research and Sponsored Project,* University of Michigan, Ann Arbor, Michigan, 2014. https://orsp.umich.edu/sites/default/files/resource-download/proposal-writers-guide-final.pdf (Accessed on September 6, 2021).
12. Barrett, E. *Hints for Writing Successful NIH grants. https://cihr-irsc.gc.ca/e/documents/ig_guide_for_new_pis_e.pdf (Accessed on September 9, 2021).* (Accessed on September 6, 2021).
13. Kraicer, J. The Art of Grantsmanship. https://www.hfsp.org/node/5761 (Accessed on September 7, 2021).
14. Bourne PE, Chalupa LM (2006) Ten simple rules for getting grants. *PLoS Comput Biol* 2006; 2(2): e12..
15. *Handbook on National Ethical Guidelines for Biomedical and Health Research involving Human Participants.* 2018 https://ethics.ncdirindia.org//asset/pdf/Handbook_on_ICMR_Ethical_Guidelines.pdf). (Accessed on September 7, 2021).
16. *Proforma for Submission of Project Proposals on Research and Development*, Programme Support. https://dbtindia.gov.in/sites/default/files/Proforma_R&Dnew.pdf. (Accessed on September 7, 2021).

CHAPTER

9 Writing a Research Protocol for Non - Communicable Diseases

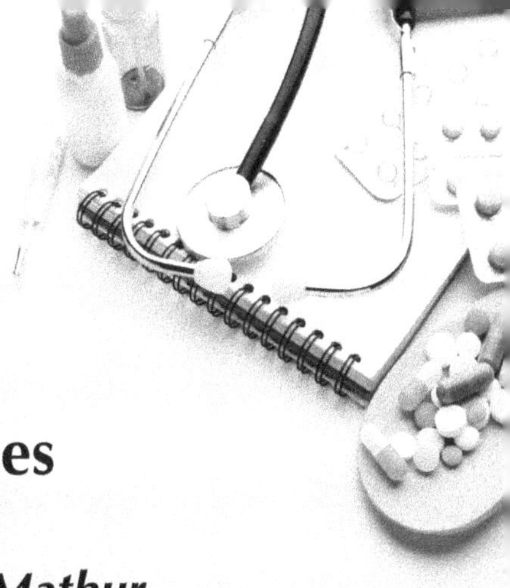

Vani Srinivas and Prashant Mathur

1. Overview

Non-communicable diseases (NCDs), also known as chronic diseases, refer to a group of health conditions such as cardiovascular diseases (CVDs), stroke, cancers, chronic respiratory diseases (such as chronic obstructive pulmonary disease and asthma), diabetes and many more. They have complex aetiology, multiple risk factors, incurability, long latency, and progress relentlessly over the lifetime if unchecked and not treated appropriately. They may result from a combination of infectious, genetic, physiological, environmental and behavioural factors. [1]

They are responsible for substantial morbidity, premature mortality and poor quality of life. NCDs kill 41 million people each year, equivalent to 71% of deaths globally. Each year, more than 15 million people die from an NCD between the ages of 30 and 69 years, of which 77% are in the low- and middle-income countries (LMIC) and 85% are premature deaths [2]. In India, NCDs are estimated to account for 63% of all deaths. In the year 2016, a total of 5.9 million deaths were attributed to NCDs. Approximately 23% of the population in the age group of 30-70 years is at risk of premature death due to NCDs [3].

Rapid globalization, urbanization, increasing exposure to harmful factors, reduced prevalence of protective factors, ageing population along with social determinants are the key underlying causes of NCDs. These expose individuals to modifiable behavioural risks like tobacco use, unhealthy diet, lack of physical activity, alcohol use, air pollution, stress etc.

Over time, increasing proportions of the population (across all age groups) experience overweight and obesity, raised blood pressure and raised cholesterol, which subsequently increase the occurrence of CVDs, diabetes, cancers and chronic respiratory diseases. Fortunately, a large proportion of NCD risk factors are preventable which could reduce the magnitude of related diseases. Most of the common risk factors lie outside the health sector (Figure 9.1) [4]. These require interventions by non-health sectors (agriculture, education, food industry and transport etc.) to control underlying determinants of NCDs. They are established at young ages and progress into and throughout adulthood in the absence of corrective measures taken for their avoidance.

Once the disease is established, for further prevention and control of complications and deaths related to NCDs, a robust health system response in terms of improved coverage, equitable access and quality care is required to manage acute and chronic cases. The Health system and community also need to plan for long term rehabilitation services and palliative care. Thus, chronic disease prevention and control help people to live longer, healthier lives.

To address the huge burden of NCDs, appropriate research is an essential component of NCD prevention and control programs. It can provide evidence on causation, prevention and better clinical management of NCDs. Evidence-based health promotion strategies focusing on children, adolescents and vulnerable populations can significantly reduce the burden in the near future.

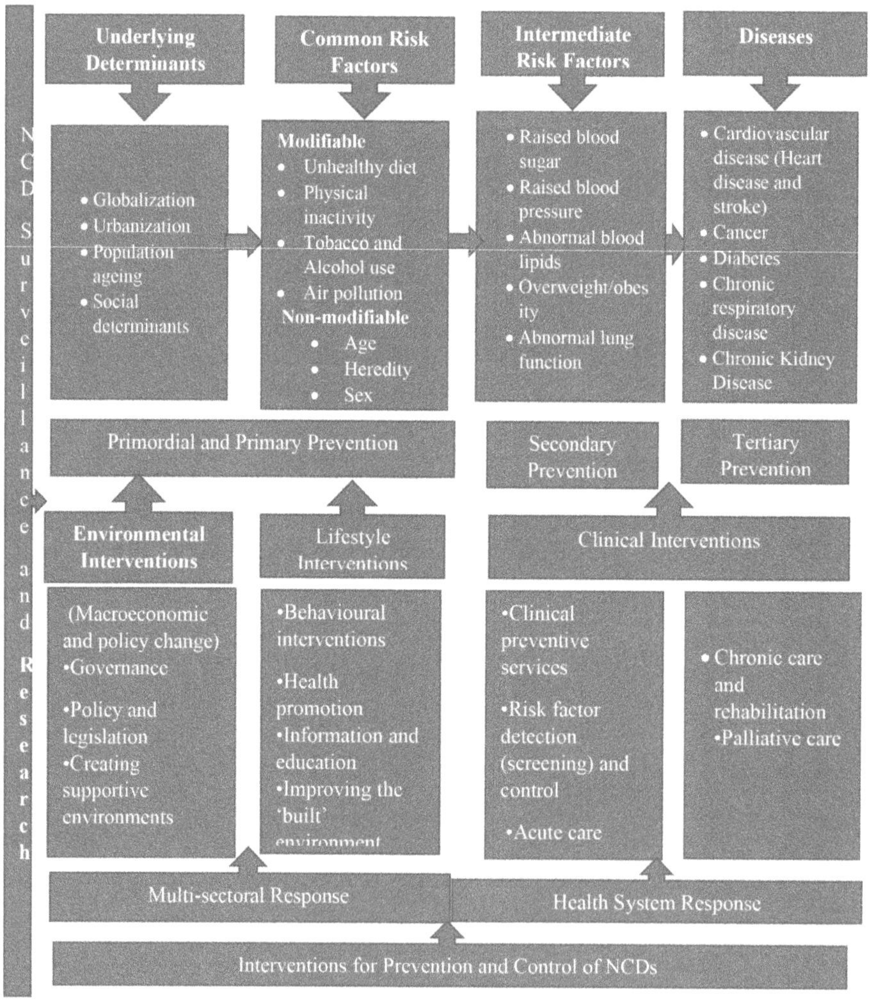

Figure 9.1: Causation Pathway and Approach for Prevention and Control of NCDs

Source: Adapted from WHO document *"Western Pacific Regional Action Plan for non-communicable diseases. World Health Organization (2013)"*

The results of research can be utilized for developing evidence-based policies, public health programs, academic programs and implementation strategies which can eventually contribute to improving health, saving lives, improving workforce participation, countries' economic productivity and limiting the financial burden of unexpected health costs on individuals and their families. [5]

The goal of NCD research is to generate evidence for reducing the burden and avoid premature deaths. To overcome the burden of NCDs, the government has developed an action plan. India is the first country to develop specific national targets and indicators to reduce the number of premature deaths from NCDs by 25% by 2025. The national framework outlines 10 targets and 21 indicators. These targets focus on reducing the burden of risk factors and increasing the access to care for those suffering from NCDs. [6]

2. Approach to NCD Research

Based on the need and response for NCD prevention and control activities, knowledge gaps must be identified and research questions should be framed to address them. Research focusing on strategies for health promotion and its interventions like health education and communication can provide evidence for reducing the burden. Other areas of focused research can be addressed such as strategies for increasing the trained health workforce, clinical trials for new drugs, diagnostics and digital health for health records, and continuum of care. Such results can provide evidence for strengthening of health systems. NCD studies can be on measuring the burden of risk factors and evaluating interventions under various NCD programs. The evidence on the impact of interventions can support a programmatic decision on scaling up good interventions and discontinuing less effective ones [7].

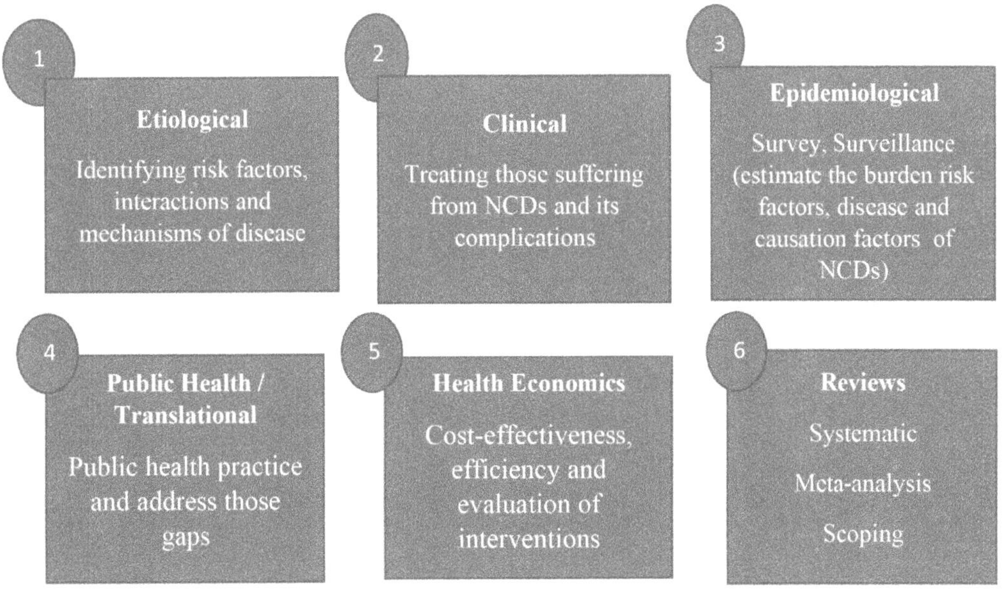

Figure 9.2: Key Domains for NCD Research

3. Domains of NCD Research (Figure 2)

Etiological:

Etiology is to understand the basis of diseases, their interactions, mechanisms and pathways. Avoid research to merely reconfirm well-known facts, but undertake it to either re-confirm their role in our settings, find newer information on them or new discoveries not yet known.

Clinical

Clinical is to address gaps in the knowledge needed to treat those suffering from NCDs and their complications. This could include finding applications of diagnostics, drugs, procedures, treatment algorithms, etc. to improve clinical outcomes.

Epidemiology

Epidemiology is to better define the problem, its distribution and determinants.

Public Health and Translational

These are questions which arise from public health practices and address those gaps. They include operational, implementation research, program evaluation and policy research. Health system research addresses clinical and public health matters including not only public health systems but the private and not-for-profit systems and alternative health systems. Translational Research is any type of research that leads to knowledge translation. Help to translate the available knowledge and make it useful for practise and/or policy to improve health and effective health services.

Health Economics

These include studies on cost-effectiveness, efficiency and evaluation. They help in the use of appropriate technology and tools on a large scale with maximum impact. They also guide in resource allocation and better utilization of finances are achieved.

Reviews:

The major ones are systematic reviews and meta-analyses. Also, scoping reviews help in developing better research protocols.

4. Types of NCD Research (Study Designs for NCD Research)

Based on an appropriate research question, the researcher can consider (Table 9.1) the following study designs.

Table 9.1: Study designs suitable for NCD research. [8]

S. No	Type of Study	Unit of Study
1.	**Observational Studies**	
i.	***Descriptive Studies***	
a	Cross-sectional	Individuals
b	Ecological	Populations
ii	***Analytical Studies***	
a	Case-control	Individuals
b	Cohort	Individuals
2.	**Experimental Studies**	
a	Randomized Controlled Trial	Individuals
b	Community Trials	Communities
3.	**Review from Published Studies**	
a	Systematic Reviews	Secondary Data
b	Meta-analysis	Secondary Data

Broadly the study designs that can be considered for NCD research can be observational or experimental. In observational studies, the researcher observes the various characteristics in a sample of the population by not intervening in the course of the disease or outcome of the study. The observational studies can be descriptive or cross-sectional or analytical. NCD related surveys, i.e., descriptive or cross-sectional studies, can help to estimate the burden of NCDs and their risk factors e.g. prevalence of diabetes, hypertension, COPD and various cancers can be conducted by this method. Need assessment can also be done for health care related to NCDs by using cross-sectional studies. For these descriptive or cross-sectional studies, no comparison groups are required. The analysis of the result can help in generating the hypothesis for the next level of studies. In cross-sectional studies, the cause and effect are studied at the same time.

The analytical observational studies can be retrospective (case-control) or prospective (cohort and retrospective cohort studies) to study the NCD risk factors. These methods compare groups of individuals for differences in exposure or outcome. Thus, these methods require a control or comparison group e.g. if the researcher is planning to conduct studies on hypertension, then high intake of salt is associated with hypertension (based on the finding of a descriptive study). Further analytical studies can be planned to assess the cause-and-effect relationship. A case-control or cohort study can be planned to understand the causes or risk factors of hypertension.

While conducting case-control studies, cases (have hypertension) enrolled will have the disease and the controls will not have the disease (no hypertension). In this type of study, the outcome would have happened at the onset of the study and exposure to the risk factor/s, e.g. salt will be assessed between the cases (hypertension) and controls (Normal blood pressure i.e., Normotensive). Information about the exposure (salt intake) can be assessed by taking a history and/or from records. Thus, this study design is relatively simple except that it is backward-looking (retrospective) based on the exposure histories of cases and controls. The conclusions are drawn by comparison of exposure to risk. However, the cases and controls have to be selected carefully and the selection criteria for the cases should be defined well in advance e.g., level of blood pressure/stage of disease or duration of disease or the cut-off reading of blood pressure in this hypothetical example. To a large extent the cases and controls should have similar characteristics other than the disease and the risk factors being investigated.

If the researcher plans to conduct a cohort study to understand the risk factors/causes of hypertension, the study should begin with a group of individuals/population or individuals free of disease (no hypertension) but who have certain characteristics or attributes relevant to the study (exposed group) with others who do not have those characteristics (unexposed group). This group will be followed up over a period of time till they develop the disease i.e Hypertension (outcome of the study). The comparison will be made between the two groups, who had exposure to excess salt (excess salt intake per day) and another group with less exposure to salt (limited intake of salt per day). The data can be collected by interview surveys with follow-up procedures or medical records monitored over time or medical examinations and laboratory testing or record linkage etc. Multiple diseases associated with high intake of salt (risk factor) can be observed in the cohort study over a period of time.

An experiment is the best epidemiological study design to prove causation. In experimental designs, the researcher or investigator tries to manipulate the given condition through an intervention. The researcher can plan a clinical trial to check the effectiveness of a new drug e.g. drug "Y", a new antihypertensive is better than X (already existing/best treatment/ drug already available). For conducting a clinical trial, the researcher needs to identify the appropriate reference population, also known as the target population (e.g., patients with primary/essential hypertension), to whom the finding of the study is generalizable (applicable). Careful choice of the outcome variable, the sample selection, allocation process and the statistical analysis procedures are essential for the success of the experiment. The subgroup of participants can be selected by specific inclusion (e.g. those with primary hypertension in the age group of 30 to 60 years etc) and exclusion criteria (those with secondary hypertension and above the age of 60 years and less than 30 years). To overcome selection bias, the most commonly encountered in health science experimental research, by which evidence of effectiveness (new drug, diagnostic/devices/any intervention e.g., Health education) is measured, is the randomized, controlled, double-blind clinical trial, commonly known as an RCT, can be considered. The following NCD related studies can be considered by RCT:

i. Drugs for prevention, treatment or palliation
ii. Clinical devices such as the use of medicated stents versus non- medicated stents for angioplasty procedures in diabetic patients with ischemic heart diseases
iii. Interventions with different categories of health personnel, e.g. doctors versus nurses, for increasing the care for routine services for NCDs;
iv. medical counselling as an intervention by doctor versus nurses for adherence to continue the NCDs drugs
v. Interventions with diet, exercise and change of other lifestyle habits
vi. NCD related risk-factor trials, e.g. proving the aetiology of a disease e.g use of coconut oil and occurrence of coronary artery diseases
vii. Hospital services, e.g. Integrated versus non-integrated, acute versus chronic care of NCDs
viii. Communication approaches, e.g., face-to-face communication for quitting tobacco versus pamphlet distribution for tobacco de-addiction

5. Community Intervention Trials (CITs)

In this type of study, the communities are randomized rather than the individuals. Communities selected for entry to the study have to be as similar as possible, especially since only a small number of communities will be selected. Very often, blinding is not possible in these types of studies, and contamination (information/health education intervention from one community i.e., intervention community can be adopted by the members of the control community) and co-interventions become serious problems.

Following studies for NCDs can be considered by CITs

i. Evaluating the need for a service, i.e. community diagnosis for Diabetes, Hypertension, COPD and Cancer (assessment or evaluation of needs)
ii. Evaluating the design of a health service (design evaluation); i.e., NCD care from primary to tertiary level
iii. Evaluating the performance or efficiency of the process of delivery of the services (efficiency or process evaluation) e.g., Continuum of care for DM and hypertension approach of the health system for NCD care
iv. Evaluating the effectiveness and impact of the programme or procedure (effectiveness or impact evaluation) e.g., studies to evaluate the population-based screening (PBS) for NCDs and the impact of PBS on detection of new and less complicated cases of NCDs in the community
v. Relating the outcome to the input and constraints of the programme (system evaluation), including cost-benefit analysis e.g., studies to assess the impact of reduction in risk factors of NCDs (tobacco reduction) and its impact on reducing premature deaths from oral and lung cancers etc

Already published articles can be considered for systematic and meta-analysis review.

A systematic review uses standardized methods to select and review all relevant studies on a particular topic to eliminate bias in critical appraisal and synthesis of pooled results e.g. all the studies with the effect of a particular group of anti-hypertensives (e.g., calcium channel blockers) to reduce blood pressure can be considered in the literature search and recommendations can be based on the analysis of the pooled results of all the studies. All systematic reviews may not consider meta-analysis.

***Meta-Analysis Review*:** It is a statistical technique available for pooling of results of several independent studies that have examined the same issue e.g., Randomized Controlled Trials (RCT) on particular group of drugs can be considered and interpreting the results based on the conclusion of results of all selected studies using statistical technique. This can be based on systematic reviews.

6. Format of NCD Research Protocol [9, 10]

A research protocol is an action plan of thoughts of the investigator/s. It's a detailed plan explaining all the essential components of the study and how the study will be carried out. The format depends on the potential sponsors, funding agency or university/educational institute. However, a generic format requires the following essential components:

Title of the Research Project:

The research title can be based on the overall objective of the study and study population. The title may convey the idea about the area of Research and the Methodology to be used. The first study of the NCDs can be the descriptive study to estimate the disease burden. It can be done in a hospital, specified geographical region or at an individual's workplace. For example, if the researcher is planning to conduct a study on hypertension, he/she needs to decide who will be the study participants i.e., age criteria, gender and locality/setting etc. Based on the information, the researcher can write the title of the study as "Estimating the prevalence of hypertension among young medical professionals working in a tertiary care hospital in X city". Or the title of the study can be "Cross-sectional survey to estimate the burden and causes of hypertension in Y community".

The study title should be compact, appropriate, precise, attractive, self-explanatory and informative. It should be able to convey the essence of the proposal and indicate the objectives laid down later. It is recommended that you keep the title within 12-15 words.

Name and Designation of Investigators:

Mention the name of the Principal Investigator (PI) and Co-Investigator(s) (Co-PI) and Email address along with their designations and the name of the institute of affiliation. The co-investigator team must include all the people who are experts in the subject with skills and knowledge required for the successful conduct of the study. They would also be equally responsible for the conduct and outcomes of the study. All should be ready to devote dedicated time and efforts to complete the research. Multi-centric studies will require site investigators who will provide the overall implementation of the research at their place and under their guidance and supervision.

Background information of the proposal

A good literature search is the key for writing the background of any research as it will be wise to undertake the study for which the relevant gaps have been identified. While writing the background, attention should be drawn to the positives, negatives and limitations of the studies which have already been published. The most recent publications on the related topic of the research can be quoted along with information on the knowledge Gaps. The overall aim of writing the background is to convey the importance of the topic, the existing gaps/ lacunae in the literature, the purpose of the study and the overall benefits of the proposed study results. The background should logically end with the aims and objectives of the study. Thus, it should be precise and focused.

Hypothesis

A research hypothesis is a tentative statement that can be tested by the scientific study design. The research Hypothesis is stated at the beginning of the study. It should be very clear and specific. The association between the exposure or intervention and the outcome can be considered as the hypotheses statement.

If the study involves determining the association between two observations or variables, it is essential to mention the hypothesis. A null hypothesis is a statement that there is no actual relationship between the variables (H0 or HN) or an alternative hypothesis suggests a potential relationship or difference between the variables that the researcher may expect (H1 or HA). The above literature synthesis will help in arriving at stating the hypothesis. However, there is no need to mention the hypothesis for observational studies.

Aims and Objectives

The aim of the study should be very precise and clear. It describes what you would like to see as achieved through the study. This is derived from the study questions/ hypothesis. The objective/s of the study helps to achieve the stated aim. They may be divided into primary and secondary objectives. Primary objectives are the target that the Investigator is aiming at, while secondary ones are additional study points. The commitment of the study is to achieve the primary objectives. One should be able to get the answers to the questions through the study methods described subsequently. Details of each objective that will finally lead to the achievement of the goal should be stated. The objectives should be SMART: Specific, Measurable, Achievable, Relevant and Time-based. It's recommended to avoid too many objectives of the study. They should be stated in action verbs that illustrate their purpose i.e. "to describe, to compare, to verify, to determine, to reduce, to calculate, etc."

Methodology

The methodology section of the protocol should describe all the details pertaining to the conduct of the research. It should describe what type of study design will be used, where and when the study will be conducted, who will be the study participants, how will they be selected, what criteria will be used to select the participants, method of data collection, details of data instruments, data analysis and ethical consideration related to the study.

- ***Study Design:*** Based on study objectives, an appropriate study design should be selected (refer Table 9.1). A study design is a scientific approach to acquire the answer to the proposed objectives of the study. Appropriate selection of the study design is very important to obtain reliable and valid scientific results. It also determines the methods that will be used to collect and analyse the data.
- ***Study Setting*:** It describes in detail where the study will be carried out. It may be institutional settings like hospitals, clinics, schools, industry or residential locality or in the community or more than one setting.
- **Study Duration:** Mention the time period needed for planning and preparing the study, collecting the data, analysing the data and writing the report.
- ***Study Population:*** Describe the target population/study participants to be included in the research. Give details of the study subjects and all aspects of the selection procedure.
- ***Inclusion and Exclusion Criteria*:** Proper definition of eligibility, inclusion (gender, age and clinical stage) criteria i.e. give details which can be included in the study, exclusion criteria (age and stage of disease, gender in study), i.e. give details that will not be included in the study. In the case of clinical trials, the discontinuation criteria of the study subjects should be stated.
- ***Sampling*:** Describe how you will select the study population - randomly or purposively. The allocation of subjects to study arms and control arm for the clinical trials should be explained. If it is a randomized clinical trial, describe in detail the blinding and randomisation processes.
- ***Sample Size:*** Sample size calculation is another very important aspect of a good proposal. Without understanding the concept, the study results may not be interpreted. Sample size calculation is essential for economic and ethical reasons. Different formulas will be used to calculate the sample size based on the study design. It is recommended to mention all the assumptions used for calculating the sample size. Mention the prevalence level, confidence interval level and acceptable range of results used for the calculation of sample size.
- ***Intervention details:*** For studies involving intervention, complete details of proposed intervention should be given. Here, all the activities and actions should be recorded and thoroughly explained in their order of occurrence.
- ***Data collection tools*:** Based on the study design, data collection tools can be in the form of questionnaires for surveys. For clinical studies, details of symptoms, signs and findings of clinical examinations, essential investigations and final diagnosis should be a part of the data collection tool. Details of laboratory investigations and

the standard methods which will be used for estimation can be described in this section of the protocol.

- *Data collection procedure:* Describe how the data will be collected - by in-person interview in survey forms or self-administered digital data entry on mobile or tablets, e-mail or by post.
- ***Quality Control of data collection and Data Analysis (software):*** Describe how the collected data will be entered, along with the measure to assure quality checks, cleaning and analysis of the final data set. Mention the type and version of the software which will be used for analysis.

7. Ethical Considerations

For all the studies involving human subjects, the investigators must be well-versed in the ethical requirements of the study so that they are addressed in the protocol. A letter of approval from the Institutional Ethics Committee (IEC) should be enclosed with the research proposal. Guidelines for IEC for human studies should follow the National Ethical Guidelines for Biomedical and Health Research Involving Human Participants. These guidelines are issued by the Indian Council of Medical Research (ICMR). All other relevant guidelines/regulations/statutory requirements must be adhered to. The Investigators must identify the ethical challenges in their proposal and address them. This will help to develop a better proposal and save time of the Ethics Committees. All research proposals need to be submitted to the Ethics Committee for approval. The investigator cannot decide on 'no need for Ethics Committee approval' as it may seem like a low-risk research. Multi-centric studies will require ethical approval of all sites.

8. Administrative Approvals

For clinical trials, permission from the Drugs Controller General of India is essential. Import of equipment will also require the approval of a competent authority. For studies requiring foreign collaboration in India, ICMR-Health Ministry Screening Clearance (HMSC) is mandatory. All the research funds should have administrative approvals, must follow the institutional policy and all documents should be available for audit. After completion of the study, all documents should be archived for years specified by the funder.

9. Budget Required

Based on the type of study and its requirement, the proposed budget can be included in the proposal in a tabular format. It should cover subheadings like human resource/staff, material/ equipment required, cost of laboratory investigations, sample transportation, cost of communications, consumables, funds to compensate for patient's/participant's wage loss, purchase of computer, software etc. all need to be included along with the number of items and unit cost. The justification for the need for each item should be provided. The budget should be realistic, not too high nor too low. Reviewers are able to judge the funds requested and the scientific work proposed.

10. Outcome

Always write the expected outcome of the research in the protocol. This will be based on the objectives of the study. Describe how the results of the study will be useful and contribute to new knowledge or would overcome the existing knowledge gap in the particular subject. A strong outcome will help the project reviewers to determine the value addition of the research proposed.

11. Referencing

Referencing can be defined as a method of acknowledging and recognizing someone for his or her work that the researcher would have used in his/her research to back and support his/her idea. Referencing is also called citation. A reference usually includes the author's name, date of publication, name and location of the publishing company, title of the journal or name of the book, title of the research or chapter's name, and DOI (Digital Object Identifier).

In the research protocol, referencing is done at two levels - the first level is in the text (background, method section or discussion etc.) the reference is given for the information quoted from other researchers. This is called "in-text citation"; and, the second level is a detailed reference provided at the end of the document in the form of a list.

Referencing is an extremely important aspect of the research protocol. A proper citation will enable the readers to follow any reference of interest and original source of information. There are different standard methods used for referencing. These methods are called referencing styles or citation styles. Various referencing styles differ in terms of formatting, use of punctuation and the order of information; such differences occur at both the levels of referencing i.e. in-text citation and in reference list. Based on the recommendation of the funding agency where the research protocol is being submitted, the researcher can use the appropriate referencing system. Failure to provide reference or to acknowledge the idea/work of other researchers falls under the category of plagiarism. The two most commonly used citation systems i.e. Vancouver System and the Harvard System are detailed below:

i. Vancouver System (Journal Article)

Mention the following while listing the reference:

Author(s) – Family name and initials

Title of the article

Title of Journal – Abbreviated publication year, month, day (month & day only if available); volume (issue); page

e.g. Mathur P and Shah B Research Priorities for Prevention and Control of Non-communicable Diseases in India. Indian J Community Med. 2011 Dec; 36 (Suppl 1): S72-7. doi: 10.4103/0970-0218.94713.

ii. Harvard system

Mention the following while listing reference by the Harvard System:

Author of the article - Surname, Initial (s)., (Year)

Title of the article

Journal title

Volume in bold (Issue), page range

e.g. Mathur P and Rangamani S. (2020). COVID19 and non-communicable diseases: Identifying research priorities to strengthen public health response. Int J NonCommun. **5**, 76-82.

12. Annexures

Along with the research protocol, some additional documents are submitted in the form of Annexures:

1. Informed Consent Form (English/local language)
2. Letters from the Ethics Committees
3. Study Questionnaire/s
4. Case Record Forms (CRFs)
5. Budget Details
6. Curriculum Vitae (CV) of the Principal Investigator and Co-Investigator/s and their role in the study. It will ensure that the role of each Investigator is well defined.

13. Report Writing

It is essential to develop a report or manuscript after completion of the research. Identify the target peer-reviewed journal printed/online/electronic media for publication. The manuscript can be an original article, review article or letter to the editor. A manuscript write-up should have an abstract, introduction/background, methodology, result, discussions and conclusion sections. While submitting a manuscript, the researcher should follow the guidelines of the targeted journal. The research report can be generated in similar sections and the Executive Summary which is the most important component of the report summarizes the findings of the research.

14. Sharing Results with Study Participants

The overall findings of the research should be shared with the study participants, not the individual findings. It is recommended that after the completion of the study, the final analysis is completed and reports are generated, the researcher can decide and plan for sharing of results. Using non-technical/simple language, the scientific findings can be conveyed and for some studies after sharing the findings of the results e.g. NCD research, the participants may change the behaviour in the desired way e.g., reduce intake of salt to reduce hypertension. In clinical trials, the results can be shared in two different groups i.e., control and intervention groups separately. After completion of the trial, if required, the control group can be given the same treatment as the intervention group.

15. Dissemination

After the study is completed, the researcher can develop a scientific manuscript or report and plan for dissemination of the findings of the research. Identifying the key audience for dissemination is essential. If the research findings are very important and have public health importance, a press release can be planned for dissemination. Using non-technical language and simple words the scientific findings can be communicated to the mass media (television or newspapers). Other ways of dissemination of research can be peer reviewed journals as scientific publications or presenting at a scientific forum (conference/workshop/seminar/symposium).

16. Other Aspects of Research

Advocacy

Researchers initiating studies in a new area of medicine or unfamiliar topics generally face difficulties in enrolling study subjects. To overcome fear and anxiety of community members or potential research participants, it is essential to have an open and transparent discussion, public engagement and advocacy with relevant key stakeholders. Advocacy with community leaders and other stakeholders will help in understanding the objectives of the research and build trust in the researcher. Engaging the general public through advocacy also helps in accepting the biomedical and health research findings.

Responsibility Towards Funder

A researcher is responsible for conducting the research as per the terms and conditions of the funding agency. It is recommended that the scientific and ethical approvals are completed before the funds are released. The researcher should be in regular touch with the funder and communicate the implementation and progress of the ongoing research on a regular basis.

A researcher should utilize the funds and keep accountability of all the expenses as per the agreed terms and conditions with the funder. Based on the agreed policy with the funder, the researcher should submit regular reports and financial expenditure statements.

Research Integrity

Plagiarism means taking someone else's work or ideas and projecting or informing or claiming it to be of yours. Even rewriting another person's ideas or work in your own words by just reordering or rearranging or substituting the words i.e. paraphrasing, is still considered plagiarism. While conducting research, it is essential that the researcher avoids plagiarism. One of the ways to avoid plagiarism is to appropriately quote the reference or quote the sources, if the researcher has used information from other researcher/s or others' ideas. Source of information or citation should be mentioned as per the requirement of the journal/educational institute. Researchers can also avoid plagiarism by directly quoting another person's written or spoken words and putting these words and/or sentences in quotation marks.

It is essential that researchers are true to themselves, to their institute and to society. Based on existing knowledge, the research should be carried out in a fair manner, and the results of the research should never be manipulated. Both positive and negative findings of the research should be communicated. Thus, value and benefits of research are dependent on the integrity of the researchers who have a significant social responsibility to prevent misconduct and misuse of research. It is the responsibility of all team members involved in the research to maintain high standards of ethics and integrity of research at all times.

17. Conclusion

Writing a research proposal is an art which develops as one writes more and gets experience. Failures should not discourage, rather they should strengthen the resolve. Sound knowledge of the subject of research proposed is essential. A clear understanding and inclusion of each research proposal's administrative/financial requirements are as important as the science it contains. A good research proposal is half the work done!

References

1. Center for Disease Control and Prevention (CDC). Introduction to NCD Epidemiology. Facilitator Guide. Atlanta, GA: 2013.
2. World Health Organization. Non- Communicable Diseases Fact Sheet. World Health Organization. 2018 Available on https://www.who.int/news-room/fact-sheets/detail/noncommunicable-diseases. Assessed on 9th August 2021.
3. World Health Organization. Non- communicable Diseases (NCD) Country Profiles. India. 2018
4. World Health Organization. Western Pacific Regional Action Plan for non-communicable diseases. 2013
5. World Health Organization. Saving lives, spending less: A strategic response to non-communicable diseases. 2018
6. Ministry of Health and Family Welfare. Government of India. National Multisectoral Action Plan for Prevention and Control of Common NCDs (2017-2022). Revised Oct. 2017.
7. World Health Organization. A Prioritized Research Agenda for Prevention and Control of Non-communicable Diseases. 2011

8. World Health Organization. Health Research Methodology A Guide for Training in Research Methods. Second Edition. World Health Organization Regional Office for the Western Pacific Manila. 2001
9. Jundi A Al- and Sakka S. Protocol Writing in Clinical Research. Journal of Clinical and Diagnostic Research. 2016;10(11): ZE10-ZE13
10. World Health Organization. Development of Research Proposal on Communicable Diseases. Report of an Informal Consultation Kolkata, India, 23-24 December 2010. World Health Organization 2012.
11. References/Bibliography Vancouver Style. The University of Queensland, Australia. Available at https://guides.library.uq.edu.au/referencing/vancouver/reference-list

CHAPTER

10 The Art and Science of Scientific Writing

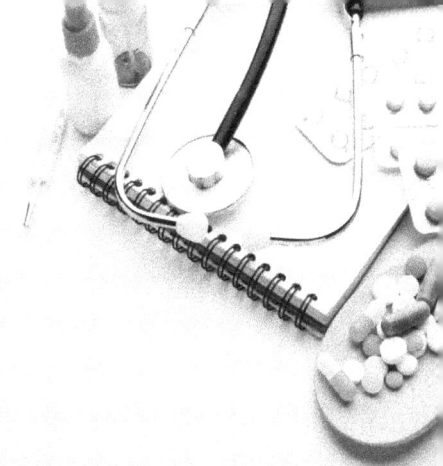

Renu Bharadwaj

"Whatever you dream, begin it, for boldness has power, magic and genius."

Goethe

1. Introduction

The basic purpose of scientific writing is not the mere presentation of information but rather its actual communication. It does not matter how elegantly an author might have converted all the right data into sentences and paragraphs; it matters only whether a large majority of the reading audience accurately understands what is written. [1] Therefore, in order to understand how best to improve writing, we would do well to understand better how readers go about reading it.

Scientific writing is important as the publication of research results has become the measure used by all disciplines to gauge a scientist's level of success. [2] Each researcher must decide why he wants to write about his research. Publication plays an integral role in his academic career. Research done in small bits by various sScientists can be read and built upon by others and thus increase the body of scientific knowledge available to the world. Occasionally, scientists have the urge to prove that conventional wisdom is mistaken!

Historically, scientific writing in English started in the 14th century. [3] The Royal Society established this practice. Its founder member Thomas Sprat wrote on the importance of plain and accurate description rather than rhetorical flourishes in his *History of the Royal Society of London*. Subsequently, Robert Boyle emphasized the importance of not boring the reader with a dull, flat style. [4] Over the years, scientific writing has evolved into a Science and an Art.

Make writing easier by planning before one writes and knowing the target audience of the paper can make it more impactful. However, it can be a major challenge to find time to write. Most professional writers recommend setting aside 20 minutes every day to write and plan before one writes. Only the best and the most practiced can effectively squeeze it in between other work.

2. What, Where and How Before Writing

If the editors cannot work out a single take-home message from the article and its importance, they will reject the paper outright. Readers should know throughout the article: where they've come from, where they are now and where they are heading.

It is important to first choose a journal and write for that journal's audience. This can usually be done by checking the references of your work to see in which journals the research you are citing mainly falls. Select a journal that is indexed on some database: Medline, PubMed, EMBASE, SCOPUS, EBSCO Publishing's Electronic Databases, SCIRUS etc. The type of paper you are planning to write will also affect your decision i.e., Empirical Research, Review Paper or Brief Report. Not all journals publish all types of articles. Ensure that the journal you are selecting publishes the type of study you are planning to write.

Having selected the journal, it is important to study the journal's author guidelines and then make sure the guidelines specific for the type of study conducted have been followed. To give a few examples:

- CONSORT Guidelines for Randomised Control Trials [5]
- PRISMA for Systemic Reviews [6]
- STROBE for Observational Studies [7]
- STARD for Studies of Diagnostic Accuracy [8]
- MIAME for Microarray Data [9]

Read and follow the journal's author guidelines and style guide also. Before starting to write keep in mind what the audience already knows about the topic and what they want to now know by doing enough reading on the subject.

The "IMRAD" structure is the format encouraged for the text of observational (i.e. retrospective/descriptive) and experimental (i.e. randomised controlled) studies by the "Uniform Requirements for Manuscripts Submitted to Biomedical Journals."

The IMRAD structure is shown in Figure 10.1.

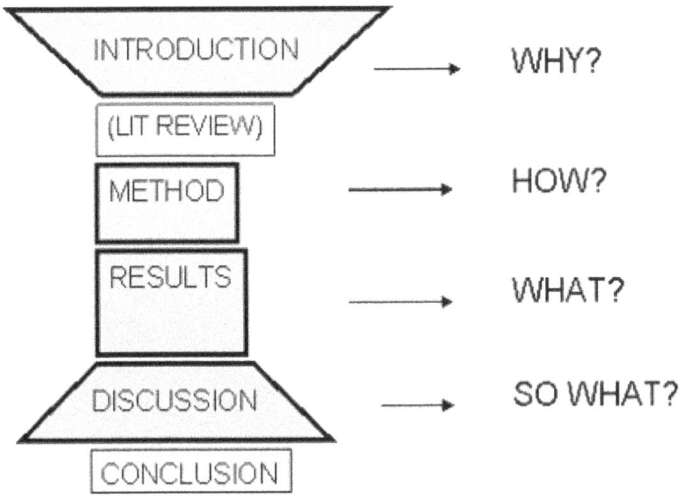

Figure 10.1: The IMRAD Structure

Figure 10.1: Source: Swales, J and C. Feak (2000) English in Today's Research World: A Writing Guide, Michigan: Ann Arbor

IMRAD stands for Introduction, Methods, Results And Discussion. It basically covers the Why, How, What and So what of the article?

In which order should the article be written?

The article is not recommended to be written in the order of IMRAD. Then in which order should it be written? The **'Methods'** is what should be written first. They are also fresh in the Rresearcher's mind as he has just completed the project. They are crucial in the editorial Triage Process. It is extremely common for editors to reject a paper because authors used the wrong method to answer their questions. Give enough details so that a qualified reader could repeat the study. If the methods section is "thin on details" editors will worry that the authors are hiding something.

3. Quantitative Study

Quantitative research is a way to learn about a particular group of people known as a sample population. Using scientific inquiry, quantitative research relies on data that is observed or measured to examine questions about the sample p

opulation. Quantitative Research gathers a range of numeric data.

Divide the Methods section into 6 subheads/paragraphs:

- Design
- Sample
- Intervention

- Outcomes Measures
- Data Analysis
- Ethics: Informed Consent & IRB Approval

Design

Clearly state the design used:

- Observational or Interventional [10]
- Prospective or Retrospective
- Controlled or Uncontrolled
- Cohort Study, Cross-sectional Survey or Case-controlled Study [11]

For Randomized Controlled Studies, it is important to state how exactly the randomization was done ex: randomized numbers in sealed envelopes and what was the unit of randomization e.g. individual patients or GP practices.

Sample

The sample size chosen and how it wasdetermined (including the power of calculation) for the study must be clearly mentioned. How the participants were recruited needs to be mentioned and how did the authors ensure they were representative of the population under study. This needs to be followed by Inclusion and Exclusion Criteria.

Intervention

Discuss the intervention studied and how was the control group selected.

Outcome Measures

The outcomes measured need to be mentioned, especially the Primary and Secondary outcomes. The validated tool used for the same needs to be specified and how was the bias reduced.

Data Analysis

The statistical methods used to analyze data need to be specified.
E.g. Odds Ratio to assess risk factors for a disease.
If software like Statistical Package for Social Sciences (SPSS) has been used, it needs to be mentioned.

Ethics

That informed consent of participants has been taken and the name of the Ethical Committee which approved the project before commencement needs to be mentioned.

4. Qualitative Study

It is a process of inquiry that seeks an understanding of phenomena within their natural setting. It focuses on the "why" rather than the "what" of the phenomenon.

While going through such a study the editor will focus on:

- Appropriateness of the study question for a qualitative study
- Ethical considerations

Appropriateness of Methodology

Firstly, was a Qualitative approach suitable for the study?
E.g. Qualitative: What stops people from using mosquito nets over their beds?
Quantitative: What proportion of people in Delhi use mosquito nets over their beds?

Sample Size

The Sample Size must be appropriately determined and clearly mentioned.

Ethical Considerations

The study must have been given approval by the Institutional Review Board (IRB), and Informed consent must have been taken. Both these facts need to be clearly mentioned.

Data Analysis

Methodology of the research needs to be mentioned clearly.
After completing the methodology of the study, the next thing to write is the Results.

Results

This part should contain facts and nothing but the facts. The results of the study need to be mentioned clearly using words and numbers. They should be organized around the Primary and Secondary outcomes of the study as listed in the **Methods Section**. It is advisable to use tables and figures for the main numbers. However, do NOT duplicate information in the text and tables.

Tell a quick visual story as a graph wherever possible. Keep the graphs simple. Make the various groups easy to distinguish by using contrasting colours or signs such as triangles and squares. Circles vs squares are not easy to distinguish. There are various types of graphs: Line graphs, scatter graphs, Histograms, box plots, survival curves etc. However, a word of caution 'Keep it simple!' If the graph looks very complex, maybe the information belongs in a table.

Discussion

Now that the results are ready, it is time to discuss what they mean. Do not write an expansive essay. Start the discussion with a single sentence that states your main findings and discusses the interpretation based on key findings mentioning supporting evidence in the results. Do not overstate the importance of the findings; readers will come to their own conclusions. Avoid a long rambling discussion. In the subsequent paragraphs, compare your results with previous studies on the subject. Mention the strengths and limitations of the current study then discuss the interpretation of your secondary endpoint if any, and how it compares with other similar studies.

Relate your study to what has already been found. Mention how your study fits into what is already known. If it does not, why it offers a different conclusion definitely needs an explanation. Discuss what this conclusion means. Mention any unexpected findings and what is the Hypothesis generated at the end of the study. The last paragraph should be reserved for the summary of the study, its conclusions, significance and implications. There should be a mention of unanswered questions and areas of future Research. What did your Research not address? Avoid using the cliché; more Research is needed.

Introduction

The last thing to write is the Introduction of the article, as this is where the attention of the reader is grabbed and held. It is important to draw them immediately to the crucial issue of the paper. However, to keep it readable, it must be kept short about 2 to 3 paragraphs. It must set the scenario in which the research was done, the state-of-the-art of the scenario rather than describe everything known on the topic. Cite the best current evidence from systematic reviews.

The opening sentence must take the reader straight to the issue. The first paragraph must contain the most important details of the issue. Give a summary of the controversies and the best evidence for them. Then explain why it matters to doctors, patients, policymakers or researchers. Explain why further research is needed and end with a crisp and clear research question. Were there any controversies you were trying to address? Explain what new or innovative techniques you planned to use without giving away the results or conclusions here.

Abstract

Finally, it is time to write the Abstract. Many journals base their decisions on the Abstract alone, but sadly many authors write the Abstract as an afterthought! It should be a concise standalone piece with a clear message. It must accurately reflect the full text of the paper. It must clearly mention as to why the study was done, how was it done, what was found in the study and what were the conclusions of the study.

Many journals require a structured Abstract that must be written as per the journal's requirements with an introduction, materials and methods, results and a conclusions section and within the word limit prescribed by the journal.

The ***keywords*** must be mentioned below the Abstract. The focus should be on only 3-4 keywords which best reflect the study. The keywords are picked up by search engines.

Highlights of the study

Many journals require 3-4 highlights of the study to be mentioned. These are 3-4 words which best reflect what the study has done or approached. Again, these are picked up by the search engines when a researcher is performing a review on the subject and so are very important.

Title

This should be compelling, concise and informative. It should contain the most important words related to the topic and entice the reader without giving away the punch line. At the same time, it cannot be over-sensationalized. Some journals now insist on including study design in the title.

A bad title example is:

"The amazing effect of the use of mosquito nets on the prevalence of malaria!"

A better title would be:

"A Randomized Controlled Trial of the efficacy of insecticide-treated mosquito net use for the control of malaria."

References

All references referred to in the article should be cited in the text of the article and listed at the end.

Cite the references accurately while preparing the manuscript. Restrict yourself to the key ones only. It need not be a composite Bibliography.

References can be cited by various methods e.g. Harvard, Vancouver created by the Institute of Electrical and Electronics Engineers, Oxford, Chicago (American Psychological Association, APA) style, etc.

The first three are the commonly used ones in most medical journals [12].

(A) Harvard

In-text Citation:

This consists mainly of the authors' last name and the year of publication (and page numbers if it is directly quoted) in round brackets placed within the text.

Reference List

The reference list should be placed alphabetically by the last name of the first author of each work. Only the initials of the authors' given names are used. There is no full stop and space between the initials. Last name comes first.

(B) Vancouver Style

In-text citation:

References are indicated using a number in square brackets [1] in the order of appearance in the article.

Reference List

This is displayed at the end of the article, providing full details of all references cited in the text. References are listed in numerical order and in the same order in which they are cited in the text (not in alphabetical order). Only the initials of the authors' given names are used. Full stops are placed between the initials. The author's last names come after the initials.

(C) Oxford Style

In-text citation:

This consists of two parts:

The first is a Superscript number in the text and the second is a note at the bottom of the page (footnote). Notes are numbered sequentially, beginning with 1 in superscript, throughout each article, chapter or paper. Author›s given name or initial before the last name (e.g. John Smith) then cite the title, place of publication, publisher, date of publication, the page reference. If the same work is referred to again in the footnotes, only the author's last name and the page number(s) are used. If more than one work by the same author is referred, use the author's last name, then a short title and page number(s).

Reference list

References are listed in alphabetical order by the author's last name. If you have cited more than one work by the same author, you should arrange them by date.

References with no author are ordered in the reference list alphabetically by the first significant word of the title.

Use only the initials of the authors' given names. Use full stops with no spaces between the initials. Last name comes first.

Before writing out the references refer to the instructions to the authors of the journal you are writing for and see their style for writing references and accordingly write the references as per the style of the journal

Acknowledgements

People who have helped with the research but have not been given weightage as authors, can be acknowledged in this section.

Author Contributions

Specify which author helped with planning the project, execution of the project, writing of the paper etc. in short, who did what.

Competing Interests

Clearly mention here for e.g. if any of the authors have shares in the company of the drug being evaluated. If funding has been given by a company for the research, by anyone who might have interest in the end result of the research then it must be clearly mentioned.

Funding

All funding sources of the project need to be mentioned.

5. The Basics of Scientific Writing

Having finished with the infrastructure of the Scientific article, lets go back to the basics of bcientific writing. Whatever you write, ensure it is written to engage the reader and not to bore them. Avoid long words and sentences. There should be an average of 20 words in a sentence and never longer than 50 words. Cut out unnecessary adjectives. Avoid passive tense. Avoid jargon and use short and simple words. Avoid double negatives such as "Leptospirosis is not uncommon in this area".

Never use short forms without having given the full form first. Make the presentation crisp and not unnecessarily "wordy" e.g. 'Most' can be used instead of 'A majority of…'

Paragraph Structure

The first sentence of each paragraph captures the main message. A topic sentence should be followed by supporting sentences. Explicit relationship must exist between sentences. Provide continuity across sentences and set up expectations about what is coming next. Once you have checked all this, your manuscript is all ready to go.

What is the first thing an Editor looks at when you submit your manuscript?

Your covering letter!

Don't waste this opportunity to "sell" your work and don't write something dull:

"Please consider this manuscript for publication in your esteemed journal."

Clearly write and tell the editor why they should take your work seriously and why it would be of interest to his readers.

What does the editor look at next?

The Editorial Triage.

The Editorial Triage

- Is the article within the journal's interest?
- Does this article have a clear message?
- Is it original?
- Is it important?
- Is it true?
- Is it relevant to the readers of the journal?

You will get Published if

- You picked an important Research Question
- You used the right method to answer it
- You wrote a short, clear account of the study that followed a tight structure
- You used effective writing to convey your message clearly

It is rare that you get accepted at the first submission. Once you have cleared the Editorial Triage, the article goes to the Reviewers, who may/will request revisions. Incorporate the reviewers' suggestions fully into the revised manuscript and address all their concerns in your rebuttal letter. Address the rebuttal letter to the editor. Unfortunately, the road is not always so smooth and much to your dismay, you get a REJECTION letter.

Why do Journals Reject your utterly groundbreaking, brilliant work?

Often it is because the paper was so poorly written and structured that the editor simply couldn't fathom its meaning.

Editors are human beings and they get impressed by papers that are short, easy to read and contain a clear message.

6. Common Reasons for Rejection

- Too wordy; too long; text difficult to follow
- Not of interest to the readership of the journal
- Plagiarism
- Copy editor issues – grammar, spelling, format
- Content incomplete, insufficient or out-of-date
- Study limitations not well stated;
- Conclusions do not fit the data
- Emotionalism: 'getting carried away';
- No evidence to support statements
- Authorship not fully stated
- Pre-publication use of data

However, Rejection is not the end of the world. 'Try, Try, Try again!' If you genuinely think that your research is important, well done, well written and deserves to reach the journal's audience, you can write an appeal letter to the editor. The other alternative is to use the comments of the journal to send an improved version of the paper to another journal and I am sure you will succeed in publishing.

"For as long as there is a dream there is hope. The key to success is making your dreams come true".

References

1. George Gophen & Hudith Storm *"The science of scientific writing*" American Scientist jan 2018
2. *Noble, Keith. "Publish or perish: What 23 journal editors have to say". Studies in Higher Education. 1989;* ***14*** *(1): 97.*
3. Irma Taavitsainen, Päivi Pahta (11 March 2004), *Medical and scientific writing in late medieval English*, ISBN 978052183133
4. Joseph E. Harmon, Alan G. Gross (15 May 2007), "On Early English Scientific Writing", *The scientific literature*, ISBN 9780226316567
5. Schulz KF, Altman DG, Moher D, For the CONSORT group2010" *Updated guidelines for reporting parallel group randomised trials*" Ann Int Med 2010;152(11):726-32
6. Matthew J Page, Joanne E McKenzie,Patrick M Bossuyt,et al "The PRISMA *2020 statement: an updated guideline for reporting systematic reviews*" *BMJ* 2021;372:n71
7. Von Elm E, Altman DG, Egger M, Pocock SJ,et al "Strengthening the reporting of Observational studiesin Epidemiology(STROBE) Statement: guidelines for reporting observational studies" Ann Intern Med. 2007: 14798):573-577

8. Bossuyt PM, Reitsma JB, Bruns DE et al For the STARD Group STARD 2015: "*An updated List of Essential Items for Reporting Diagnostic Accuracy Studies*" BMJ 2015;351h5527
9. Ron Edgar and Tanya Barrett" *NCBI GEO standards and services for microarray data*" Nat Biotechnol. 2006 December; 24(12): 1471–1472
10. Thiese MS. "*Observational and interventional study design types; an overview". Biochem Med (Zagreb)*. 2014;24(2):199-210.
11. Song JW, Chung KC. "Observational studies: cohort and case-control studies". *Plast Reconstr Surg*. 2010;126(6):2234-2242.
12. Robert Trevethan & Michela Betta (2017*)" Academic Referencing on University Library Websites. A Call for Clear, Coherent and Correct Categorisation",* Journal of the Australian Library and Information Association, 2010; 66:1; 50-67

CHAPTER

11 Good Laboratory Practices

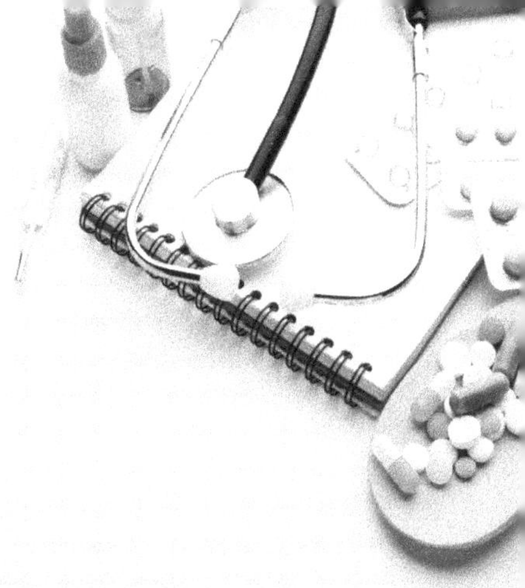

Megha Joshi

1. Introduction

Good laboratories must produce accurate, precise and timely results. Accuracy is how close your laboratory result is to the true value, whereas, precision is how reproducible your result is over time. However, not very long-ago medicine was subjective and the diagnosis intuitive. The maximum a physician could say about the lab investigation would be "why not just repeat it? Better send it to another laboratory". These feelings of a physician were universal, but they were not without reason. The reliability and repeatability of the investigations were very poor and there was considerable inter-laboratory variation. Equipment was often outdated, of poor quality and ill-maintained. Most operations were manual. The concept of SOPs (Standard Operating Procedures) was alien to majority of the labs.

However, medicine changed imperceptibly. Laboratory investigations started getting more weightage in patient management as the quality of lab reports improved. Today, modern medicine is evidence-based and heavily dependent on laboratory results. This puts a lot of responsibility on laboratories. Investigations have to be reproducible and inter-laboratory difference minimum. Quality control is now the buzzword, and to achieve good QC and QA both internal and external checks are in place.

2. Evolution of Regulatory Laws

It was globally recognized that poor and erratic laboratory services adversely affected not only medical practice but also National Health Programs. New Zealand was the first nation to recognize the problems and enacted laws to standardize laboratory services in 1972. Later most of the developed nations enacted similar laws. Today, in the US the laboratories are governed by two laws - CLIA 67, CLIA 88 and CMS (Center for Medicare and Medicaid Services). All laboratories performing testing must be registered with CMS and obtain a CLIA license. In India, labs are governed by ISO 15189.

Tests under CLIA are classified as waived and non-waived. Waived tests are simple tests that do not require Proficiency Testing (PT). Non-waived tests (moderate and high complexity tests) require PT three times a year with five samples for testing. Proficiency Testing or PT is the evaluation of participant performance against pre-established criteria by means of inter-laboratory comparison. If PT does not exist for a test, the laboratory must develop some method to assess performance twice a year. Laboratories performing non-waived tests are subject to inspection every two years by CMS or a deemed provider such as CAP (College of American Pathologists). Most of the labs in the USA are CAP accredited. In India, the accreditation body is NABL (National Accreditation Board for Testing and Calibration Laboratories). Unfortunately, only 1% of labs are NABL accredited.

3. Essential Components of a Good Laboratory

1. Space
2. Common Lab practices
3. Instruments/Equipment:
4. Technical Personnel
5. Medical Director
6. Data Management
7. Accreditation

Space

A lab must have adequate, open, well-ventilated space, preferably air-conditioned. The floor should be impervious and chemically resistant. There should be separate chemical/biological hoods, one-two sinks, a shower (desirable) and separate preparation and common instruments rooms. There should be a separate area for a reception counter. Offices should be totally separated from the labs. Fire hazard equipment has to be functional and in position. Every lab should have a first aid kit. Specialized labs for example, labs for tissue culture, cytogenetics, immunology and molecular biology have special requirements. The lab must be well connected with the adjoining buildings.

Common Lab Practices

Principles of good hygiene should be followed. A culture of safety is of paramount importance. No food or drink should be allowed inside the labs. Proper laboratory attire should be used at all times by everyone. There should be proper storage for hazardous chemicals and facilities for disposal of waste. Chemicals and reagents should be properly labelled. Avoid working alone. internal and external cross-checking of QA (Quality Assurance) and QC (Quality Control) should be conducted periodically.

Depending on the volume and cost of test, it may be advisable to send a particular test to a reference laboratory. Continuous evaluation of send-outs is required, as a change in volume of a particular test may justify bringing the test in. The automation in Molecular Testing makes it easy to bring in sophisticated tests (push-button technology/testing). Barcoding, voice recognition, automation, auto verification and delta checks can make laboratory practices safe. Computerized order entry, less human touch points, electronic medical records, scanning barcodes rather than manual entry eliminates errors introduced by transcription and clerical mistakes. It is desirable to outsource maintenance to authorized firms so that the instruments are properly maintained.

Instruments/Equipment

While buying instrumentation for any section of the laboratory, time should be spent researching what is available, what is cost-effective in the long run and what will work in your set-up. It is always good to ask experts in the field and visit other laboratories which have used the equipment and be convinced of the right choice. The right equipment and right personnel with the right expertise are keys to success. In today's world, where medicine is getting more molecular and genetic, it is preferable to incorporate the latest technological advances of Flow Cytometry, FISH, PCR and next-generation sequencing. Every instrument must have a log book to keep information on its users and services and maintenance records.

Technical Personnel (The right person for the right job)

Adequately trained and knowledgeable staff is irreplaceable. Labs should have technologists performing routine tests, however, specially trained personnel is desirable for specialized tests/procedures. For example, for Immunohistochemistry (IHC), hire someone who is especially trained in this discipline. He/she can also oversee the lab functioning including validation of new antibodies and also train staff. Subspecialty expertise is now routine in pathology laboratories. Recognition of this facet in the practice of pathology is important. For example, now surgical pathologists do not feel comfortable signing out hematopathology as advances in FLOW, FISH and classification of leukaemias and lymphomas is way too complex to be managed by a surgical pathologist. The same applies to other specialized technology, particularly for molecular and genetic medicine.

Medical Director

The medical director should be well qualified. Generally, he is a MD Pathology or a PhD who can handle and supervise all areas of the Laboratory and be responsible for the accuracy and timeliness of all laboratory results. One way of supervising all sections of a laboratory and being reassured of the quality of the laboratory should be to evaluate Proficiency Testing (PT) results. The job is made easy in many laboratories wherein the medical director is required to verify and sign all PT results produced by all sections of the laboratory. He/she is responsible for periodic inspection and accreditation of the lab. He/she should ensure that the lab is subject to periodical inspection by authorized bodies.

Data Management

In the past labs would get samples for analysis that were all entered in the inward register and the results entered in suitable forms were dispatched and recorded in the outward register. Today, computers have made inroads in all walks of life and laboratories are no exception. Almost all equipment is computerized. Every lab procedure generates a lot of data. So much data is generated that handling it manually is almost impossible. Also, the labs must have an excellent retrieval system. Currently, data management is done by senior lab managers. Future labs would need a Data Manager - an expert in Information Technology to handle the data that is generated.

Accreditation

Accreditation has to be conducted by an authorized agency. In the US, CAP is the most popular accreditation organization. CAP accreditation program involves in-person, unannounced inspections every two years and a thorough self-inspection in the interim period. The inspections are by peers and performed by volunteers. A key ingredient of the accreditation program is proficiency testing of almost every analyte tested in the laboratory. Check samples with unknown values provided by the CAP are sent 3-4 times a year and should be run the same way as a test sample. The unknown check samples usually test analyte values in the low, high and intermediate ranges. Collaboration between different laboratories regarding the results of check samples is strictly prohibited. All technicians and pathologists have to participate in the evaluation of check samples. Individual and group results have to be submitted to the CAP in a timely fashion. A laboratory with over 20-30 recurrent deficiencies is considered not to be functioning well. If a laboratory fails PT greater than 80-90%, it has to stop testing the particular analyte and perform remedial action.

To summarize, good laboratory practices is a culture of safety, consistency and diligence. Subscribing to a quality control/proficiency testing program can ensure the accuracy and precision of results. Research laboratories as well as clinical laboratories need validation of their results.

Additional Reading Material

1. In further Pursuit of Excellence, 75 years, 2021 College of American Pathologists, ISBN 978-1-941096-60-4
2. Clinical and Laboratory Standards Institute. Nonconforming Event Management, 2nd ed. CLSI guideline QMS11-ED2. Clinical and Laboratory Standards Institute, Wayne, PA; 2015.
3. Department of Health and Human Services, Centers for Medicare and Medicaid Services. Clinical laboratory improvement amendments of 1988; final rule. Fed Register. 2003(Jan 24): [42CFR493.1249]
4. ISO International Standard 15189: Medical laboratories—Particular requirements for quality and competence. Geneva: International Organization for Standardization, 2003

5. Narayanan S. The preanalytic phase. An important component of laboratory medicine. Am J Clin Pathol. 2000;113:429-452
6. Renner SW, et al. Wristband identification error reporting in 712 hospitals. A College of American Pathologists' Q-Probes study of quality issues in transfusion practice. Arch Pathol Lab Med. 1993;117:573-577
7. Title 45 – Code of Federal Regulations – Parts 160, 162, and 164, Health Insurance Reform: Security Standards; Final Rule, Federal Register, Published Feb. 20, 2003.
8. Winkelman JW. How fast is fast enough for clinical laboratory turnaround time? Measurement of the interval between result entry and inquiries for reports. Am J Clin Pathol. 1997;108:400-405
9. Clinical and Laboratory Standards Institute. Training and Competence Assessment; Approved Guideline. 3rd ed. CLSI Document QMS03-A3. Clinical and Laboratory Standards Institute, Wayne, PA, 2009.
10. Occupational Safety and Health Administration. Exit routes, emergency action plans, and fire prevention plans: standard, 2002 [29CFR1910.38]

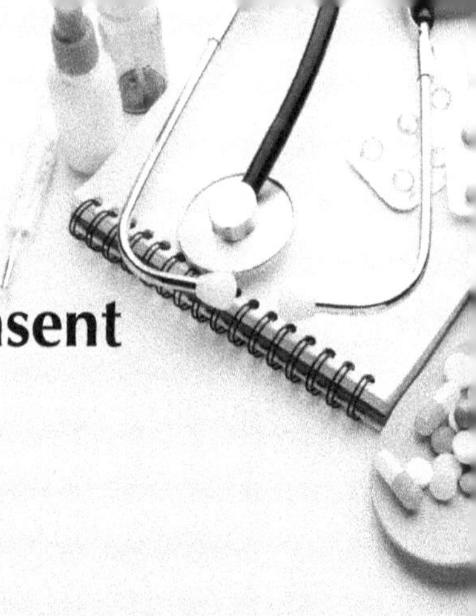

CHAPTER

12 Designing Informed Consent Proforma

Shreerang Joshi

1. Introduction

Biomedical research has gained prominence all over the world today, especially against the backdrop of the Chinese Covid-19 Viral Pandemic. A large number of diagnostic tests, prognostic investigations as well as treatment protocols have been proposed for combating this disease. Due to the severity of this disease and its ability to invade vast swathes of geography and populations, most countries have allocated huge amounts of money for research into it.

All this has put patient safety, their consent and rights on the backburner. Measures like mandatory diagnostic tests, empirical remedies, quarantine regulations, vaccines and related documents like Vaccine passports and Vaccine E-passes all indicate that governments have temporarily put the collective societal good before individual rights and liberties. For example, the RT-PCR Test and the Vaccination Certificate have become symbols of State control over society. As things stand today, for even common day-to-day activities like going to a Mall, travelling by train or bus (leave alone air travel), a suitable RT-PCR test report and/or Vaccination Certificate is almost mandatory.

However, this transient phase in biomedical science should not take us away from the basic principles of involving subjects in our research endeavours. Informed consent is a single pillar on which biomedical research stands.

Informed consent is the procedure through which a mentally competent subject after having received and understood all the research related information voluntarily provides his willingness to either participate or provide his body fluids/tissue samples for a clinical trial or experiment.

2. History

The concept of Informed Consent first came into focus after World War-II, when reports of experiments on prisoners and concentration camp inmates by Nazi doctors surfaced. It became obvious that the subjects in the experiments i.e. concentration camp inmates, were either oblivious to what they were going to face or had no choice even if they were aware of the ghastly fate that awaited them.

Initially, the emphasis was on being able to consent and be free from coercion. Next came the Helsinki Declaration in 1964, where the guiding principles on ethical issues in biomedical research were highlighted. These were periodically revised, the last being in 2008.

The formulation of research policies for Institutions was first addressed in the Belmont Report in 1979. The formation of Institutional Ethics Committees to oversee biomedical research was encouraged around this time which later became the norm.

The Common Rule formulated in the USA in 1991 emphasized that no research would be conducted without informed consent. It further stated that no researcher would be allowed to force a patient to sign a waiver of his legal rights, and no researcher, sponsor, institution or intermediaries would be exempted from liability for negligence.

In general, there are four components of informed consent:

1. Decision capacity of patient and absence of coercion
2. Documentation of consent
3. Disclosures to the patient about risks, benefits, costs, compensatory mechanisms, Rights and exit clauses and his voluntary acceptance of the same
4. Disclosures about the competency of the team conducting the research

The HIPAA (Health Insurance Portability and Accountability Act) of 1996 about the security of patient data and protection of patients' privacy has now been superimposed on the above four aspects.

Finally, as the importance of Data Banks became obvious, it was imperative to have international norms for Patient's data protection, as well as anonymization of the data.

The European Union General Data Protection Regulation of 2018 laid down clear guidelines for informed consent.

3. Medical Research Ethics Guidelines

Generally, in India we follow the guidelines laid down by the Indian Council of Medical Research (ICMR). In 2020, Dr Mathur et al came out with the mandate that Ethics Committee guidelines must be followed while designing proforma for Informed Consent for any medical research, be it in vivo or in vitro. The prominent principles, as clearly stated in these ICMR guidelines, are:

1. Respect for the patient (Autonomy)
2. Benefits and Risks clearly outlined to the patient (Information)

3. Non-malfeasance (Do no harm)
4. Justice (Right to opt-out of research, compensation for untoward fallouts of therapy)

As we try to understand more about informed consent for biomedical research, it becomes clear that there is nothing like a Universal Informed Consent format for any medical research or procedure. For a long time the focus was on the protection of the researcher or the research institution from criminal or civil liabilities. Patient data protection, protection of patient against sharing of data or publishing it without the patient's consent was never addressed or was taken for granted.

For long, patients had to sign blanket consent forms with lots of fine prints and totally alien terminologies, not unlike what many financial institutions and investment agencies use.

This is not so any longer. In fact, in a recent ruling in 2021, the Hon. Supreme Court of India specified that printed consent forms with even legally correct wording would have only a limited value.

4. Informed Consent

So, what are the essential features of an Informed Consent Form that should be signed by the patient, his guardian (for minors) or a representative?

1. It should clearly outline what the patient is consenting to and the full estimated pathway of treatment. The patient should be made fully aware of the following:
   (a) Doctors want to cure or alleviate his suffering and are not merely experimenting on him
   (b) The clear purpose of the procedure or use of specific technology and how it will help overcome the shortcomings of existing treatment modalities
   (c) All records will be maintained with a level of confidentiality as specified in the HIPAA
   (d) Consent has specifically to be taken for publishing his data, photographs, operative videos or post-operative results in authentic publications
   (e) The principles of anonymization of medical data will be followed in letter and spirit. Any private data which is unrelated to the research project will not be published, released or used for any other purpose
   (f) Details of the procedure must be clearly mentioned in a language and at a level that the patient understands. The more uneducated the patient, the greater is the clinician's responsibility to come down to his level and explain. If required, the language used in the consent form can be as low a level as Class 7th in school

2. If the research involves the use of materials that may offend the socio-cultural sensibilities of the patient, it should be specifically avoided or the patient excluded

from the study. For example, the use of rat-tail collagen matrix for cartilage tissue culture. Here it is preferable to use a synthetic substitute.

3. If the procedure involves some danger to the patient's life or body part, the consent form must clearly mention so, and the patient's consent must specifically be taken for the risks involved. In such cases, the patient has a right to clearly know the following:
   (a) Measures taken to avoid these dangers
   (b) Possible measures to alleviate suffering, should the precautions fail
   (c) Fixing of responsibilities of treating doctor or institute in terms of monetary issues of all kinds, indemnity of doctor and vicarious responsibility of the institution
   (d) In case treatment is based on in vitro studies, as is frequently the case, fixing of responsibilities of the in vitro researchers

All these cannot form the contents of the main format for informed consent. They can be included as a separate consent form.

The aspiring researcher will not fail to notice that a lot of the above-mentioned facets of Informed Consent were sacrificed at the altar of general societal good during the Covid-19 Pandemic.

To be somewhat fair to the researchers in the Covid-19 disease:

1. The Pathogenesis and disease course were largely unknown, especially the systemic effects, since this was a once-in-a-century phenomenon
2. The disease markers were largely unknown, so the investigations in the initial stage of the disease were unclear, resulting in many unwanted deaths more so in a totally low-risk section of the population
3. The shrill propaganda wars in social media and knee jerk reactions of health authorities forced the researchers to somewhat abandon the basic tenets of research. In a majority of cases, especially drug therapeutic research to counter the pandemic, even the patients were desperate enough to sign any document in the hope of saving lives

Having seen the exception, let us now peruse the norms:

Medical research can be broadly classified into:

1. Applied Research, with its myriad variety of procedures, treatment modalities like drugs and use of a variety of existing or new technologies
2. Basic Research fields like Nano-technology, Molecular Biology, Drug Synthesis etc

Frequently, both these inevitably merge into each other or are complementary to each other. Basic research remains abstract until an application can be found to make it worthwhile.

Original or basic medical research can involve the following:

1. Trying to link apparently unrelated patient body parameters to a disease process, e.g. D-Dimer Test during Covid-19, the discovery of 'Disease Markers'
2. Micro or Nano level research into a disease process, e.g. Genome mapping of viruses
3. Micro or Electron Microscopic analysis of a patient's cells, disease-causing organisms or vectors
4. Use of revolutionary technologies like 3-D Printing and Synthetic Molecules

To start with all these are in-vitro studies. The level of Informed Consent required here is very basic. It is needed because the patient may be donating a body fluid or tissue for analysis. Here the most important issues are confidentiality of patient records and anonymization of patient data.

Applied medical research can involve the following:

1. Addressing a specific disease or medical issue or intra-therapy problem, e.g. Pain relief modalities, control of Diabetes, Hypertension and Cardiac Dysfunction
2. In vivo use of any new technology, e.g. Interventional Radiology, Post-amputation Prosthetic Design, designing hi-tech implants like intra-ocular lenses, Cardiac stents and, of course, Joint Replacement implants
3. In vivo use of a totally new drug or molecule. Contrary to hope, this is now evidently a rare phenomenon. Very few drugs in recent times have turned out to be the wonder drugs or panacea that they promised
4. In vivo use of already existing drugs or molecule or technology with or without modification in a new usage area (for example, use of a drug for Pulmonary Hypertension for treating Erectile Dysfunction in males).

Here, the level of consent required is extensive, as outlined earlier.

5. Process of Informed Consent

1. The patient is given all information about what the research or new procedure or treatment involves in a language and at a level that he understands
2. The benefits and risks of participation are clearly explained to him
3. His right to opt-out of the research process at any stage is also clearly explained to him
4. Reasonable alternate treatments with their pros and cons are clearly outlined to him so he can make an informed choice
5. Risks of non-participation are also clearly outlined to him
6. The language used throughout the form is at the level of a local student of class 6th/8th

Challenges

1. Religious or socio-cultural influences
2. False expectations of guaranteed cure in the patient's mind
3. False perception of equating research modality with definitive treatment
4. Obtaining the cooperation of Children/Minors even after the guardian's consent

5. Vulnerable people and patient groups, e.g. Poor patients in government/free hospitals being coerced to participate under the threat of denial of existing treatment

6. Exceptions

There are very special situations when empirical therapies are necessary. As in the present pandemic, the general societal good may override patients' rights. This is called 'Emergency Research'.

Following situations may involve Emergency Research and hence the dilution of the format of informed consents:

1. Life-threatening situations necessitating the use of previously untested modalities
2. Available treatments to save lives are unproven or unsatisfactory
3. Collection of valid scientific information crucial to determining the safety and efficacy of the new treatment
4. Participation in the research holds out the prospect of direct benefit to subjects or society, e.g. New vaccines
5. Clinical investigation cannot be practically carried out without a waiver of consent

All these will apply to the emergency use of newer treatment modalities in pandemic situations. However, additional responsibilities for the researchers will then include consultation with community representatives and governments, public disclosure before the start of the study and after its conclusion, protection and anonymization of patient data in accordance with the HIPAA and establishment of independent Data Monitoring Committees.

The consent form is customized to the research project. The language used in preparation of the form should be at the level of a local student of class 6th/8th. This is then signed by the patient himself/herself or his/her guardian in the case of minors. A link is provided of WHO templates for either clinical trials or clinical research as an example. However, it must be emphasized that the consent form is project specific. https://research-compliance.umich.edu/informed-consent-guidelines

Additional Reading

1. Dankar FK, Gergely M, Dankar SK. Informed Consent in Biomedical Research. Comput Struct Biotechnol J. 2019;17:463-474. doi: 10.1016/j.csbj.2019.03.010. eCollection 2019.
2. Mathur R, Swaminathan Soumya National ethical guidelines for biomedical & health research involving human participants, 2017: A commentary Indian J Med Res 2018;148: pp 279-283 DOI: 10.4103/0971-5916.245303
3. Church GM, Personal Genome Project Molecular Systems Biology (2005)1:2005.0030https://doi.org/10.1038/msb4100040
4. European General Data Protection Regulation (GDPR 2018); https://gdpr-info.eu Federal policy for Protection of Human subjects; http://www.hhs.gov/orhp/human subjects/common rule
5. C. Ervine; Directive 2004/39/EC Macmillan Education, UK London (2015)
6. HIPAA: Health Insurance Portability and Accountability Act of 1996 (HIPAA) Public Law 104-191

CHAPTER

13 Good Clinical Practice Ethical and Scientific Standard for Clinical Research Conduct

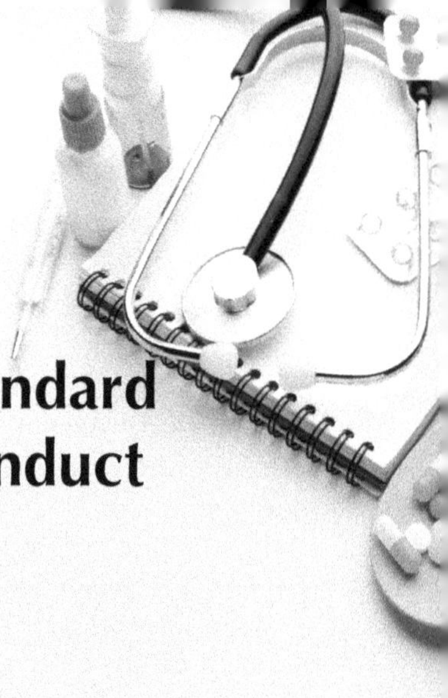

Arun Bhatt

1. Introduction

Good Clinical Practice (GCP) is an international ethical and scientific quality standard for clinical research, which encompasses all aspects of clinical research conduct. GCP guidelines are E-6, one of the efficacy guidelines released by the International Council for Harmonisation of Technical Requirements for Pharmaceuticals for Human Use (ICH). The guidelines laid down principles and prescribed processes for designing, conducting, recording and reporting trials that involve the participation of human beings. GCP is a standard for design, conduct, performance, monitoring, auditing, recording, analysing and reporting of clinical trials that provides assurance that the data and reported results are credible and accurate and that the rights, integrity and confidentiality of trial participants are protected [1].

In India, GCP guidelines were formulated by the Indian regulatory authorities - Central Drugs Standard Control Organisation - based on ICH-GCP [2]. Compliance to GCP is mandatory for clinical trials of Investigational Products (IP) – a pharmaceutical form of an active ingredient or placebo being tested or used as a reference in a clinical trial - that are intended to be submitted to regulatory authorities. However, the principles and practices of GCP essentially provide ethical and scientific frameworks for all types of clinical research.

2. Evolution of ICH-GCP

The ethical principles of GCP have their origins in many guidelines on the ethics of clinical research. Some of the most well-known landmarks are:

- The Nuremberg Code
- Declaration of Helsinki
- The Belmont Report

The Nuremberg Code

During the Second World War, there was gross and criminal exploitation of human participants during medical experimentation. The major consequence of this was the setting up of the Nuremberg War Crime Trials, in which the ethical violations during the conduct of medical research were examined and an ethical code- a set of directives for human experimentation was established in 1947 [3]. The Nuremberg Code was the first international guideline which described the basic principles of ethical behaviour in the conduct of human experimentation. The focus of the Nuremberg Code directives is on:

- Clinical Researcher's responsibility:
  - Conduct of research by scientifically qualified persons
  - Designing experiment/study based on adequate animal experimentation and knowledge of natural history of the disease
  - Research/experiment beneficial for the society
  - Degree of research/experiment risk is not more than the importance of the problem to be solved by the experiment
  - Avoidance of research with a high risk of death or disabling injury
  - Prevention of all unnecessary physical and mental suffering and injury of research participants
  - Protection of research participants against injury, disability or death
  - Stopping the experiment if there is a likelihood of harm to the research participant by the continuation of the experiment
- Research participant's rights
  - Voluntary consent essential
  - Freedom to stop participation during the experiment

Declaration of Helsinki

The World Medical Association developed the Declaration of Helsinki (DOH), which describes ethical principles for physicians conducting medical research involving human participants [4]. Since its release in 1964, DOH guidelines have been revised from time to time in line with evolving scientific and ethical norms.

Major recommendations of DOH 2013 are:

- The duty of physicians involved in medical research is to protect the life, health, dignity, integrity, right to self-determination, privacy and confidentiality of personal information of research participants
- Medical research to be conducted only by individuals with the appropriate ethics and scientific education, training and qualifications
- Medical research is conducted only if the objective's importance outweighs the risks and burdens to the research participants

- Careful assessment of predictable risks and burdens and foreseeable benefits to human research participants
- Special protection for vulnerable groups and individuals participating in the research
- Ethics Committee reviews and approvals of the research protocol before initiation of the study
- Voluntary informed consent from research participants
- Informed consent for the collection, storage and/or reuse of research using identifiable human material or data
- Provisions for post-trial access for all participants who need an intervention identified as beneficial in the trial
- Registration of research study in the publicly accessible database before recruitment of the first subject
- The researchers must make public the results of their research on human participants

The Belmont Report

The US National Commission for the Protection of Human Participants of Biomedical and Behavioural Research was set up in response to the Tuskegee Syphilis Study scandal in 1974. This was a study of natural history of the progression of Syphilis in which treatment for the disease was withheld from impoverished African American men in Alabama. This study began in 1932 and was stopped in 1972 when the media exposed the ethical violations in the conduct of the study in a vulnerable population. The commission prepared the Belmont Report in 1979, which identified the fundamental ethical principles that should guide the conduct of research with human participants [5]. These are:

- Autonomy or respect for persons:
    - o Research participants have autonomy in decision making
    - o Research participants with diminished autonomy are entitled to protection.
- Beneficence - maximize possible benefits
- Non-malfeasance – avoid harm
- Justice - fairness in the distribution of benefits of research to participants from all education and socioeconomic – low or high - strata

These principles are applicable to the key research concepts of:

(a) Informed Consent
(b) Assessment of Risks and Benefits
(c) Selection of Participants

3. Evolution of Indian GCP

Indian GCP guidelines[2] have been evolved with consideration of ICH-GCP and National Ethical Guidelines for Biomedical and Health Research Involving Human Participants issued by the Indian Council of Medical Research (ICMR). [6]

ICMR guidelines discuss the following major ethical issues in Biomedical and Health Research:

1. Benefit-Risk Assessment
2. Informed Consent process
3. Privacy and Confidentiality
4. Distributive justice
5. Payment for participation
6. Compensation for research-related harm
7. Ancillary care
8. Conflict of Interest
9. Selection of vulnerable and special groups as research participants
10. Community engagement
11. Post research access and benefit-sharing

ICMR guidelines give specific recommendations for an ethical approach for:

- Responsible Conduct of Research
- Ethical review procedures
- Informed Consent process
- Vulnerability
- Clinical trials of drugs and other interventions
- Public Health Research
- Social and Behavioural Sciences Research for Health
- Human genetics testing and research
- Biological materials, Bio-banking and Data-sets
- Research during Humanitarian Emergencies and Disasters

Compliance to Indian GCP is mandatory for clinical trials of new drugs for regulatory approval [7]. Academic clinical trials of new drugs and biomedical and health research studies should be conducted in accordance with the ICMR guidelines [7].

4. ICH-GCP Guidelines

The ICH-GCP Guidelines include:

- Glossary - covers the definition of all terms discussed in the guidelines
- Principles – describes the fundamentals of GCP (Table 13.1)
- Responsibilities of Institutional Review Board (IRB)/independent Ethics Committee (IEC), investigators and sponsors
- Clinical Trial protocol contents
- Investigator's Brochure (IB)
- Essential documents

Table 13.1: Fundamentals of GCP

Ethics	• Ensure balance of foreseeable risks and inconveniences vis-à-vis the anticipated benefits to the trial participant and society • Most important consideration - rights, safety, confidentiality and well-being of the trial participant • IRB/IEC approval prior to initiation of the trial • Freely given informed consent obtained from every participant prior to clinical trial participation • A qualified physician responsible for medical care and medical decisions for the treatment of participants • Protection of confidentiality of participants' records
Science	• Adequate pre-clinical and clinical information on IP • Scientifically sound and detailed clinical trial protocol
Competence of the study team	• Everyone involved in conducting the trial to be qualified by education, training and experience to perform his or her respective tasks
Documentation	• All clinical trial information to be recorded, handled and stored in a way that allows its accurate reporting, interpretation and verification
Quality	• Manufacturing, handling and storage of IP in accordance with Good Manufacturing Practice (GMP) • Systems with Standard Operating Procedures (SOP) to cover all essential steps in the conduct of clinical trial

As GCP covers all stages of the clinical study from design to reporting, it applies to all stages of clinical study – before the initiation of the study, during the study and after the completion of the study.

Key Documents

Key documents for a clinical research study are:

- *Protocol:* It is a document that describes the objectives, design, methodology, statistical considerations and organization of a trial [1]. The protocol for an interventional clinical trial of Investigational Products (IP) should include [1].
    - Background information with rationale
    - Study objectives and purpose
    - Study Design
    - Selection and withdrawal of participants
    - Detailed description of the methodology
    - Treatment details for IP
    - Assessment of Efficacy and Safety
    - Statistics
    - Ethics

- Quality Control and Quality Assurance
- Data handling and record keeping. This format could be modified for observational study designs.

- *Investigator's Brochure (IB):* It is a compilation of the clinical and non-clinical data on the investigational products relevant to human participants' clinical study. The purpose of IB is to facilitate the investigator's understanding of the rationale and compliance with key features of the protocol [1]. The IB also provides insight to support the clinical management of the study participants during the conduct of a clinical trial.

- *Informed Consent Document (ICD):* This includes Patient Information Sheet (PIS) and Informed Consent Form (ICF).

  - PIS describes the rights and responsibilities of the participants [1]:

  (a) Right to Information

  - o Research Study – description of experimental nature, purpose, duration of participation, number of participants
  - o Trial treatments and the probability of random assignment to each treatment
  - o Trial procedures
  - o Risks - reasonably foreseeable risks or inconveniences to the participants
  - o Benefits
  - o Alternative procedures or treatments
  - o Any new information relevant to the participant 's willingness to continue participation in the trial
  - o Contact details of
    - IEC member for further information regarding the trial and the rights of trial participants, and
    - Investigator/site team to contact in the event of a trial-related injury
  - o Termination of the subject's participation - Foreseeable circumstances and/or reasons

  (b) Right to Confidentiality

  - o Protection of confidentiality of records identifying the participant

  (c) Right to Compensation

  - o Compensation and treatment are available to the participant in the event of trial-related injury
  - o Compensation for participation

  (d) Right of Withdrawal

- Withdraw from the trial at any time without penalty or loss of benefits to which the participant is otherwise entitled

(e) Responsibilities of the Participants

- Compliance with protocol procedures, treatment, follow-ups, laboratory tests
- Permission for direct access to the participant's original medical records for the sponsor's monitoring, the auditors, the IRB/IEC and the regulatory authorities

  - The ICF is meant for documentation of the consent. The participant confirms his/her voluntary participation by signing and dating the ICF. If the participant is not capable of understanding the PIS e.g. Minors or severe dementia patients, his/her Legally Acceptable Representative (LAR) would sign and date the ICF. If a participant is unable to read or if a LAR is unable to read, an impartial witness should be present during the entire informed consent discussion and should sign and personally date the ICF. The investigator or a person designated by the investigator who conducted the informed consent discussion should sign and date the ICF.

  - *Clinical Study Agreement (CTA):* A written, dated and signed agreement between sponsor and investigator and/or institution that sets out any arrangements on delegation and distribution of tasks and obligations and financial matters.

5. Responsibilities for GCP Compliance

The stakeholders responsible for ensuring compliance to GCP Guidelines are [1]:

- **Sponsor:** An individual, company, institution or organization which takes responsibility for the initiation, management and/or financing of a clinical trial [1]
- **Investigator:** A person responsible for conducting the clinical trial at the a trial site [1]
- **Sponsor-Investigator:** An individual who both initiates and conducts, alone or with others, a clinical trial and under whose immediate direction the IP is administered, dispensed or used by a subject.[1] The obligations of a sponsor-investigator includes both those of a sponsor and an investigator
- **IEC:** An independent body whose responsibility is to ensure the protection of the rights, safety and well-being of human participants involved in the trial and to provide public assurance of that protection by reviewing study-related documents [1]

GCP guidelines are applicable for all stages of a clinical study, from design to reporting. Hence, it is important to discuss the obligations of stakeholders for each stage.

5a. Before initiation of the clinical phase of the study

Sponsor

In the planning stage before the study formally starts, the sponsor plays the most important role in setting up the clinical trial. This includes several critical tasks [1]:

- Quality Assurance (QA) and Quality Control (QC) systems with written SOPs
- Regulatory approval for the clinical study, if applicable
- Preparation of study documents – protocol, ICD, Case Record Form (CRF)
- Information on the investigational product(s) – updated IB
- Selection of the investigators who are qualified by training and experience and who have adequate resources to conduct the trial properly
- CTA with the investigators/ institutions to conduct the trial in compliance with GCP, regulatory requirements and protocol
- Training of all the investigators and their teams to comply with a uniform set of standards for following the protocol, for assessment efficacy and safety, and for completing the CRFs
- Compensation to participants for trial-related injuries as per regulations
- Confirmation of review approval/favourable opinion by IRB/IEC
- Manufacturing, packaging, labelling and coding IP in accordance with applicable regulations
- Supply an investigator/institution with the IP after obtaining documentation of approval from IEC and regulatory authorities
- Instruct the investigator/institution on handling and storage of IP and documentation of the process

Investigator

Before the initiation of the clinical phase, the investigator's main responsibility is to get the site ready for the study. This includes the following tasks [1, 7]:

- Documented evidence of the investigator's qualification, education, training and experience to assume responsibility for the proper conduct of the trial
- Develop site SOPs for the conduct of the clinical trial
- Compliance with the protocols, GCP and applicable regulatory requirements
- Familiarity with appropriate use of IP as described in the protocol and IB
- Delegation of significant trial-related duties to qualified and trained team members
- Training of team members about the protocols, IP and trial-related duties and functions
- Demonstrate potential for recruiting the required number of suitable participants
- Have sufficient time and adequate facilities to conduct and complete the trial properly
- Obtain written and dated IRB/IEC approval/favourable opinion for the trial protocols, written ICF, consent form updates, participant recruitment procedures, and any other written information to be provided to participants
- Obtain and document informed consent in compliance with the applicable regulatory requirements and conformity to GCP and the ethical principles of DOH

IEC

In the stage before initiation, IEC's vital responsibility is to review the study documents and opine about approval. For this purpose the IEC should [1, 6, 7]:

- Ensure protection of the rights, safety and well-being of the research participants
- Have SOPs for:

  1. Determining composition and quorum
  2. Handling Conflict of Interest
  3. Scheduling and Conducting Meetings
  4. Type of Review – exempted, expedited, full
  5. Reviewing study documents
  6. Documenting decisions
  7. recording minutes

- Have a reasonable number of members who collectively have the qualifications and experience to review and evaluate the study proposal
- Ensure training of members in human research protection, GCP and regulatory requirements
- Should be registered with CDSCO and ICMR
- Review documents

  1. Trial protocol and CRF
  2. ICD in English and local language
  3. IB
  4. Participant recruitment procedures – advertisements
  5. Investigator's current Curriculum Vitae
  6. Payments and compensation available to participants
  7. Investigator Undertaking, if applicable
  8. Regulatory permission, if applicable
  9. Documentation of clinical trial registration
  10. CTA between the sponsors, investigator and institution, if applicable
  11. Insurance Policy for study participants

- Review risks, benefits, science, medical aspects and ethics as per GCP and regulatory requirements
- Special attention to trials that include vulnerable participants
- Document decision – approval, modifications of study, disapproval or termination/ suspension of any prior approval, the documents reviewed and the conditions of approval

5b. During the Clinical Conduct of the Trial

Sponsor

During the clinical conduct, when the participants are enrolled in the study, the sponsor's major focus is to ensure the quality of clinical trial conduct, the safety of study participants and data integrity[1]. The essential tasks are [1, 6, 7]:

- Focus on trial processes and data essential to ensure human participant protection and data integrity
- QC to ensure that all data is reliable and has been processed correctly
- Conduct ongoing safety evaluation of the IP
- Promptly notify the investigator and the regulatory authorities of findings that could adversely affect the safety of participants, impact the conduct of the trial, or alter the IEC's approval to continue the trial
- Expedite the reporting of Serious and Unexpected Suspected Adverse Drug Reactions (SUSARs) to all investigators, IECs and to the regulatory authorities
- Submit all safety updates and periodic reports to the regulatory authorities as required by applicable regulatory requirements
- Comply with all regulations applicable to Serious Adverse Events (SAEs)
- Ensure monitoring of the trial to verify that:
    - o The rights and well-being of the human participants are protected
    - o The reported trial data is accurate, complete and verifiable from the source documents
    - o The conduct of the trial follows the approved protocol with GCP and the regulatory requirements
- Maintain records that document shipment, receipt, disposition of IP
- Ensure IP accountability
- Perform audits to evaluate trial conduct and compliance with the protocol, SOPs, GCP and regulatory requirements
- Take prompt action to secure compliance from the investigator
- Perform a Root Cause Analysis and implement appropriate corrective and preventive actions, in case of significant non-compliance

Investigator

During the clinical phase, the investigator's responsibility is to ensure human protection and assure data integrity[1].

Important activities include [1,7]:

- Conduct the trial in compliance with the protocol approved by the regulatory authorities, IEC and GCP
- Obtain and document informed consent in compliance with the applicable regulatory requirement(s) and conformity to GCP and to the ethical principles of DOH
- Inform the participant or the LAR in a timely manner if new information becomes available that may be relevant to the participant's willingness to continue in the trial
- Report to IEC any protocol deviations/changes increasing the risk to participants or likely to have a significant impact on the conduct of the trial
- Comply with all regulations applicable to SAEs

- Report SAEs to the regulatory authorities, the IEC and the sponsor in the stipulated time
- Medical care of trial participants for any adverse events and SAEs
- Report all SUSARs and new safety information to IECs
- Ensure that source data is attributable, legible, contemporaneous, original, accurate and complete
- Ensure that data reported on the CRF is consistent with the source documents
- Ensure and document IP accountability at the trial sites
- Use IP in accordance with the approved protocol
- Submit Progress Reports of the trial status as per the frequency requested by the IEC

IEC

During the clinical phase, the IEC's main responsibility is to guard the safety of study participants. This would necessitate [1, 6, 7]:

- Ongoing review of the clinical trials based on periodic study progress reports from investigators
- Review and act on reports of:
    - Protocol deviations
    - Changes increasing the risk to participants
    - Changes significantly affecting the conduct of the trial
    - All SUSARs
    - New safety information
- Comply with all applicable regulations to SAEs
- Examine measures taken for medical management of SAEs
- Ensure compensation for research-related injuries, if applicable

5c. After Completion of the Trial

Sponsor

After the completion of the trial, the sponsor's main responsibility is to complete data analysis and prepare a clinical trial report. This includes the following activities [1]:

- Close all findings, data queries and audit observations
- Document completion of all activities required for trial close-out
- Copies of essential documents to be held in the appropriate files
- Perform data processing and management
- Conduct statistical analyses
- Prepare clinical trial report and provide to the regulatory agency as required
- Document the final accounting of IP received at the site, dispense to participants, return by the participants and return to sponsor
- Document destruction of unused IP
- Retain all sponsor-specific essential documents in conformance with the applicable regulatory requirements

- Promptly inform the investigators/institutions, IEC and the regulatory authorities about premature termination or suspension of the clinical trial
- Be prepared for regulatory inspection

Investigator

After completion of the study, the important responsibility of the Investigator is supporting the sponsor in data management and closing the study. This would include:

- Respond to all findings, data queries and audit observations
- Ensure IP accountability for the site and return unused supplies to the sponsor
- Inform IEC about completion of the trial
- Provide summary or final study report of the trial's outcome to IEC
- Report premature termination of the study to IEC and if required, to regulatory authorities
- Inform the trial participants about the premature termination of the study and assure appropriate therapy and follow-up
- Maintain all essential trial documents as per GCP and regulatory requirements
- Be prepared for Regulatory Inspection

IEC

After completion of the trial, the IEC's role is to:

- Receive the clinical study report
- Retain all relevant records for the period required as per the regulatory requirements

6. Essential documents

Documentation is the heart and soul of GCP compliance. Essential documents are those which individually and collectively permit evaluation of the conduct of the trial and the quality of the data.[1] GCP guidelines lists the essential documents for documentation of all processes during each stage of a clinical study which should be filed in the trial master files at the investigator site and at the sponsor's office.

These essential documents are vital in demonstrating the compliance of the investigator and the sponsor with the standards of GCP and regulatory requirements. These documents are audited by auditors and inspected by the regulatory authorities as part of the process to confirm the validity of the trial conduct and the integrity of the data collected [1].

7. Conclusions

The success of a clinical research study rests on ensuring human protection and data integrity in the planning and conduct of the study. The clinical research physician should be aware and comply with the GCP principles and processes in conducting all clinical research studies.

References

1. European Medicines Agency International Council on Harmonisation. Guideline for good clinical practice E6(R2) Step 5 London, United Kingdom 2016
2. Central Drugs Standard Control Organisation. Good Clinical Practices for Clinical Research in India 2001
3. Nuremberg Code. Trials of War Criminals before the Nuremberg Military Tribunals under Control Council Law No. 10, Vol. 2, pp. 181–182. Washington, D.C.: U.S. Government Printing Offce, 1949. https://history.nih.gov/display/history/Nuremberg+Code Accessed 31 Aug 2021
4. Declaration of Helsinki: ethical principles for medical research involving human participants. Fortaleza: World Medical Association. 2013; https://www.wma.net/policies-post/wma-declaration-of-helsinki-ethical-principles-for-medical-research-involving-human-participants/ Accessed 31 Aug 2021
5. The National Commission for the Protection of Human Participants of Biomedical and Behavioral Research. The Belmont report: ethical principles and guidelines for the protection of human participants of research. Washington DC: Department of Health, Education and Welfare; 1979. https://www.hhs.gov/ohrp/regulations-and-policy/belmont-report/read-the-belmont-report/index.html Accessed 31 Aug 2021
6. Indian Council of Medical Research. National Ethical Guidelines for Biomedical and Health Research Involving Human Participants 2017
7. Central Drugs Standard Control Organisation. New Drugs and Clinical Trials Rules 2019

CHAPTER

14 Designing a Clinical Protocol

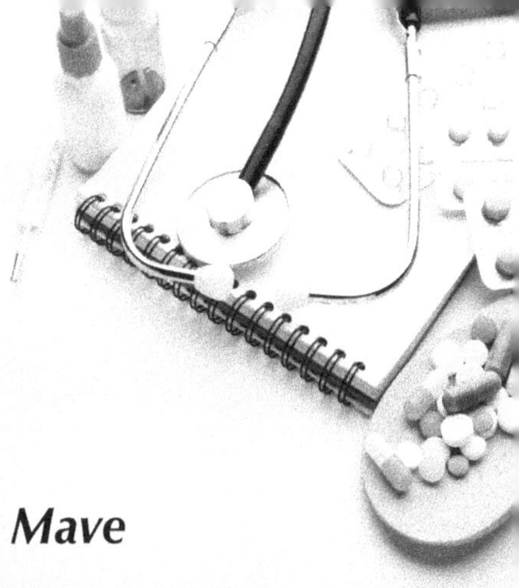

Priyanka Raichur and Vidya Mave

1. Introduction

Clinical research involves the study of the effectiveness and safety of medicines, devices and treatment regimens. It is intended for human use and broadly covers investigations of new diagnostics, prevention and treatment regimens or strategies. Furthermore, clinical research may assess interventions to relieve symptoms of a disease. It has been categorized by the United States National Institute of Health (US-NIH) as follows [1]:

Patient-oriented Research

This involves research conducted with human participants (or on the material of human origin, such as tissues, specimens and cognitive phenomena) where an investigator (or colleague) directly interacts with them. *In Vitro* studies that use human tissues but cannot be linked to a living individual are not considered patient-oriented research. This type of research encompasses the evaluation of mechanisms of human disease and therapeutic interventions and includes clinical trials or development of new technologies.

Epidemiological and Behavioural Studies

This involves the investigation of cause, frequency and distribution of diseases in the population and application of behavioural sciences on human subjects. Behavioural research helps to evaluate and understand the impact of human behaviour on health outcomes and designs interventions aimed at modifying the health-related behaviour.

Outcomes and Health Services Research

This involves the evaluation of outcomes and effectiveness of Public Health Interventions and Health Care Delivery [1].

Clinical research may also involve exploration of epidemiology and pathogenesis of diseases and is administered by a clinical research team. A clinical research team includes clinical investigators, laboratory personnel, pharmacists, counsellors and the data management team. Further, research studies can be undertaken by a single institution or it can be a collaborative effort between multiple sites within and between countries. To ensure that uniform procedures are followed it is essential to have a written protocol that outlines the research hypothesis, objectives, eligibility criteria and all the procedures involved in conducting the research study. A clinical research protocol is a written plan of procedures for any research activity involving human participants.

2. Need for Clinical Research Protocol

A written set of procedures and guidelines documented in a clinical research protocol provides a roadmap to different teams involved in conducting a research study. This is especially critical for multicentric trials as it provides a uniform framework for all sites. Importantly, this helps to minimize variability between sites and ensures uniformity and integrity of the data collected.

A Protocol is a prerequisite document for regulatory and ethics approval of clinical research. However, in many instances, a concept sheet is developed as an initial step, particularly to apply for funding. The concept sheet provides an overview of the plan for conducting the research project, including the background, objectives, hypothesis, study procedures, statistical considerations and study outcomes. The concept sheet often forms the basis for the development of a full clinical protocol after funding is secured. Publication of a clinical protocol ensures sharing of knowledge which has the potential for replicability of the methods and transparency of the research methods. Clinical research protocol is required for the conduct of the research and is used by clinical investigators, funders, ethics and regulatory authorities, health care professionals and journals.

In this chapter, we aim to provide tools to design a sound clinical research protocol.

3. Steps in Conducting a Research Study

The process of research begins by defining a research problem. This is initially a vague idea and can be developed further by conducting an extensive literature review. Essentially, the literature search helps to outline the current knowledge and identifies the knowledge gaps. Once a clear research gap or a problem is identified, formulation of a hypothesis becomes the next step. The overarching research goals and objectives are then developed to prove or disprove the hypothesis.

After a hypothesis and objectives are defined, the research design appropriate to meet the objectives is formed. The research design describes the type of studies (case-control, observational or clinical) and includes the detailed methodology and procedures. The proposed methodology and procedures should help to achieve the proposed objectives.

Having a well-written and comprehensive protocol defining the study hypothesis, objectives and procedures is an essential part of the research process. After a protocol is developed and all the regulatory approvals are obtained, the next steps include the development of Case Report Forms (CRF), training of the study personnel, conducting the research, collection of data, analysis of data, interpretation and inference of results (Figure 14.1).

4. Essential Components of a Clinical Trial Protocol

A clinical research protocol is a comprehensive document that describes the research question, the scientific rationale behind the research, the hypothesis, specific aims and objectives, ethical considerations and all procedures of the research study from recruitment of participants to publication of the study results.

Many funding organizations such as the Indian Council of Medical Research (ICMR), Department of Biotechnology (DBT), Department of Science and Technology (DST), corporate foundations, and the US-NIH may require specific templates which incorporate all the procedures as per the requirements of International Conference on Harmonisation (ICH) Guidance for Industry, E-6 Good Clinical Practice (GCP): Consolidated Guidance (ICH-E6) [2]). While templates for designing a research protocol may vary across different institutions, the essential components remain the same. The section provides a framework for designing a clinical research protocol.

5. Title Page for Clinical Protocol

The title page must include the full title of the study, an acronym (if applicable), the protocol version and the names of the Principal Investigator (PI), the sponsor, and the funder. The title page must clearly mention the current version of the protocol.

The title of a protocol should be clear, concise and indicate the study design, the phase of the trial, setting and population and for clinical trials the drug/product under investigation or the specific intervention. Every version of the protocol must be clearly numbered and dated, as the protocol is expected to undergo review and changes throughout the development process. Each time a protocol undergoes an amendment, a summary of changes from the previous version must be listed as an appendix or as the initial pages in the protocol. Additionally, the version and date should be added as a header throughout the document, so that each page reflects the current version of the protocol. The title page must be followed by the Table of Contents and a List of Abbreviations. In addition, page numbering is recommended to help rapidly identify sections during the protocol implementation.

Protocol Team and Contact Information

The contact details of the key personnel, including the Principal Investigators, Site Investigators, Trial Managers, Data Managers, Trial Physicians, Clinical Monitoring Team and Trial Statisticians should be listed. This should include the full name, degree, title, role in the trial, name of institution, address, phone number and e-mail. These details provide a point of reference for the staff conducting the trial.

Statement of Compliance/Investigator Statement/General Statement

This is a requirement of the US-NIH and includes a statement template that is signed by the principal and site investigators. This statement is an undertaking by each investigator that they will be responsible for conducting the trial in accordance with the protocol and applicable ethical and regulatory requirements.

Protocol Summary

This includes a short description of the study including the design, setting, population, sample size, randomization for clinical trials, duration, objectives and the main outcomes. The study schema may be represented as a table, a flow chart or a process diagram to illustrate the snapshot of the trial on a single page.

6. Introduction of the Protocol Topic

This section provides the background and rationale for conducting the research. It includes a description of the research problem, the epidemiology and public health importance, a description of the intervention being investigated, a review and discussion of the existing literature and the need for the study. The rationale for the use of an investigational drug/ device or an intervention should be clearly defined with sound scientific evidence. The known potential risks and benefits should also be described using existing literature or from the package inserts. The hypothesis for the study should be stated in this section.

Study Objectives

The Study Objective is an active statement about how the study is going to answer the specific research question [3]. Every study usually has one primary and multiple secondary objectives. These objectives must be expressed as Statement of Purpose (e.g., to assess, to determine, to evaluate) and include both a general (e.g., feasibility, efficacy, safety) and/or specific purpose (superior or non-inferior) [2].

Study Design and End-point

A detailed description of the Study Design including the type of Research - Descriptive or Analytical, should be illustrated in this section. In a clinical trial (blinded/open-label/ placebo-controlled) the phase, the number of study arms, single or multicentric and details of the intervention need to be detailed here. Study End-points are measurements or observations that help to assess the effect of the study intervention or variable. There are several study end-point variables. Generally, clinical trials have two major endpoints - Safety and Efficacy which are measured using clinical and laboratory observations and measurements. Study End-x`points should always correspond to the study objectives and hypotheses being tested.

7. Participant Enrolment and Withdrawal

This section provides detailed guidance to the Recruitment and Retention of Trial Participants.

Study Population

This should include a detailed description of the inclusion and exclusion criteria. The demographic characteristics for inclusion which includes age and sex should be defined. If the inclusion criteria includes a population with a certain disease then clear definitions must be used to define the disease. The exclusion criteria must be mentioned considering the risk of intervention in case of clinical trials.

Appropriate laboratory cut-off points must be clearly stated for recruitment of participants and prohibited medications should be listed clearly for exclusion. Inclusion and exclusion criteria must be mutually exclusive, and the same criteria should not be listed as both inclusion and exclusion criteria. Additionally, statements on the provision of written consent and assent, willingness and ability to participate and appropriate use of contraceptive methods must be included.

Recruitment and Retention Strategy

This section describes the target sample size, recruitment sites, anticipated accrual rates and source of participants. For studies with long-term follow-up periods strategies for retention of trial participants should be described. A statement on the recruitment of vulnerable populations may be included in this section.

Participant Withdrawal and Premature Study Termination

A list of reasons for withdrawal and termination should be defined. This could either be participant or investigator-initiated withdrawal. Procedures for handling withdrawals including follow-up and data collection of withdrawn participants should be described in addition to a discussion of replacement of withdrawn participants with additional enrolments. In some cases, due to safety, data integrity or funding issues, a study may be prematurely terminated. The anticipated reasons may be outlined here with a description of the procedures for informing the ethics and regulatory authorities.

8. Study Intervention

This protocol section should describe in detail the intervention including study agents or behavioural intervention. As per the US-NIH definition, a Study Agent may be a

Drug (including a biological product), Imaging Agent or Device subject to regulation under the Federal Food, Drug and Cosmetic Act that is intended for administration to humans and which has been or has not yet been approved by the Food and Drug Administration (FDA).

All details relating to the use of the study agent in the trial, including formulation, appearance, dosing, preparation, administration, packaging, labelling, acquisition, manufacturer, shipment, storage requirements, etc. should be described in this section. Specific instructions related to weight-based dosing, dose adjustments, modifications and adherence measures should also be described here. An important component is the description of study agent accountability procedures including the amount and frequency of drug shipments, tracking of each dose dispensed and returned and procedures for handling unused medications.

9. Study Procedures and Schedules

This section includes a description of the schedule of visits, procedures at each visit and allowable window periods for those visits (**Table 14.2**). In this section, all study procedures and evaluations done as part of the research are detailed including clinical history, physical examination, randomization procedure, laboratory evaluations, imaging, questionnaires, counselling procedures, assessment of adherence, etc.

The Consenting Process is a vital step in any clinical trial and the method of consent should be clearly defined in the protocol including consenting of illiterate participants, the requirement of a witness, assent, audio or video consenting. Assent is consenting by a mature child (generally 12 years or older) in appropriate language commiserate with his/her age, in addition to obtaining parental consent. Details of procedures at every visit, including screening, enrolment, follow-up, premature discontinuation, protocol-directed additional visits, unscheduled visits and final visits should be described. **Table 14.2** depicts a template for the schedule of evaluations summarizing all the procedures required at expected visits and allowable window periods. Additional descriptions of procedures including storage and handling of specimens, imaging, detailed description of consenting procedures, etc. may be described in the Manual Of Procedures (MOP).

10. Safety and Adverse Event Reporting

Adverse Event Reporting is a critical component in conducting a clinical trial as it helps in the assessment of safety of the investigational agent. Detailed definitions of adverse events, serious adverse events and the steps for recording and reporting such events should be clearly outlined in the protocol. Protocol-specific reporting requirements, timelines, procedures for reporting, steps to be taken, including dose interruptions or modifications are outlined here. The definitions for describing severity, expectedness and relation of the event to the investigational agent should be clearly mentioned in the protocol. The time period for event assessment and follow-up also need to be defined.

An independent safety oversight including a Data Safety Monitoring Board (DSMB) and a Safety Monitoring Committee (SMC) should be considered for a clinical trial. The type of safety oversight along with responsibilities for the oversight of safety in the study, frequency of meetings, composition of SMC or DSMB, frequency of interim data review, final data analysis and method of reviews should be clearly identified.

11. Monitoring Procedures

Periodic monitoring is needed while a research study is ongoing to ensure that the trial is being conducted as per the currently approved protocol, GCP and applicable regulatory requirements. Monitoring ensures that the rights and well-being of the study participants are being protected and the reported trial data is accurate, complete and verifiable with the source documents. The process of monitoring, frequency, type, who will conduct the monitoring, etc. needs to be described here. A separate detailed Clinical Monitoring Plan may also be referred in this section.

12. Statistical and Analysis Plan

The Statistical Tests to be used and the Analysis Plan should be well described in the protocol. The study hypothesis, sample size estimation, analysis of data-sets, description of statistical methods, type of tests to be used, how the results will be presented, plan of analysis for primary and secondary safety and efficacy end-points, etc. should be clearly defined in statistical terms. A description of procedures to reduce bias should also be included in this section where randomization and masking procedures can be explained.

13. Source Documents and Access to them

This section lists all the essential documents which need to be maintained throughout the conduct of the research study as per the ICH-E6 and regulatory requirements [4]. This includes a comprehensive list of essential documents, including the Investigators Brochure, all versions of the protocol and MOP, Informed Consent Forms, Case Report Forms, signed agreements between involved parties, insurance statements, adverse events, etc. The protocol should define who will have access to these documents and the measures to be taken to protect the confidentiality of the study data. The complete list of essential documents which need to be maintained can be found at the ICH website. (https://database.ich.org/sites/default/files/E6_R2_Addendum.pdf).

14. Quality Management

This includes Quality Assurance (QA) and Quality Control (QC). Each clinical research site should have a detailed Standard Operating Procedure (SOP) and Clinical Quality Management Plan (CQMP) outlining the quality management procedures including frequency of review, generation of quality reports, measures to reduce errors and corrective action plans. QA includes measures to check that all procedures are being conducted as per the protocol and GCP requirements. For example, documentation of Informed Consent Process to ensure that procedures are conducted as per the Schedule of Evaluations, etc also needs to be outlined. QC checks include data checks for CRF completeness, source versus CRF entry, data entry errors, etc.

15. Ethics/Protection of Participants

This includes a statement on the guiding ethical principles being followed by the study. Each participating site must provide for review and approval of the protocol and supporting documents by an appropriate Institutional Ethics Committee (IEC) or Institutional Review Board (IRB). Approval of both the protocol and consent forms must be obtained before the enrolment of participants. Each version of the protocol and consent forms must have EC/ IRB approval prior to implementation.

This section should also describe in detail the procedures for obtaining and documenting the informed consent from the study participants. A blank template of all the consent/assent forms which will be used for consent of the research participants should be added in the Protocol. Steps taken to maintain the confidentiality of data, who will have access to data, use of identifiers, delinking patient information with data, data sharing guidelines especially for Genomic Studies, security measures for physical and electronic records, etc. must also be described. An important component is also describing what will be done with stored specimens when applicable. The intended use of stored specimens, both planned and future use including provision for consent, duration of storage of specimens and documentation of laboratories where the specimen will be analyzed should be clearly outlined in the protocol.

16. Data Handling and Record Keeping

Data Collection and Management Responsibilities:

This section describes the type of data captured (electronic or paper forms), timelines for data completion and entry, key responsibilities and record keeping requirements. A detailed Data Management Plan may be referred which includes responsibilities and procedures for data handling and record keeping, CRF completion guidelines, coding for CRF and data entry and procedures for data monitoring.

Retention of Study Records:

The protocol should clearly mention the duration for which the study documents need to be stored as per applicable regulatory requirements. It is a good practice to mention the method of long-term storage of study documents (electronic or paper copies).

17. Protocol Deviations

Plans for detecting, reviewing and reporting deviations from the protocol should be described.

18. Publication and Data Sharing Policy

The Publication and Authorship Policies should be defined in the protocol. An Executive Committee overseeing the decisions related to authorship should be described.

19. Study Administration

This describes the governance of the study and the leadership structure. These include committees such as Trial Steering Committee (TSC) and Trial Management Group (TMG). The composition, role and frequency of meetings should be outlined.

20. Conflict of Interest Policy

This section should include a description of how the study will manage actual or perceived Conflicts of Interest (COI).

21. Literature References

All relevant literature and publications referenced in the text should be listed using a standard prescribed format. The International Committee of Medical Journal Editors (ICMJE) format is preferred by many sponsors including ICMR, DBT, DST and the US-NIH [5].

22. Appendices

Appendices may include a summary of changes from previous protocol versions, severity grading documents, coding for clinical events and medications, etc.

23. Publication and Registering a Clinical Protocol

It is a good practice to publish a research protocol. Publication of a research protocol creates a scientific record of the research methodology used and enhances the transparency of Research.

Some regulations mandate the registration of clinical trials in a public trials registry, such as the ClinicalTrial.gov in the United States and the Clinical Trial Registry India (CTRI) for trials conducted in India [6, 7].

Links for Protocol Templates

1. US NIH: https://grants.nih.gov/policy/clinical-trials/protocol-template.htmWorld Health Organisation: https://www.who.int/groups/research-ethics-review-committee/recommended-format-for-a-research-protocol/
2. ICMR: http://www.nirrh.res.in/wp-content/uploads/2019/08/06-Templates-for-protocol-Other-submissions.pdf

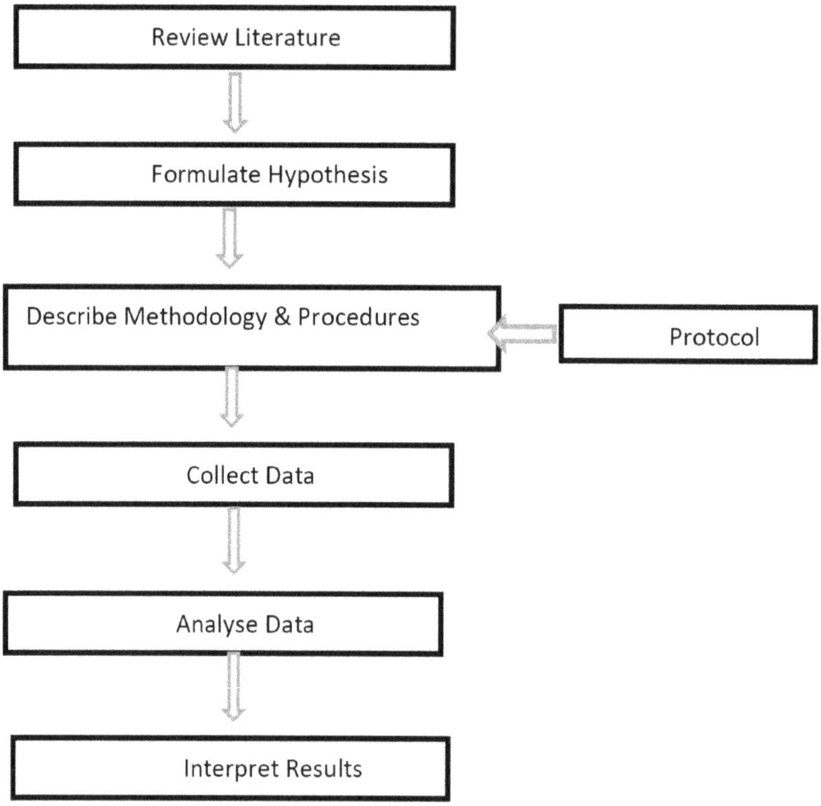

Figure 14.1: Steps in Conducting a Research Study

Table 14.2: Schedule of Events

Procedures Study Window (+- _ weeks)	Enrolment/ Baseline	Follow up (Visit 2) Week __	Folloup (Vist) Weekn	Unscheduled Visits	Premature Study Discontinuation	Final Visit
Informed Consent	X	X				
Demographics	X					
Medical History	X		X		X	
Anthropometry	X	X	X		X	
Randomisation*		X				
Laboratory Investigations **	X		X		X	X
Storage Specimen		X	X		X	X

Procedures Study Window (+- _ weeks)	Enrolment/ Baseline	Follow up (Visit 2) Week __	Folloup (Vist) Weekn	Unscheduled Visits	Premature Study Discontinuation	Final Visit
Radiological Evaluations	X					
Other Procedures as appropriate	X	X				
	*For Clinical Trials: Add Footnotes as appropriate					

References

1. NIH Definitions | Office of Research on Women's Health [Internet]. [cited 2021 Sep 28]. Available from: https://orwh.od.nih.gov/toolkit/nih-policies-inclusion/definitions
2. Protocol Templates for Clinical Trials | grants.nih.gov [Internet]. [cited 2021 Sep 28]. Available from: https://grants.nih.gov/policy/clinical-trials/protocol-template.htm
3. Farrugia P, Petrisor BA, Farrokhyar F, Bhandari M. Research questions, hypotheses and objectives. Can J Surg [Internet]. 2010 [cited 2021 Sep 28];53(4):278. Available from: /pmc/articles/PMC2912019/
4. ICHGCP-Essential documents for the conduct of a clinical trial - ICHGCP [Internet]. [cited 2021 Sep 28]. Available from: https://ichgcp.net/8-essential-documents-for-the-conduct-of-a-clinical-trial
5. ICMJE | Recommendations | Preparing a Manuscript for Submission to a Medical Journal [Internet]. [cited 2021 Sep 28]. Available from: http://www.icmje.org/recommendations/browse/manuscript-preparation/preparing-for-submission.html
6. Home - ClinicalTrials.gov [Internet]. [cited 2021 Sep 28]. Available from: https://clinicaltrials.gov/
7. Clinical Trials Registry - India (CTRI) [Internet]. [cited 2021 Sep 28]. Available from: http://ctri.nic.in/Clinicaltrials/login.php

CHAPTER

15 Genetics in Medicine

Shubha Phadke

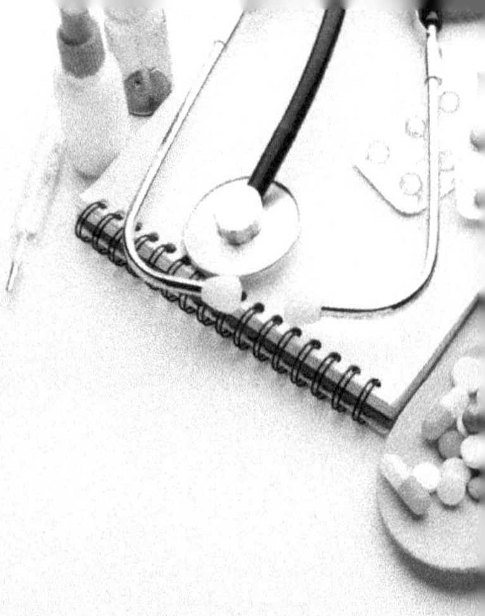

Genes, which are composed of Deoxyribonucleic Acid (DNA), are basic to the biology of animals and plants. *Genetics* is a diverse subject dealing with the variations and heredity of all living organisms. The genes are responsible for the development of an organism from a Zygote. Mammals including human beings, receive a set of genes (in the form of 23 chromosomes) from each parent. These carry information about the growth, development and functioning of various organ systems in the body. Variations in the genetic material in the form of DNA sequence variations or organization and copy numbers of genes lead to genetic disorders and genetic susceptibility to diseases. With the knowledge of genes and their variations and techniques to study them, many applications have been developed in the diagnosis and management of patients and families with genetic disorders. This has led to the development of a separate medical speciality known as Medical Genetics.

1. History of Medical Genetics

Human genetics is the study of variations and heredity in human beings. The part of human genetics related to the study of human genetic variations for the practice of medicine is *medical genetics*. This is almost synonymous to *Clinical Genetics*, i.e. Applications of genetics in patient care. Identification of the correct number of chromosomes in human beings, the concept of genetic counselling and prenatal diagnosis are the first important milestones in the establishment of medical genetics (Table 15.1).

Table 15.1: Landmarks in the History of Medical Genetics

Year	Scientist	The 'Milestone'
1865	Gregor Mendel	Particulate inheritance
1866	Langden Hayden Down	Mongolian idiocy (Down syndrome)
1946	Roberts	First genetic clinic in the UK
1947	Sheldon Clark Reed	Coined the word 'Genetic Counselling'
1949	Linus Pauling	Electrophoretic abnormality of Sickle Hb
1953	James Watson and Francis Crick	DNA structure
1956	Tjio and Levan	46 chromosomes in man
1959	Jerome Lejeune	Trisomy 21 as the cause of Down Syndrome
1966	Breg and Steel	First prenatal chromosomal analysis
1966	Victor McKusick	First edition of Mendelian inheritance in man—Catalogues of autosomal dominant, autosomal recessive and X-linked phenotypes
1970	Hargobind Khorana	First gene synthesized in vitro
1977	Sanger, Maxam and Gilbert	Method of DNA sequencing
1978	Kan and AM Dozy	First DNA diagnosis
1985	Jeffreys	DNA fingerprinting
1985	Ward	Fluorescence in situ hybridization
1991	Barton	Enzyme replacement therapy for Gaucher disease
1997	Solinas-Tolodo	DNA Microarray (Array Comparative Genomic Hybridization)
2009	Celera Genomics and NIH-USA	Human genome sequenced
2009	Sarah Ng and Jay Shendure	Exome sequencing identifies the cause of a monogenic disorder
2010	Marina Cavazzana-Calvo	Successful gene therapy for Beta thalassemia
2011	Bamshad and Shendure	Exome sequencing in clinical diagnosis
2019	Novartis	FDA approved gene therapy for spinal muscular atrophy

With the development of easy techniques of chromosomal analysis, clinical genetics got established and many families could be helped by prenatal diagnosis. In the 1980s, the DNA techniques to sequence genes established diagnostic tests for monogenic disorders. Inventions of polymerase chain reaction and automated sequencing simplified genetic diagnosis and research in the area of identification of genes causing monogenic disorders.

The development of genomic techniques, namely array comparative hybridization and massively parallel sequencing (next generation sequencing) caused a paradigm shift in the diagnostic approach for genetic disorders.

2. The Classification of Genetic Disorders

The disorders caused by abnormalities of genetic material, genes and chromosomes are labelled as genetic disorders. Deoxyribonucleic acid (DNA) is compactly arranged along with histone and non-histone proteins, the combination of which takes the shape of chromosomes. The sequence of DNA coding for a protein or a polypeptide is labelled as a gene. Some genes code only for RNA which is not translated to a protein. The controllers of gene expression may be close to the gene or far away from the gene in concern. Traditionally, genetic disorders are classified as chromosomal disorders and monogenic disorders based on the etiological genetic defect in chromosomes or a gene.

However, it is obvious that the gene/genes are parts of a chromosome and deletion or duplication of small parts of a chromosome beyond the resolution of traditional karyotyping can lead to birth defects. These are now grouped under contiguous gene syndromes, as a segment of a chromosome harbouring many genes, is deleted or duplicated. On the other hand, a change in one or a few nucleotides of a gene can lead to diseases and these monogenic diseases follow the Mendel's laws of genetics, hence also known as Mendelian disorders. Beta-thalassemia and sickle cell disease are the commonest Mendelian disorders. Figure 15.1 shows representative examples of genetic disorders and techniques used to detect the causative genetic abnormality.

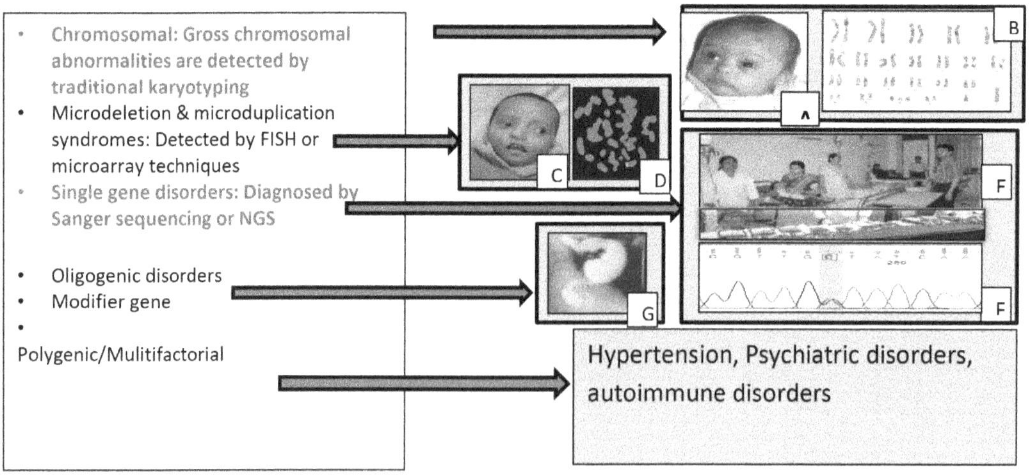

Figure 15.1: Genetic disorders and diagnostic investigation- [A] An infant with Trisomy 21 [B] A karyotype showing trisomy 21- 47,XY,+21 [C] A child with Wolf Hirschhorn syndrome due to deletion of the terminal part of the p arm of chromosome 4 [D] Fluorescence in situ hybridization showing only one signal for 4p confirming deletion on one chromosome 4 [E] Patients with thalassemia major on hyper-transfusion therapy [F] Sanger sequencing showing common mutation - c.92+5G>C in HBB gene for beta-globin in heterozygous form [G] Imaging study showing Hirschsprung disease

In addition to these classical genetic disorders, most disorders have some genetic component in their etiologies in the form of susceptibility of resistance due to a combination of variations in many different genes. These disorders are known as multi-factorial disorders as many known and unknown genetic and environmental factors contribute to the disease and its outcome with treatment. Table 15.1 shows the population-based prevalence vs family data about common multi-factorial diseases indicating the genetic contribution of the disease.

Table 15.1: Common Multi-Factorial Disorders

Multi-factorial Disorder	Population Prevalence	Prevalence in the first-degree relatives of a patient	Known gene contributing to the causation of the disease [Representative]
Cleft lip	About 1 per 1000 live births	3 to 5%	*IRF-6*
Meningocele	About 5 per 1000 live births	5%	*MTHFR*
Crohn disease	2 per 1000	10%	*NOD-2*
Schizophrenia	Lifetime prevalence of approximately 1%	10%	*NRXN-1, PRODH*

Other than these diseases, diabetes, hypertension, and ischemic heart disease are heterogeneous disorders with complex etiological factors. It has been understood now that the susceptibility to infectious diseases and response to drugs are also partly governed by genetic factors. Some malformations like Hirschsprung disease need variations in more than one gene to develop and hence, an oligogenic group of disorders is being identified. For single-gene disorders, multiple affected members in a family may have different severity or phenotype of the disease indicating the effect of other modifying genetic and non-genetic factors in the development of the disease. This is true as no gene works in isolation, but is usually a part of a pathway or a metabolic cycle with complex steps and interactions. The existence of modifier genes is getting attention as they may help in developing drug therapies.

3. Clinical Presentation of Genetic Disorders

There are about 22000 genes in each human being and they code for a much higher number of proteins. Variations in DNA sequences of any of these genes are known to cause genetic disorders, with more than 6000 being documented till date <https://www.omim.org/statistics/geneMap>. These include disorders or traits of all organ systems of the body e.g. anaemia in beta-thalassemia, immunodeficiency disorders, short stature due to involvement of bones in skeletal dysplasia, intellectual disability due to various single gene disorders or chromosomal disorders. Some genetic disorders like Marfan syndrome have the involvement of many organs like dislocation of the lens, aortic root dilatation, tall stature, dural ectasia, etc. due to pleiotropic effects of the gene. Some other genetic disorders like lysosomal storage disorders have manifestations in different systems of the body as the protein (enzyme in this case) is required in many organs while some genetic metabolic disorders have varied manifestations as the metabolites produced due to derangement affect effect the brain and other organs. Some disorders have characteristic clinical features making clinical diagnosis easy (Figure 15.2). Table 15.2 shows some examples of monogenic disorders.

Chromosomal disorders are due to imbalances of many genes on the deleted or duplicated chromosome and chromosomal segment and are usually associated with neurodevelopmental disorders like intellectual disability, and autism with or without major or minor structural birth defects. Another group of disorders due to genetic aetiology is cancers. Most cancers have DNA defects in somatic cells and DNA based testing is becoming the most important part of diagnosis and prognostic evaluation. Specific therapies based on genetic defects have led to a paradigm change in the management of cancers. About ten per cent of cancers are familial and due to inherited germline mutations in cancer susceptibility genes. Identifying such families e.g. familial carcinoma breast or retinoblastoma is a must as family members can be provided genetic testing and management for improving the outcomes.

Table 15.II: Manifestations of monogenic disorders, some with clinical features overlapping with non-genetic disorders

Disorder	Mode of Inheritance	Clinical **features - Phenotype**	
		Similar to genetic or non-genetic disorders	**Characteristic** features
Maple syrup urine disease	AR	Encephalopathy, seizures during neonatal period	Smell of urine
Fragile X-syndrome	X-linked	Intellectual disability, seizures	Macro-orchidism, long face with prominent mandible
Metachromatic leukodystrophy	AR	Spasticity in legs	Loss of milestones after one year, progressive course
Tuberous sclerosis	AD	Seizures, Intellectual disability	Adenoma sebaceum on face, tubers seen in neuroimaging, hypo/hyperpigmented patches

Note: AR – Autosomal recessive, AD – Autosomal dominant

The clinical features of genetic syndromes may be overlapping with non-genetic disorders. It is important to be aware of genetic disorders and consider them in differential diagnoses in appropriate clinical situations. The family history drawn in the form of a pedigree may provide a clue to the possibility of genetic etiology of similarly affected family members (Figure 15.2) or consanguinity [https://medicine.uiowa.edu/humangenetics/resources/how-draw-pedigree]. However, for many patients with genetic disorders there may not be similarly affected family members. Also, it is important to note that not all genetic disorders manifest at birth or are congenital. Similarly, not all congenital disorders or familial disorders are genetic.

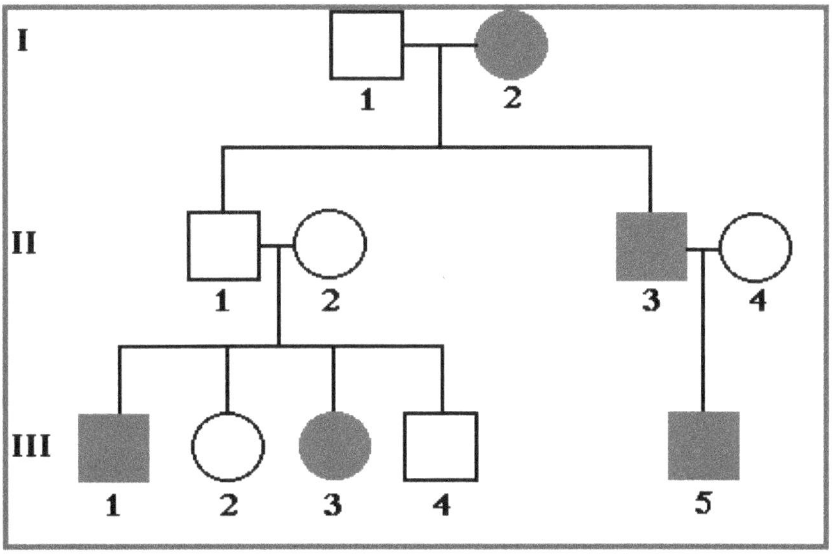

Figure 15.2: A pedigree showing autosomal dominant inheritance with a skipped generation suggesting incomplete penetrance for the disorder in the family. Individual II-1 must be a carrier of genetic mutation as his mother (I–2), a son (III-1) and a daughter (III-3) are affected with the disorder. Hence, individuals, III-2 and III-4 may be carriers of the disease-causing mutation even if they are not showing disease phenotype.

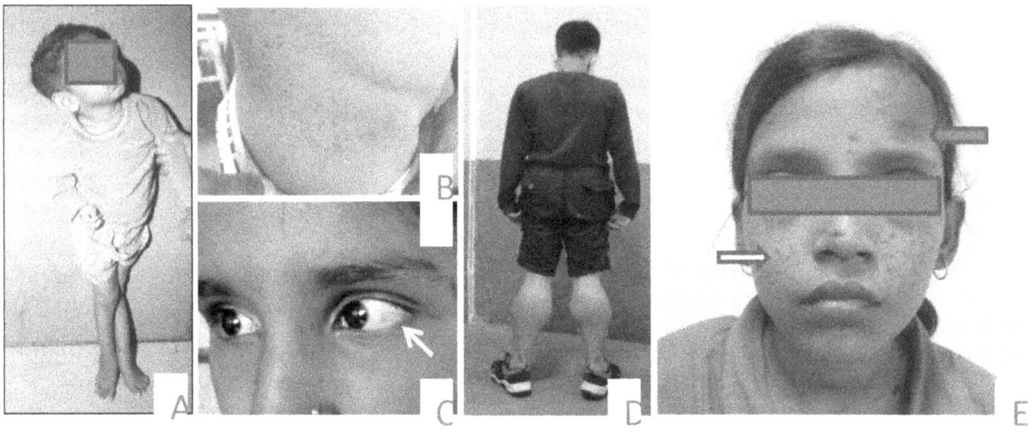

Figure 15.3: Characteristic features of common monogenic disorders

[A] A child with Metachromatic Leukodystrophy showing spasticity in lower limbs similar to cerebral palsy [B] Angiokeratoma in a boy with Fabry disease [C] Telangiectasia on the sclera of the eyes in a girl with Ataxia Telangiectasia [D] A boy with Duchenne muscular dystrophy – Note hypertrophy of calves [E] Adenoma sebaceum on face (bold arrow) and Shagreene patch (thin arrow) characteristic of Tuberous Sclerosis

The clinical presentations requiring genetic evaluation are listed below:

1. Congenital malformation: Lethal or non-lethal, isolated or multiple, prenatal or postnatal.
2. Stillbirths/perinatal deaths with or without malformation.
3. Developmental delay or intellectual disability or autism or other developmental disabilities with or without malformations, facial dysmorphism and/or neurological deficit.
4. Neurodegenerative diseases present as a focal neurological deficit, ataxia, spasticity, hypotonia, seizures or psychomotor regression.
5. Myopathies and muscular dystrophies.
6. A neonate or an infant with acute sickness, failure to thrive or jaundice or recurrent episodes of vomiting, acidosis and/or convulsions.
7. Ambiguous genitalia or abnormalities of sexual development like primary amenorrhoea and delayed puberty.
8. Infertility and poor obstetric histories like recurrent spontaneous abortions and foetal losses.
9. Proportionate or disproportionate short stature.
10. Childhood deafness.
11. Known monogenic disorders like thalassaemia, Wilson disease, haemophilia A, mucopolysaccharidosis, retinitis pigmentosa, epidermolysis bullosa, Huntington chorea, etc.
12. Down Syndrome and other chromosomal disorders.
13. Familial cancers or cancer-prone disorders.
14. Relatives of an individual having a structural abnormality of a chromosome or chromosomes.
15. Any unusual disease of the skin, eyes, bones or unusual facial features.
16. Any disease which is familial.
17. Exposure to a known or possible teratogen during pregnancy.
18. Consanguineous marriage.
19. Advanced maternal age.
20. Carrier of a genetic disorder.
21. Positive screening test for a genetic disorder.

4. Diagnosis of Genetic Disorders

Suspecting a genetic disorder is very important for all clinicians to start an appropriate evaluation. Drawing a pedigree is the first and simplest step in the approach to a possible genetic disorder. The history taking, clinical examination is similar to any other clinical speciality. An astute clinician with good observation and communication skills can be a good clinical geneticist. Examination of family members for subtle clinical findings of a genetic disorder can go a long way in making a diagnosis and giving the risk of recurrence. The diagnosis of genetic disorders does not always need DNA based diagnosis, diagnosis of beta-thalassemia major is complete by estimating foetal haemoglobin level while gold standards for diagnosis of lysosomal storage disorders and haemophilia A are enzyme levels and coagulant activity of factor VIII respectively. However, many genetic disorders need DNA based genetic tests to identify mutations. Examples of such diseases are Duchenne muscular dystrophy, spinal muscular dystrophy, and Huntington chorea. These disorders do not have biochemical or imaging tests. The identification of DNA mutation is important not only for confirmation of the diagnosis of the proband (affected individual in the family) but also for genetic counselling, prenatal diagnosis and pre-symptomatic diagnosis of the family members. Nowadays, Such DNA based testing is also used for population-based screening tests.

The genetic tests are mainly divided into techniques to evaluate chromosomes and single genes. Table 15.III describes the techniques briefly.

Table 15.III: Advantages and limitations of various cytogenetic & molecular techniques

Technique	Indications	Limitations
Traditional karyotyping: Available easily. Evaluates all chromosomes in one go	A child with a chromosomal abnormality, Down syndrome, Turner syndrome, hypogonadism, ambiguous genitalia, intellectual disability, and malformations.	Low resolution. Needs live cell Reporting time of 2 to 3 weeks
Fluorescence in situ Hybridization (FISH)* Uses probe in the region of interest.	Can detect sub-microscopic microdeletion syndromes like 22q deletion, Williams syndrome	Can look at only one or few regions of the genome at one time.
Cytogenetic Microarray Whole-genome hybridization with array of probes. Very high-resolution chromosomal analysis as compared to karyotype	Should be offered to all cases with intellectual disability, pre or postnatal malformation. Can detect minute chromosomal abnormalities (known as copy number variations -CNVs) anywhere in the genome	In about 1% of cases, some CNVs detected may have uncertain significance
Sanger sequencing Get to know sequences of 200 to 800 base pairs in one go.	It is used to identify small deletions/ duplications and point mutations which are the most important causes of monogenic disorders	Cannot detect large deletions which are usually seen in patients with Duchenne muscular dystrophy, spinal muscular atrophy
NGS based exome sequencing (WES) High thru put sequencing; can sequence all genes or many genes in one go and hence cost and labour effective as Sanger sequencing for many genes may take a long time and will be costly	Indicated in diagnosis of the proband with a disease known to be caused by a very large gene or the causative genes can be many (e.g. retinitis pigmentosa, myopathies) or a phenotype which can not give any clue to the causative gene (e. g. Intellectual disability) and the disorder in concern is likely to be autosomal or X linked recessive, the parents can be tested for carrier status of the disorder in concern	Interpretation is a challenge. May detect variations of uncertain significance or information about other disease causing genes for which the test had not been done.

Note: * Other molecular cytogenetic techniques like quantitative fluorescent PCR (QF PCR), multiplex ligation probe amplification (MLPA), etc are devised to suit various indications in diagnostics and research. NGS – Next Generation Sequencing

The principles of each technique need to be understood so that the appropriate investigation can be ordered and results interpreted correctly from the perspective of the clinical scenario. For clinically homogeneous phenotypes like beta-thalassemia, there can be any one or two mutations in HBB gene of more than 350 reported to date. This is true for most monogenic disorders as hundreds of mutations are known in each disease-causing gene. Very few diseases like achondroplasia and progeria are known to be caused by only one mutation. For some diseases like Duchene muscular dystrophy, large deletions in the DMD gene are common. These cannot be detected by Sanger sequencing and the MLPA technique need to be used.

Presently, Next-Generation Sequencing (NGS)-Based Testing is replacing all tests and it is soon expected to become one test for all. It can be done as soon as the child is born or is in utero. The whole-genome data thus generated can be interpreted for pre-symptomatic diagnosis as the patient develops some diseases throughout his/her lifetime. NGS based testing has opened up many diagnostic options which were thought to be impossible.

5. Treatment of Genetic Disorders

Even before DNA based genetic diagnosis, genetic disorders were successfully treated by various methodologies as shown in Table 15.IV

Table 15.IV: Traditional treatments of genetic disorders

Strategy of Treatment	Diseases	Comment
Diet modification to limit a specific component	• Phenylketonuria • Galactosemia	• Phenylalanine restricted diet • Avoidance of milk and milk products
Removal of the offending agent	• G6PD deficiency • Porphyria	• Avoidance of drugs like primaquine, etc. • Avoidance of drugs like phenobarbitone, etc.
Avoidance of triggering factor	• Fatty acid oxidation defects • Glycogen storage disease I	• Avoid fasting • Avoid fasting
Replacement of the deficient product	• Thalassemia major • Haemophilia A • Congenital hypothyroidism	• Red blood cells • Factor VIII • Thyroxine hormone
Augmentation of deficient protein by drugs	• Crigler-Najjar syndrome II	• Phenobarbitone
Megavitamin therapy	• Sideroblasticanemia • Homocystinuria	• Vitamin B_6 • Vitamin B_6

Strategy of Treatment	Diseases	Comment
Removal of an organ	• Hereditary spherocytosis • Familial adenomatous polyposis	• Splenectomy • Colectomy
Specific drug therapy	• DOPA responsive dystonia	• Dopamine
Removal of toxic product	• Tyrosinemia	• Nitisinone (NTBC)
Organ/tissue transplantation	• Thalassemia major • Osteopetrosis Multiple epiphyseal dysplasia	• BMT • BMT • Joint replacement
Surgical treatment of malformation	• Cardiac malformation • Cleft lip	• Surgical repair • Surgical repair
Management of symptoms	• Tuberous sclerosis • Conduction defects of heart	• Anticonvulsants • Pacemaker implantation

The twenty first century has ushered in many novel treatments and showing great hope for genetic disorders which are rare and many were untreatable. Recombinant DNA technology made many recombinant products available for replacement therapy like growth hormone, enzyme replacement therapy. Enzyme replacement therapy is now available for lysosomal storage disorders like Gaucher disease (Figure 15.4), Mucopolysaccharidosis type I & II, Pompe disease, and Fabry disease. The results are impressive though enzymes cannot cross blood-brain barrier and are not effective in cases with CNS involvement. Other new drugs developed use different strategies (T Table 15.V).

Table 15.V: Novel Strategies of drug therapies for monogenic disorders

Disease	Drug	Strategy
Cystic fibrosis with a mutation affecting the gating function of the protein	Ivacaftor	Potentiate the activity of *CFTR*
Phenylketonuria is due to mutations which lead to misfolding of the protein	Sapropterin	Acts as a chaperon help a misfolded protein to gain some of its function
Plexiform neurofibroma in Neurofibromatosis (NF1)	Selumetinib	Inhibits RAS MAPK pathway which is hyper activated in NF1
Proteus syndrome	Miransertib (in clinical trial)	Inhibits AKT

New therapies for two other monogenic disorders need special mention due to their strategies and dramatic, life changing outcomes. This includes approved gene therapies for sickle cell disease, beta thalassemia and spinal muscular atrophy. For spinal muscular atrophy, two other drugs are approved by FDA and these work on RNA modification. Nusinersen is an antisense oligonucleotide modulating SMN2 splicing and increasing functional SMN protein. These successes in gene therapy and gene modification strategies provide great rays of hope for many other monogenic disorders.

6. Genetic Counselling and Prenatal Diagnosis

Diagnosis of genetic disorders is not important only for the patient but has implications for the family due to the possibility of recurrence in the family members. The process of communicating the genetic diagnosis, possible management and outcomes, risk of recurrence in the siblings or offspring and ways to avoid the recurrences by prenatal or presymptomatic testing is known as genetic counselling. Genetic counselling is an important part of the management of genetic disorders. Preventing recurrences by prenatal diagnosis and termination of pregnancy if the fetus is affected with the disorder is acceptable to many families at risk of serious disorders with the poor outcome or difficult treatment. Various invasive and non-invasive techniques for prenatal diagnosis are available. Accurate diagnosis of the proband and/or carrier parents and non-directive counselling are important pilers of successful genetic counselling.

7. Representative Cases

A few illustrative cases are discussed below to show the role of genetics in clinical practice and the power of genomic tests in diagnosis of genetic disorders which can involve any system of body and many times have clinical presentations overlapping non-genetic disorders.

Case 1: Prenatal ultrasonography at 22 weeks showed double bubble appearance suggestive of duodenal atresia. As 30% of foetuses with duodenal atresia have trisomy 21, amniocentesis was done for chromosomal analysis. It showed trisomy 21. The family decided to terminate the pregnancy as even after surgical treatment of duodenal atresia, the child with trisomy 21 will have an intellectual disability.

Case 2: Two brothers with intellectual disabilities were evaluated and diagnosed as Fragile X syndrome. Their elder sister and mother's sister were tested and found to be carriers of Fragile X syndrome. They were counselled about the risk of the syndrome in their offspring and informed about options of prenatal diagnosis.

Case 3: A neonate was detected with biotinidase deficiency on newborn screening. Immediately at 12 days of life the baby was put on 10 mg of biotin per day. Currently, at 3 years of age the child is developing normally. The treatment has to be continued lifelong.

Case 4: A consanguineous family had 2 babies who died on day one due to respiratory distress. One had talipes equinovarus. Polyhydramnios was reported. After the death of the second baby, DNA was extracted from a small piece of the umbilical cord. NGS based testing identified homozygous truncating mutation in LMOD3 gene. This confirmed the diagnosis of Nemalin myopathy in the neonate which was the cause of neonatal respiratory failure. The family was told that the risk of recurrence in the next offspring was 25% and prenatal diagnosis by doing a DNA test on chorionic villus sample at 12 weeks during the next pregnancy was an option to avoid recurrence.

Case 5: A 30-year-old woman had carcinoma breast. Her father's sister had died of carcinoma breast at 40 years of age. In addition to treatment, she was evaluated for mutations in the BRCA1 and BRCA2 genes. The mutation was identified in the BRCA1 gene. As the lady had 2 offspring and had completed her obstetric career; an option of radical mastectomy and oophorectomy was discussed with her. She informed her sisters who came for genetic counselling and opted for genetic testing for BRCA1 gene mutation.

Case 6: A family with multiple family members affected with ataxia came to notice as a young would be mother asked in the same disease can occur in her children. Her grandfather died at 70 years of age and had ataxia during old age. Her father and his brother developed ataxia around 40 years of age. Her 25-year-old brother had early signs of ataxia and her older brother was normal. She herself was 28 years old and normal. The affected father was tested for spinocerebellar ataxias of autosomal dominant types and was found to carry mutation in the gene for SCA3. This type of earlier age of onset in subsequent generations I called as anticipation. Though she does not have symptoms, she may be a carrier of the disease and can transmit the disease to the next generation. For confirmation, she will need to be tested and may find out that she also is likely to develop the disease which is untreatable. The issues of pre-symptomatic testing and prenatal testing were discussed and involve complex psychosocial issues.

Case 7: A family has a child with thalassemia major and the mother is pregnant. The family wants to know if the fetus is affected with the disease. If the fetus is not affected with thalassemia, the family wants to check HLA type of the fetus to know if the fetus is HLA matched with the child with thalassemia major. If not, the family will terminate the pregnancy. Do you think, it is ethically right?

Case 8: A seven-year-old child was brought for evaluation of short stature. She does not have any other phenotypic features. Her karyotype was 45, X. She thus, was diagnosed to have Turner syndrome and was put on growth hormone therapy.

Case 9: A ten-year-old boy with disproportionate short stature and knock knees was evaluated. Skeletal radiographs suggested the diagnosis of Morquio syndrome which is a type of mucopolysaccharidosis. Enzyme analysis confirmed the diagnosis. He was evaluated for odontoid hypoplasia which is commonly associated and needs fixation as it can cause cord compression and quadriplegia.

Case 10: A family has a 4-year-old boy with developmental delay and different-looking face. His mother had 3 spontaneous abortions. Chromosomal analysis revealed a normal karyotype of the mother and the child's karyotype showed extra material on p arm of chromosome 6 (46,XY,6p+). Molecular cytogenetics confirmed that this was from chromosome 8 (partial trisomy of 8q) and he also had partial monosomy of the terminal part of chromosome 6. Father's karyotype was 46, XY, t (6; 8) (p22; q21.3). This suggests a high risk of recurrences of a child with the chromosomal imbalance and also recurrent abortions. The options are donor sperms or pre-implantation diagnosis after in vitro fertilization with the father's sperms.

These cases highlight various ways in which genetic disorders can be present and the patients and families can be helped. In the twentieth century, genetic technologies and knowledge is rapidly increasing. The opportunities for patients' families, clinicians and researchers are immense. Everyone in medicine will need to know the basics of medical genetics, molecular vocabulary and clinical applications of genetics.

Additional Reading

1. Bedard PL, Hyman DM, Davids MS, Siu LL. Small molecules, big impact: 20 years of targeted therapy in oncology. Lancet. 2020 Mar 28;395(10229):1078-1088. doi: 10.1016/S0140-6736(20)30164-1. PMID: 32222192.
2. Amberger JS, Hamosh A. Searching Online Mendelian Inheritance in Man (OMIM): A Knowledgebase of Human Genes and Genetic Phenotypes. Curr Protoc Bioinformatics. 2017;58:1.2.1-1.2.12.
3. Nussbaum RL, McInnes RR, Willard HF. Patterns of Single Gene Inheritance. Thompson and Thompson Genetics in Medicine, 8th edition. Philadelphia: Elsievier; 2016. pp. 106-31.
4. Khan KN, Ali M, Poulter JA, McKibbin M, Inglehearn CF. Patterns of inheritance, not always easily visible. BMJ. 2013;347:f6610.
5. Thompson AA, Walters MC, Kwiatkowski J, Rasko JEJ, Ribeil JA, Hongeng S, et al. Gene Therapy in Patients with Transfusion Dependent β-Thalassemia. N Engl J Med. 2018;378(16):1479-93
6. Weiß C, Ziegler A, Becker LL, Johannsen J, Brennenstuhl H, Schreiber G, Flotats-Bastardas M, Stoltenburg C, Hartmann H, Illsinger S, Denecke J, Pechmann A, Müller-Felber W, Vill K, Blaschek A, Smitka M, van der Stam L, Weiss K, Winter B, Goldhahn K, Plecko B, Horber V, Bernert G, Husain RA, Rauscher C, Trollmann R, Garbade SF, Hahn A, von der Hagen M, Kaindl AM. Gene replacement therapy with onasemnogene abeparvovec in children with spinal muscular atrophy aged 24 months or younger and bodyweight up to 15 kg: an observational cohort study. Lancet Child Adolesc Health. 2022 Jan;6(1):17-27. doi: 10.1016/S2352-4642(21)00287-X. Epub 2021 Oct 29. PMID: 34756190.
7. Yang M, Kim JW. Principles of Genetic Counseling in the Era of Next-Generation Sequencing. Ann Lab Med. 2018 Jul;38(4):291-295. doi: 10.3343/alm.2018.38.4.291. PMID: 29611378; PMCID: PMC5895857.
8. Biesecker LG, Green RC. Diagnostic clinical genome and exome sequencing. N Engl J Med. 2014;371(12):1170
9. Ceyhan-Birsoy O, Murry JB, Machini K, Lebo MS, Yu TW, Fayer S, et al. Interpretation of Genomic Sequencing Results in Healthy and Ill Newborns: Results from the BabySeq Project. Am J Hum Genet. 2019;104(1):76-93.

CHAPTER

16 Molecular Medicine and Gene Therapy

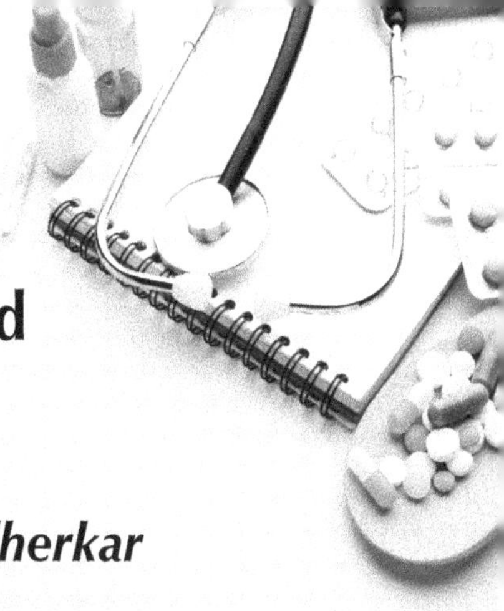

Avani Nadkarni and Rita Mulherkar

Molecular Medicine has evolved in the past few decades from our understanding of the diseases at molecular level. With the Human Genome Project, techniques for studying the whole genome and global gene expression evolved by leaps and bounds. Advances in biological sciences and computational sciences, technologies including microarray, next generation sequencing, high end computers, bioinformatics, etc., have helped in our understanding of the mechanisms of the disease and converting this knowledge into therapeutic approaches. Disease causing mutations in the genome can now be targeted by drugs, or corrected by gene therapy.

The present chapter will deal with the following:

i. Small Molecule Inhibitors
ii. Monoclonal antibodies
iii. Gene Therapy

1. Small Molecule Inhibitors

Small Molecule Inhibitors (SMI) are synthetic molecules small enough to penetrate cells passively and target important cellular macromolecules in order to block their activity. These are drugs that can easily cross cell membrane and inhibit protein-protein interactions required for survival of cancer cells and other molecules which are essential for cancer cell survival. Protein-protein interactions include ligands (which are proteins) - binding to receptors (which are also proteins). SMIs are discovered by X-ray crystallography combined with site-directed mutagenesis, where certain sites of the protein are systematically mutated to find out the regions which are required for these interactions to take place (Figure. 16.1). These regions are termed as “hot spots”. Hot spots are highly adaptive - structurally and functionally - which allows a single protein to bind to multiple partners using the same hot spot.

Most common targets of SMI are protein kinases. These are enzymes that cause phosphorylation of proteins which results in transfer of phosphate group from ATP to tyrosine, serine and threonine residues. SMIs nomenclature is such that they can be recognized from the suffix - "ib". Further tyrosine kinase inhibitors have the suffix - "tinib"; e.g., Gefitinib, Imaitinib; Proteasome inhibitors have the suffix "zomib" e.g., Bortezomib; Cyclin-dependent kinase inhibitors have the suffix "ciclib", e.g., Palbociclib, Ribociclib.

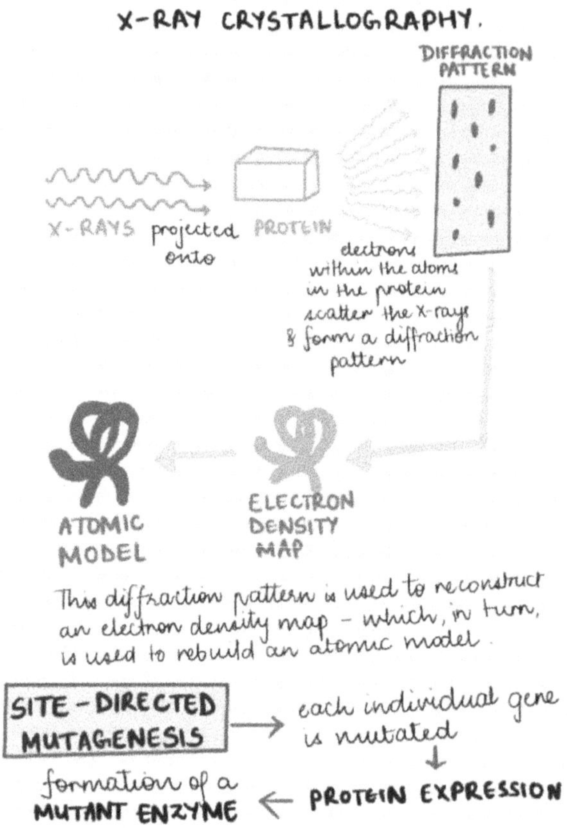

Figure 16.1: Small Molecule Inhibitors are discovered by X-ray crystallography combined with site-directed mutagenesis.

Most small molecule inhibitors act on growth factor receptors which often have tyrosine kinase activity and are therefore termed as Tyrosine Kinase Receptors (RTK). RTK can transduce extracellular signals to intracellular compartment (Figure. 16.2). RTK have 3 parts - extracellular region, transmembrane region and cytoplasmic region. Tyrosine Kinase Inhibitors (TKI) are classified into 3 groups - Type I, ATP competitive inhibitor; Type II and III, non-ATP competitors which act by causing structural changes in RTKs which modifies the TK domain in a way that prevents tyrosine phosphorylation. Examples of oncogenic RTK are - *ALK* mutations found in non-small cell lung carcinoma, colorectal cancer, breast cancer; *AXL* in lung cancer, colon cancer, breast cancer, AML, CML; *CCK4 (PTK7)* mutation in small cell lung carcinoma, breast, gastric, colon cancer, AML; *EGFR 1 (HER 1)* mutations in head and neck cancers, breast cancer, hepatocellular carcinoma; *EGFR 2 (HER 2)* mutation in breast cancer and gastric adenocarcinoma.

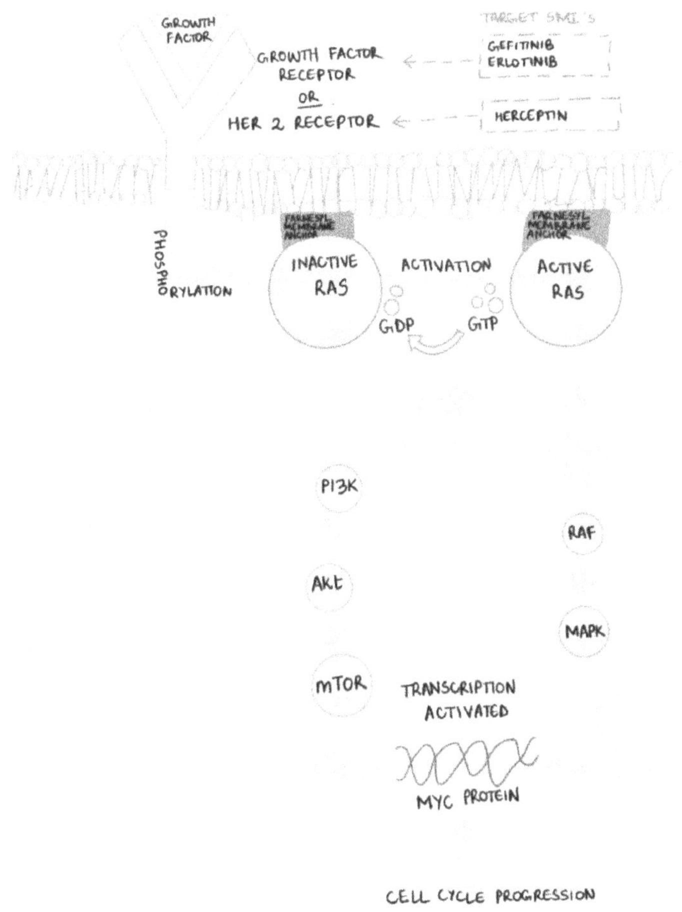

Figure 16.2: Some Growth Factor receptors have intrinsic tyrosine kinase activity. When the growth factor or ligand binds to its receptor, RTK gets activated and sets a cascade reaction - activating other signal transduction molecules (RAS, mTOR, MAPK) - ultimately leading to cell division and tumour proliferation.

Oncogenic addiction, a term introduced by Weinstein describes tumour cells that activated only specific oncogenic singling pathways to sustain survival and proliferation. The t(9;22) reciprocal chromosomal translocation causing generation of BCR-ABL fusion gene, which acts as an unregulated tyrosine kinase, is an example of one such oncogenic addiction (Figure. 16.3). And so, TKI Imatinib also known as Gleevac, was discovered in the late 1990's. It dramatically increased the 5 year survival rate of patients from 31% in 1993, to 59% in 2009, to 70% in 2016. Even though tyrosine kinase enzymes are present in most receptors, notably insulin receptors, Imatinib is specific for tyrosine kinase domain in ABL gene. It binds to the tyrosine kinase enzyme and inhibits it, but it has no activity on the underlying genetic mechanisms which led to this BCR-ABL fusion gene in the first place. Monoclonal antibodies such as Trastuzumab, against HER2 receptor in breast cancer, is particularly efficient as it utilises this concept of "oncogenic addiction".

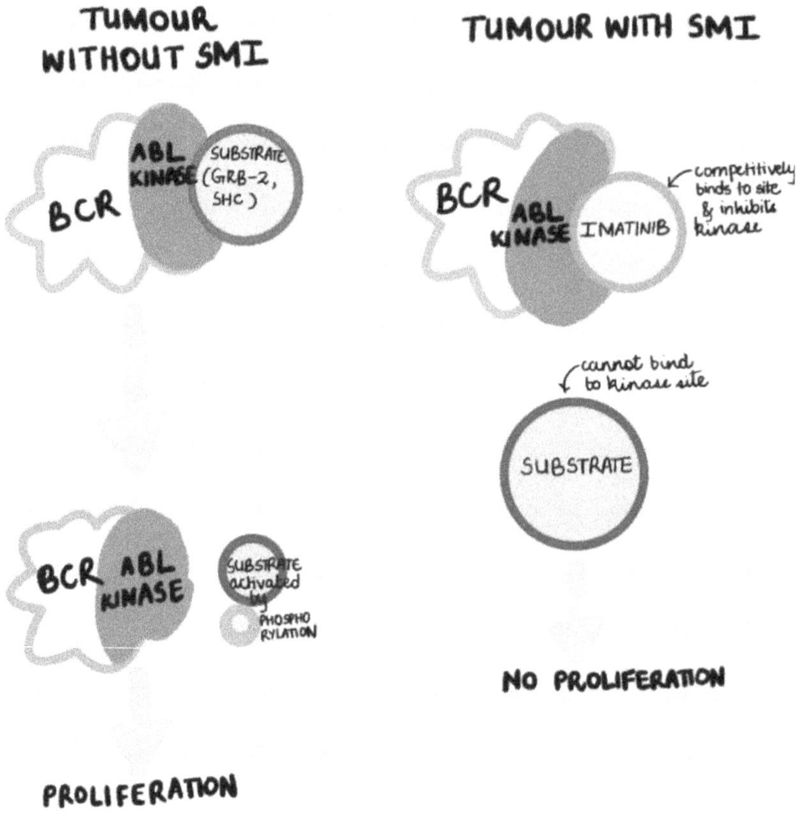

Figure 16.3: BCR-ABL is a fusion protein formed by chromosomal translocation. The substrate binds to ABL, which has kinase activity - and is activated by phosphorylation leading to cell signalling pathway activation and eventual proliferation of tumour cells. Imatinib binds to the substrate binding site on ABL kinase and hence competitively inhibits binding of substrate - therefore, no proliferation of tumour cells.

The next important discovery after Imatinib, was Gefitnib and Erlotinib - the first Epidermal Growth Factor receptor (EGFR) - tyrosine kinase inhibitor. EGFR (ErbB) is a family of 4 types of RTK which are structurally related - ErbB-1 / EGFR, ErbB-2 / HER 2 / neu, ErbB-3 / HER 3, ErbB-4 / HER 4. EGFR is usually associated in development of tumours of epithelial origin such as lung, colorectal, pancreatic, breast carcinomas. It leads to uncontrolled activation of anti-apoptotic RAS pathway. Gefitinib acts similarly to Imatinib by binding to ATP binding domain of EGFR tyrosine kinase enzyme reversibly. Hence, mutations that alter the binding site of the ATP domain, lead to resistance to Gefitinib. To combat this problem, researchers have now developed irreversible EGFR inhibitors such as Neratinib - which covalently binds to the ATP binding domain.

The term *protein homeostasis* indicates a balance between normal protein production and misfiled and abnormal protein degradation. Due to increased UV damage and other environmental factors, there has been an increase in the amount of misfolded proteins, leading to hostile intracellular conditions. The pathways that lead to this protein degradation are ubiquitin (Ub)-proteasome (26S) system and autophagy-lysosome system. Ub selectively binds to damaged proteins and this acts as a signal for the 26S proteasome to degrade the signaled protein. p53, NF-kß and ß-catenin cell signaling pathways are regulated through this protein degradation pathways. All this theory was applied clinically when Bortezomib was discovered to dramatically decrease mortality rate in patients of multiple myeloma and mantle cell lymphoma. The boron atom in Bortezomib binds the catalytic site of 26S proteasome causing inhibition of proteosomal degradation pathway and this leads to increased expression of pro-apoptotic factors such as p53, BAX and NOXA, (which would otherwise have been degraded by this proteasomal pathway) and prevents the translocation of NF-kß into the nucleus leading to reduced cancer cell proliferation and increased apoptosis. Proteosome Inhibitors (PI) also inhibit p21 and p27 degradation and hence increases expression of these two proteins that would otherwise cause cell cycle arrest.

A few decades before all these discoveries, in 1975, a peculiar soil sample was sent from Easter Island of South Pacific, termed as Rapa Nui - from this soil sample, was isolated an organism Streptomyces hygroscopicus, which gave rise to a macrolide termed as Rapamycin. This drug was originally used as an anti-fungal, but soon after its discovery, its immunosuppressant activities were detected giving rise to an entire branch of science and all these discoveries were termed as mTOR inhibitors - mammalian Target of Rapamycin inhibitors or rapalogs. mTOR is a serine/threonine-specific protein kinase which regulates cell growth and proliferation through two protein complexes mTORC1 and mTORC2. Most notable rapalogs are Everolimus and Sirolimus.

One of the most common causes of mutation is DNA damage although there are mechanisms present for repair of DNA damage, which is termed as DNA damage response (DDR). These mechanisms recognise damaged DNA, stop the cell cycle and repair the damaged DNA so it can be integrated back into the genome. The main enzymes that function in DDR are Poly (ADP ribose) Polymerase 1 and 2 - PARP1 and PARP2 enzymes. BRCA1 and BRCA2 genes are required for repair of double stranded DNA breaks by Homologous Recombination Repair (HRR) - which restores the original sequence of the DNA. Sometimes, due to repeated DNA damage or due to defects in BRCA1 and BRCA2, it can lead to deficiency of HRR and can cause other non-conserving forms of DNA repair, such as Non-Homologous End Joining (NHEJ), to predominate, and this can often lead to major alterations in the genetic sequence, even causing deletion of genetic material at times. *Synthetic Lethality* (SL) is a concept which states that a defect in one or 2 genes alone may not cause a major effect on the cell or organism but when both genes involved in DDR have a defect together, it can even lead to cell death. This concept has been discovered by geneticists almost a century ago, but in 2005 the SL interaction between PARP inhibition and BRCA1 or BRCA2 mutations was described by 2 groups, and it was first introduced in Phase I clinical trials as Olaparib and Rucaparib. Recently, Olaparib has even been approved for ovarian cancer. All these clinical trials just go to show that synthetic lethality can be used for cancer therapies.

2. Monoclonal Antibodies

Monoclonal antibodies (MAb) are proteins which recognize a specific, single epitope on an antigen and can bind to it. MAbs are made by the Hybridoma Technology and produced in animals, or in tissue culture by the recombinant DNA technology. MAbs are being used as therapeutic agents for the treatment of diseases, such as breast cancer, leukemia, asthma, macular degeneration, arthritis, Crohn's disease, and transplants, among others. They are also used as powerful tools for a wide range of medical applications such as diagnostic kits, conjugated to drugs for targeted delivery in vivo, imaging, etc.

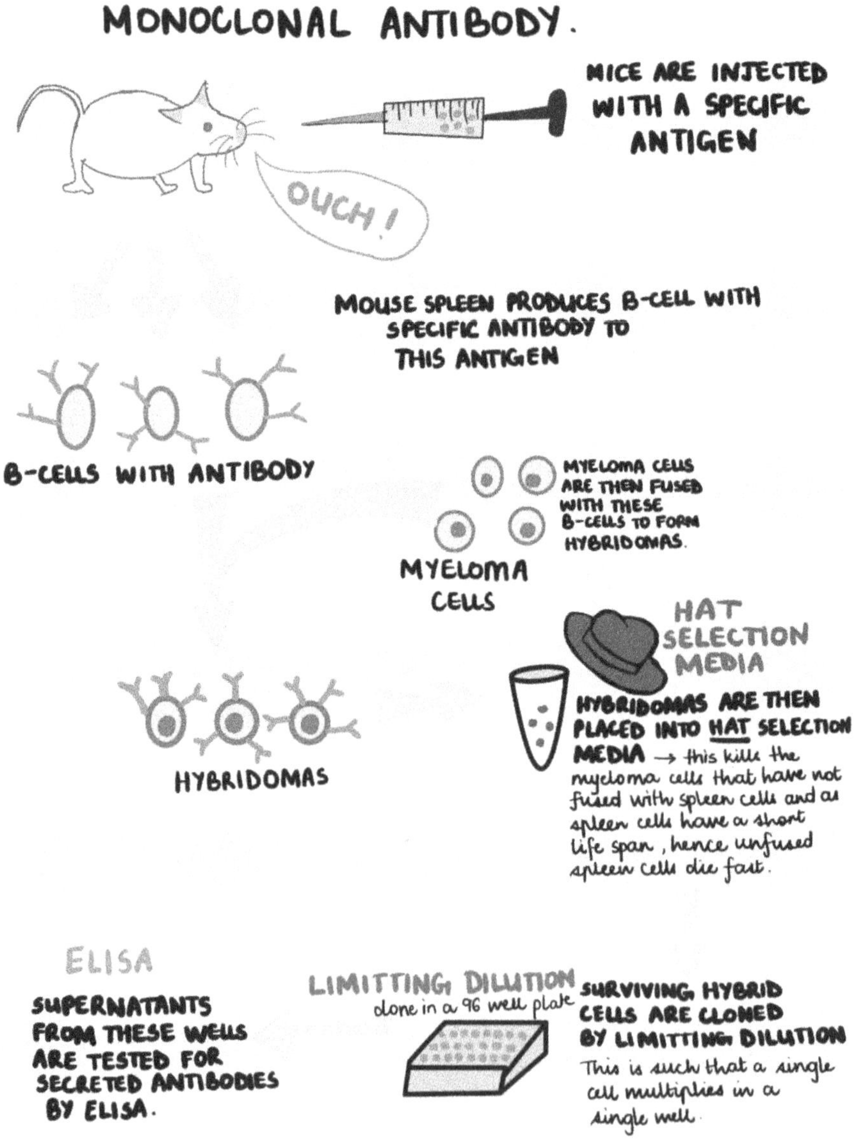

Figure 16.4: Production of monoclonal antibodies (mAb) by immunizing mice and fusing the spleen cells with myeloma cells – hybridomas, to immortalize the antibody producing cells from spleen. The hybridomas are selected on HAT medium which are screened by ELISA for specific mAbs.

Jerne, Kohler and Milstein were awarded the Nobel Prize in Physiology and Medicine, in 1984 for their discovery of the principle for production of monoclonal antibodies. They made a hybrid cell by fusing a cancerous Myeloma cell – providing its ability to proliferate continuously in culture, with a single antibody producing mouse B cell from an immunized mouse spleen – providing a single clone of antibody producing cells in culture. The hybrid cells are selected on Hypoxanthine-Aminopterin-Thymidine (HAT) selection medium. Aminopterin blocks DNA *de novo* synthesis, which is absolutely essential for cell division to proceed, but hypoxanthine and thymidine provide cells with the raw material to evade the blockage with the help of the enzyme HGPRT (the "salvage pathway"). Myeloma cells are deficient in HGPRT and hence die in HAT medium. Hybrid cells can grow in HAT medium as the HGPRT enzyme is provided by the spleen cells although the de novo DNA synthesis pathway is blocked. Myeloma cells will die as both the DNA synthesis pathways are blocked. Spleen cells cannot survive as they have a limited life span in vitro (Figure.4). This technology revolutionized immunology and gave us powerful drugs for cancer, diabetes, rheumatoid arthritis, and recently, also for COVID19.

In the beginning mouse monoclonal antibodies were used but the overall clinical outcomes were poor. This was mainly due to immunogenicity of the murine antibody. Advances in the recombinant DNA technology helped overcome these limitations. Recombinant MAb, also called as chimeric antibodies were made by fusing murine variable V(D)J gene segment of the mouse MAb to the human constant domains. These antibodies were capable of mediating antibody dependent cytotoxic response with human effector cells. The use of these antibodies reduced greatly the human anti-mouse antibody (HAMA) responses. These MAbs had the suffix 'xi' in their name, e.g., Rituximab (for treatment of CD20 expressing B cells). To reduce the HAMA response further, 'humanized' MAbs were produced. The chimeric MAbs were further humanized by selectively replacing the sequence of amino acids in the variable region with human sequences. Humanized chimeric MAbs have the suffix 'zu' or 'xi+zu', eg., Trastuzumab (for treatment of breast cancer), Otelixizumab (for treatment of rheumatoid arthritis and diabetes mellitus). A list of few of the FDA approved MAbs and their clinical use is shown in Table 16.1.

Today MAbs are being used for COVID patients. Casirivimab plus Imdevimab are recombinant human monoclonal antibodies that bind to non-overlapping epitopes of the spike protein RBD of SARS-CoV-2. US FDA issued an emergency use authorization (EUA) in November 2020 for Casirivimab and Imdevimab (REGEN-COV) to be administered together for the treatment of mild to moderate COVID-19 in adults and pediatric patients (12 years of age or older weighing at least 40 kilograms) with positive results of direct SARS-CoV-2 viral testing and who are at high risk for progressing to severe COVID-19. This includes those who are 65 years of age or older or who have certain chronic medical conditions. REGEN-COV is a recombinant human IgG1 MAb cocktail. Similarly, US FDA issued an EUA in May 2021 for another MAb - Sotrovimab which was originally identified in 2003 from a SARS-CoV survivor. It targets an epitope in the RBD of the spike protein that is conserved between SARS-CoV and SARS-CoV-2.

Table 16.1: Some of the FDA approved MAbs and indication for clinical use

MAb	Brand name	Target	Year of approval	Indication
Trastuzumab	Herceptin	HER2 / neu	1998	Breast cancer (1998) Gastric cancer (2010)
Rituximab	Rituxan	CD20	1997	Non-Hodgkin's lymphoma (1997) Chronic lymphocytic leukemia (2010) Rheumatoid arthritis (2006) Pemphigus vulgaris (2018)
Bevacizumab	Avastin	VEGF	2004	Colorectal cancer (2004) Non-small cell lung caccer (2006) Breast ERB2 negative cancer (2008) Renal cell carcinoma (2009) Glioblastoma (2011)
Nivolubmab	Opidivo	PD-1	2014	Melanoma (2015) Non-small cell lung cancer (2015) Renal cell carcinoma (2015) Head and neck squamous cell (2016)
Tocilizumab	Actemra	IL-6 receptor	2017	Rheumatoid arthritis (2017), Cytokine Release Syndrome (2017), COVID (2021)
Cetuximab	Erbitux	EGF-R	2004	K-Ras wild-type, EGFR-expressing colorectal cancer (2004), Squamous cell carcinoma of the head and neck (2004)
Adalimumab	Humira	TNF-α	2002	Rheumatoid arthritis (2002) Psoriatic arthritis (2005) Ankylosing spondylitis (2006) Juvenile Idiopathic Arthitis (2008) Psoriasis (2008) Crohn's disease (2010) Ulcerative colitis (2012) Hidradenitis suppurativa (2015) Uveitis (2018)

3. Gene Therapy

Gene Therapy is a unique treatment modality where manipulating Nucleic Acids (DNA/RNA) serves as a therapy. The nucleic acid is generally delivered via a viral or non-viral vector *in vivo* which then synthesizes the therapeutic protein. Today there are a large number of variations in the techniques with different genes, different modes of nucleic acid delivery including different viral vectors, used for Gene Therapy. Gene Therapy trials have been initiated since 1990. The first Gene Therapy clinical trial carried out in 1990, in ADA-deficient Severe Combined Immuno-Deficiency syndrome, in 2 girls was able to correct the ADA deficiency and the disease. Since then Gene Therapy for various diseases are in different phases of clinical trials.

World's first gene therapy drug to obtain a drug license in 2003 from the State Food and Drug Administration of China is Gendicine which is an adenoviral recombinant Ad-p53 gene therapy for head and neck squamous cell carcinoma. Gendicine consists of an adenoviral vector carrying wild type p53 tumour suppressor gene and is approved as adjuvant therapy along with radiation or chemotherapy. Oncorin, another product developed by Shanghai Sunway Biotech, China, is an oncolytic adenovirus that was approved by Chinese regulators in 2005 for the treatment of squamous cell carcinoma of head & neck and oesophagus.

A few therapies have recently been approved for cancer in the US, Europe and China (Table 16.2). Imlygic is the first oncolytic vector to receive approval for the treatment of advanced melanoma by the US FDA and Europe. Imlygic is a Herpes Simplex Virus 1 vector optimised in several ways which replicates only in actively dividing tumour cells causing oncolysis. It therefore promotes an immune response against released tumour antigens, and this aspect is further enhanced through arming it with the GM-CSF gene.

Although a majority of gene therapy clinical trials are for cancer, so far only one of the therapies has shown great promise and will be tested in patients in India as well. The approach called as Chimeric Antigen Receptor (CAR) T Cell – CAR-T is a therapy which has successfully cured a few leukaemia patients in the West. In this therapy, the patient's own T cells or gene edited allogenic T cells are manipulated in vitro to express a cell surface chimeric antibody against a specific antigen on the tumour cells. CARs are proteins generated by the fusion of an antigen binding domain, which is an antibody-derived single-chain variable fragment (scFv), with the T cell receptor (TCR) signalling domain CD3ζ (Figure. 5). The chimeric antigen receptor T cells are expanded in vitro and introduced back in the same patient. When the manipulated T cells are reinfused into the patient, they recognise the tumour cells and rapidly kill them.

CD19-targeted CARTs for B-ALL were the first CARTs which reported complete remission (CR) rates of 80-90% in relapsed or refractory B-cell acute lymphoblastic leukaemia (ALL), while response rates were 30-50% in chronic lymphocytic leukaemia (CLL) and NHL. The drug called Tisagenlecleucel (Kymriah), received approvals in the US FDA in 2017, and later in 2018 in the European Union, Canada, Switzerland, Australia, and Japan. Axicabtagene ciloleucel (Yescarta) was the second commercial CAR T cell therapy, approved for relapsed or refractory diffuse large B cell lymphoma (DLBCL) by the FDA as well as authorities in the EU, Canada and Switzerland.

Another approved CAR-T cell therapy is a genetically modified autologous T cell against the B Cell Maturation Antigen (BCMA) for the treatment of adult patients with relapsed or refractory multiple myeloma. It is composed of genetically modified, antigen-specific, autologous T cells reprogrammed to target cells that express BCMA through transduction with a lentiviral vector expressing a CAR targeting BCMA. The BCMA CAR is comprised of a murine extracellular single-chain variable fragment (scFv) specific for BCMA, a human CD8α hinge and transmembrane domain and the 4-1BB and CD3ζ chain T cell intracellular signalling domains. Antigen-specific activation results in CAR+ T cell proliferation, cytokine secretion, and lysis of BCMA-expressing cells.

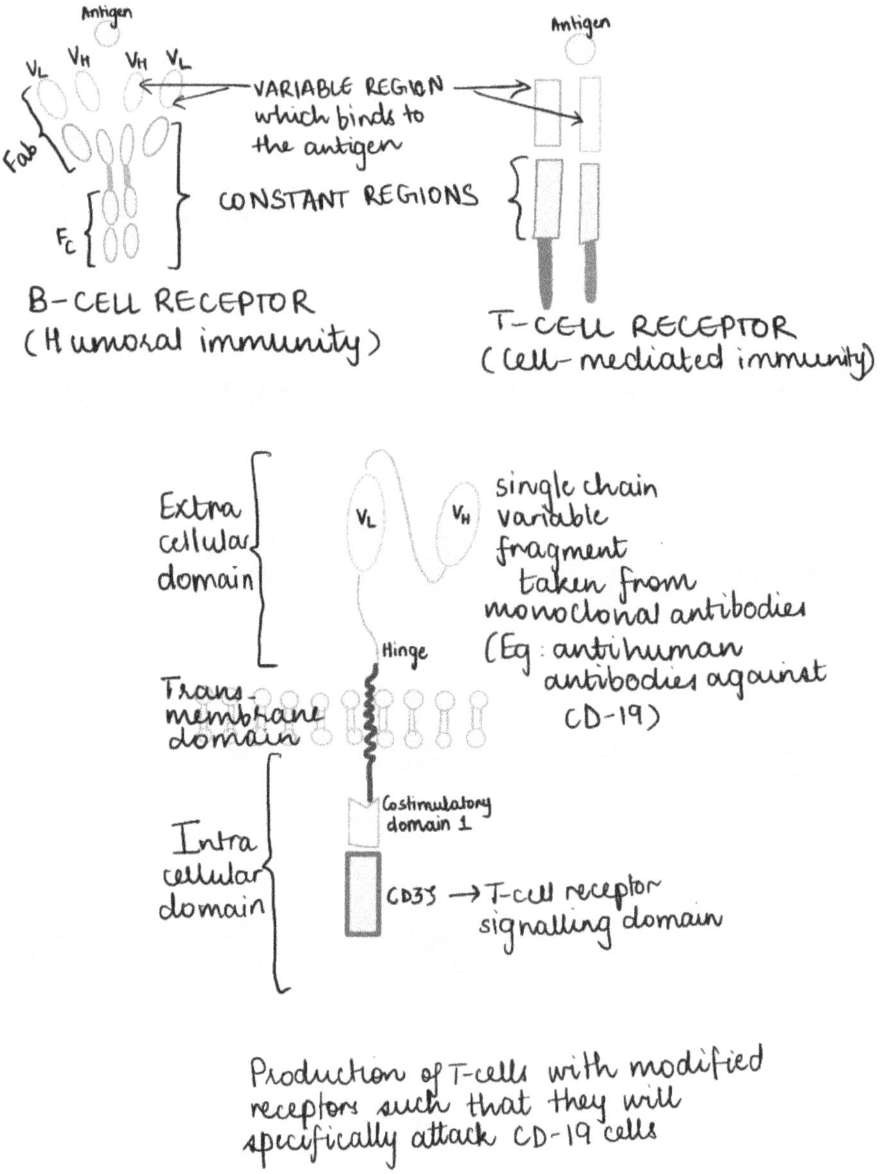

Figure 16.5: Generation of CAR-T cells specific for CD-19$^+$ expressing B cells by creating chimeric T cell receptors and transfecting the construct into T cells. Chimeric T cells are capable of attacking CD-19 expressing tumour cells.

BREYANZI is a CD19-directed genetically modified autologous T cell immunotherapy indicated for the treatment of adult patients with relapsed or refractory large B-cell lymphoma after two or more lines of systemic therapy, including diffuse large B-cell lymphoma (DLBCL) not otherwise specified (including DLBCL arising from indolent lymphoma), high-grade B-cell lymphoma, primary mediastinal large B-cell lymphoma, and follicular lymphoma grade 3B. This therapy was approved by US FDA in May 2021.

The ability to exploit new molecular tools, such as RNAi and CRISPR/Cas9, should be able to make use of some of the clinical development paradigms from earlier gene therapy trials.

Table 16.2: Gene Therapy approved drugs

Name of the gene/ vector	Name of the drug	Indication	Country in which it is approved	Year of approval	Current status
p53/ adenovirus	Gendicine	Head & Neck Squamous Cell Carcinoma	China	2003	US FDA approval awaited
Lipoprotein Lipase	Glybera	lipoprotein lipase deficiency (LPLD)	EU	2012	Withdrawn in 2017
GM-CSF/ HSV	Imlygic	Melanoma	China, EU, USA	2015	
CD19 chimeric antigen receptor – T cell	Kymriah	B cell lymphoblastic leukaemia	USA, EU	2017 / 2018	
RPE65 / AAV	Luxturna	Retinal dystrophy	USA, EU, Canada	2017/2018	priced at US$850000
ADA / retrovirus	Strimvelis	ADA-SCID	EU, USA	2016 / 2017	
CAR-T cell therapy	Yescarta	Large B cell lymphoma	USA, EU	2017 / 2018	In clinical trials in China
human SMN gene	Zolegensma	spinal muscular atrophy	USA	2019	

4. Conclusions

Molecular Medicine which includes synthetic small molecule inhibitors, recombinant monoclonal antibodies as well as gene therapy, is a new scientific discipline. With the rapidly evolving technologies, genetic errors in the disease are being identified and molecular interventions developed to correct them. The field of Molecular Medicine is rapidly evolving and benefitting mankind.

References

Trenker et al. Receptor tyrosine kinase activation: From the ligand perspective *Curr Opin Cell Biol* 2020 Apr;63:174-185

Luo et al. Principles of Cancer Therapy: Oncogene and Non-oncogene Addiction *Cell* 2009 Mar 6; 136(5): 823-837

Lu et al. Development of therapeutic antibodies for the treatment of diseases *Journal of Biomedical Science* 27:1-30 (2020)

Kumar et al. Clinical Development of gene therapy: results and lessons from recent successes. *Mol Ther Methods Clin Dev* 2016; 3: 16034

CHAPTER

17 Drug Development

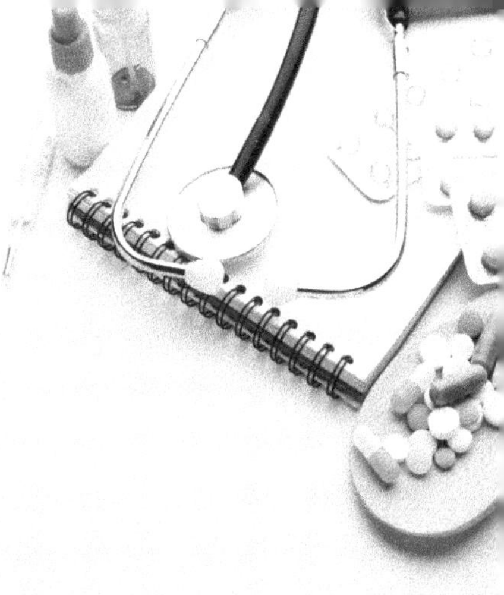

Nilima Kshirsagar

1. Introduction

Drug discovery and development is one of the most exciting, rewarding, satisfying and impactful scientific outputs from all disciplines of science. It is intellectually demanding, requiring various skills, the right knowledge, attitude and societal support. A successfully produced drug has the potential to touch/change/benefit the lives of many and change the health and socioeconomic fabric of a society. Such discoveries are lauded and rewarded by Noble prizes. India has a long history of Ayurveda, and in recent times of making and marketing generic medicines and vaccines to the whole world. In the past 20 years, India has forayed into new drug and vaccine development, and innovative products. However, there are many challenges, need for talent training, infrastructure, funding and at the same time access to affordable products. The government and Industry have come up with strategies to overcome many of the challenges. Thus, Drug discovery and development has many dimensions. This chapter provides glimpses of the past, present and what is new in this field.

2. History [1]

The history of drug discovery and development of the pharmaceutical industry and of drug regulations is intertwined, each influencing the other.

Drug Discovery

Drug discovery and its use dates back to the start of human civilization. Derived mainly from plants along with animal and mineral material, associated with religious spiritual healing, and often administered by sages or religious leaders, drugs were discovered by trial and error. Indian Ayurvedic medicine dates back to 3000-5000 years and is elaborately described in the Vedas and books authored by Charak, Sushrut and many others. Traditional Chinese medicine is also over 5,000 years old. In the West, Greek medicines were mainly derived from Egyptian and Babylonian writings while Romans extended the pharmacy practice of the Greeks.

Many of these ancient descriptions have resulted in the drugs of today. Rauwolfia Serpentina Sarpagandha of Ayurveda was meticulously studied by Dr Vakil in Mumbai in hypertensive patients and results showing efficacy were published in the British Journal of Cardiology. Reserpine, the active ingredient was isolated by the chemist in Ciba Geigy now Novartis in Basel, Switzerland. Artemisinin, the important Anti-malarial drug is derived from the Chinese plant. Artemisia Annua L (Quinghao) is described in Chinese ancient texts as useful for fever.

In the Middle Ages (around 400-1500 AD) there was a decline in Roman influence and many diseases like bubonic plague, leprosy, smallpox, tuberculosis were rampant and destroyed large populations. The Church and the Arabian medicines preserved the ancient text during this period. The foundation of the current drug discovery development was laid in the Renaissance period along with many advances made in biology, public health, hygiene and sanitation. Edward Jenner experimented with the smallpox vaccination. William Withering introduced digitalis extract from plant foxglove. Louis Pasteur discovered microorganisms and vaccinations against rabies with attenuated rabies virus. However, even at the beginning of the 20th century only a few drugs were available to mankind.

Pharmaceutical Industry [2]

The concepts of the scientific revolution of the 17th century (rationalism, experimentation) and the industrial revolution (production of goods) in the late 18th century were brought together in the Pharmaceutical Industry in the 19th century. During the early industry in Europe, Henrich Merck manufactured and sold alkaloids, in USA Beecham started the world's first factory for producing medicines, two German immigrants founded Pfizer Fine Chemicals (making painkillers and antiseptics required in world war). after his military career, Colonel Eli Lilly set-up a business, being the first to focus on research and development as well as manufacturing. Edward Squibb, as a naval doctor, found that the drugs supplied were of low quality and set-up his laboratory for quality drugs. Swiss manufacturers realized that their dyestuffs had antiseptic properties and sold them as such (they were accused of being a "pirate state" as they didn't follow patent laws laid down by the Germans!!). Bayer was also a dye maker and commercialized aspirin. (Il these eventually grew into giant pharma industries)

The interwar years saw two breakthroughs. Banting and colleagues isolated Insulin but only through collaboration with scientists from Eli Lilly that it was possible to purify and industrially produce it as an effective medicine. The Discovery of Penicillin by Alexander Fleming which was supported by the Government through international collaboration with Pfizer, Merck and Squibb which led to mass production, saving lives.

In the post-world war II period, other developments such as the social health care system NHS of UK, the booming USA economy, funding from the NHS and USA Govt helped the growth and wealth of the pharma industry. George Merck addressed the question of potential ethical conflict of making money from selling healthcare products by proclaiming that "medicines are for people.... Not for profits". The public spirited industry, however, required oversight with government regulations.

Drug Regulations [3]

The concept that the quality of medicines has to be ensured – has evolved over time. In Ayurveda descriptions of plants and seasons about when to collect and how to prepare are described. In Chinese traditional medicine that Artemisinin has to be prepared in cold water extract was described (which led to the discovery of the Anti-malarial drug and Nobel prize). Regulations for quality of medicines came into practice in the 16th century when in England the manufacturers of Mithridatium (a compound preparation of 41 components concocted by King of Pontus in 120 BC) and other medicines were subjected to supervision under Apothecaries wares Drugs and Stuffs Act. This could be seen as the start of pharmaceutical inspections. Pharmacopoeias, as we know them today, the official books on drug quality standards probably the first one, was Spanish Pharmacopoeia issued in 1581.

Regulations in modern medicine started in the 20th century. Most regulations have been issued due to some unfortunate event. In 1937, sulfanilamide elixir containing diethylene glycol (solvent) led to the death of over 100 subjects which resulted in the introduction of the US Federal Food, Drug and Cosmetics Act. The Thalidomide disaster (phocomelia in babies born to mothers taking it) led to the introduction of yellow card system for reporting Adverse Reactions and the Committee on Safety of Drugs in the UK and in the USA. Drug Amendments Act requires FDA to approve all new drug applications and demand that a new drug should be proven to be effective and safe in compliance with quality (good manufacturing practices) and registration of manufacturing establishments.

In Europe, additional efforts were made to harmonize among its member countries. In 1990 international conference on harmonization of technical requirements for registration of pharmaceuticals for human use (ICH) was set up by EU Japan and the United States with WHO, EFTA and Canada as observers. This facilitated availability for sale, of effective and good pharmaceuticals.

Ethics

While drug regulations were evolving, recognition of the downside of scientific ambition and risk to humans due to experimentation was recognized in parallel through various regulations such as the Nuremberg code, Helsinki declaration and in India ICMR guidelines for ethics in human research and good clinical (research)practices were developed

3. Steps in Drug Discovery and Development Process [4]

With this historical background, drug discovery and development occurred rapidly through the 20th century.

Discovery and development of new drugs occur with advances in knowledge, new insights into diseases, technologies to produce new drugs, tests for efficacy, safety, new effects of existing drugs innovations, trained insightful scientists, funding from industry, academia, government and suitable ecosystems which are the backbone.

Promising compounds are evaluated for safety, potential benefits, mechanism of action, pharmacokinetics, safety, interaction, variation in different populations and comparison with available therapeutic options.

Preclinical research is done using Good Laboratory Practices (GLP). Physico-chemical properties, formulations and effects on cells, tissues, organs and normal/diseased/transgenic animals are evaluated to assess safety and efficacy. Animal toxicity studies are done as per regulations depending on the route, duration and population proposed.

Clinical Research

Preclinical research is not a substitute for human studies. Clinical trials are designed to answer the specific research question, using a specific study plan – protocol and case record form and are carried out after the ethics committee and regulatory agency's permission and with the informed consent of the participant. The protocol defines the criteria for selection and exclusion of subjects, details of the product to be tested, how it is to be given and criteria for evaluation of efficacy safety.

Phase-I study is usually done on 20-100 healthy volunteers (sometimes with diseases e.g. cancer) to assess tolerability and safety. It starts with a few volunteers given a fraction of the effective dose (calculated from preclinical animal data by standard methods using a formula for calculation). The dose is successively increased till a tolerated dose is identified and given as a single dose, then as multiple doses. The effect of food, the possibility of effect on QTc Interval and the possibility of interaction with other drugs is also tested. Volunteers are carefully and closely monitored to predict the safe dose for future studies. Pharmacokinetic studies to estimate blood levels reached and elimination from the body are also done. Efficacy can also be judged to some extent in this phase by using some bio-markers/sensitive Tests. Approximately,70% of drugs move to the next phase.

Phase-II is for efficacy and safety testing which is usually done in about several hundred people with disease. Different doses are tried to come up with most optimal dose schedule i.e. effective, safe with good benefit-risk profile. Approximately, 33% of drugs go on to Phase-III.

Phase-III usually has 300 to 3000 subjects with disease. Known as pivotal study, often a comparator standard treatment is used to evaluate the benefit of the new drug. Throughout phase II and III, data on safety is captured. Approximately, 25-30% of drugs are found suitable to move to the next phase i.e. apply for permission to market the drugs.

Phase-IV is post-marketing surveillance, studies. Phases I – III studies are usually done in a few hundred or thousand patients. Side effects, which are common (occurring 1:10) or rare (occur 1:100), are captured. However, very rare side effects which occur infrequently or occur in a specific population (age, gender, genetically variant) are not known at this stage. Hence, regulatory authorities ask for post-market safety monitoring.

Regulatory authorities vary in some aspects in different countries. There is a constant attempt to harmonize regulations so that drugs approved in one country can be approved in other countries thus making them available quickly. However, due to variations in population, infrastructure, facilities, health care provision, countries demand a review of all data and at times conduct of bridging studies before granting permission.

In the COVID pandemic, to make vaccines rapidly available to the population, drug regulatory authorities gave emergency use authorization, requiring controlled distribution and administration of vaccines and capturing data on adverse events following immunization. A system for this exists in India. AEFI for immunization was given under the National program which has been expanded to include AE following the COVID vaccine immunization.

Pharmacovigilance

Globally, post-marketing adverse drug reaction data is captured through the pharmaceutical industry, health care providers and patients and is evaluated frequently by regulatory uthorities. It is aggregated by WHO collaborating centre in Uppsala, Sweden. India has a pharmacovigilance program (PvPI) which collects, analyzes and recommends to the Drug Controller for suitable action.

4. Challenges and Opportunities in Drug Development

Challenges

Control by private entities skews the drug development to profiting affecting cost and access. On the other hand, 90 % of drugs in development do not reach the market due to lack of efficacy, safety issues or lack of funding to complete a trial, failure to maintain good manufacturing protocols and follow regulatory guidelines and little or no commercial interest. It takes 7-10 years for a lead drug to reach the market due to the rigorous process required to demonstrate safety and efficacy.

The lack of reliable bio-markers is another impediment to accurate diagnosis, prognosis and effective drug development assessing dose duration of treatment for several diseases, especially of CNS eg. Alzheimer's and depression.

Indian Scenario

India is the third-largest manufacturer of drugs worldwide accounting for 10% of the global total. But it accounts for only 1.5% of the total value of drugs produced. Innovation R&D is the way forward. In the global Innovation Index as per the 2020 report, India ranked 48th. Though in the top 50, it is still below others e.g. China is 14th, Singapore is 8th.

India has an opportunity to be a global innovation hub and destination for R&D and manufacturing out-sourcing (at present this is mostly in US & Europe). With the country's strong process, chemistry skills, attractive cost value and large and diverse genetic population, it is an ideal location for cost-effective clinical research activities and novel drug trials but there are challenges.

Innovative Mind-set, Related Skills

The combination of basic research, innovation and astute observation of a prepared mind is fundamental to the drug discovery process as is illustrated by examples such as the accidental discovery of Penicillin by Alexander Fleming and Warfarin by Karl Link (investigating hemorrhagic disease in cattle) and the recent discovery and development of CRISPR/Cas9 (while investigating bacterial genome to improve yoghurt production!) illustrate this. [5]

But in India training, skills and talent are inadequate. Less than 0.5% of Indian students pursue Ph.D. Only 2.5% of higher education institutions offered Ph.D. India has 216.2 researchers per 1 million compared to 4300 in the US and 7100 in South Korea.

Clinical research ability is also low. In one survey over half the medical colleges did not have a single publication. This can be due to limited infrastructure, lack of intent, lack of incentives or clinical overwork. Studies in Gujarat, Maharashtra and West Bengal showed low awareness of clinical research among the final year medical students. There is limited expertise in designing, conducting and evaluating clinical trials, paucity of expertise for co-ordination between basic researchers, pharmacologists, clinical pharmacologists, clinicians and industry for drug development and a lack of talent that has experience for the entire product life cycle from discovery to target developing, getting regulatory approval and ultimately going to the market.

Complex Regulatory Approval Process and IPR

India Patients Act 1970 was amended to comply with the Trade-related aspects of Intellectual Property Rights (TRIPS). In October 2020, amendments were made to encourage an innovative environment. Globally, stringent rules for ensuring quality, safety and efficacy exist. India has a strong regulatory framework with the latest revision in 2019 viz New drugs and clinical trial Rules 2019. However, there are multiple Government and state ministries and departments which regulate various aspects of drug development which can be a challenge e.g. Discovery and research is under the Ministry of Science & Technology, Health & Family Welfare (MOHFW), Human Resource development and Ministry of Chemicals & Fertilizers (MOCF). Development (clinical trials, import etc.) is under the Central Drugs Standard Control Organization (CDSCO) under MOHFW, manufacturing is under the State Department of Health, Drug pricing is under MOCF, (department of pharmaceuticals) pharmacovigilance under MOHFW (Indian Pharmacopoeia Commission IPC National Co-ordinating Centre). Pharmacovigilance Program of India (NCC-PvPI) and traditional medicines are under the Ministry of AYUSH (Ayurveda, Yoga, Unani, Siddha and Homeopathy).

Financing Constraints and Limited Infrastructure

India's expenditure on R&D is 0.7% of GDP (South Korea 4.5% and even Brazil 1.3%), of this contribution by the Central Government is 45.4%, state 6.4%, higher education 6.8%, industry 41.4% (4.6% from public sector industry and 36.8% from private sector industry). Even private equity and venture financing provide only 3% of its total to pharmaceuticals.

5. Opportunities

Unmet Needs

Globally and in India there are a number of unmet needs as illustrated by a few examples below:

Infectious Diseases

Malaria, TB, HIV, AIDS and Influenza despite efforts, drugs and attempts to develop vaccines continue to cause morbidity and mortality along with social and economic burden. Novel viruses of animal origin NIPAH, SARS, Ebola and MERS cause outbreaks emphasizing the need for global preparedness. Anti-microbial resistance is projected to cause 10 million deaths per year by 2050.

Cancer

Many efforts with precision medicine and immunotherapy but still nearly one person per second death, there are nearly 10 million deaths annually.

CNS Disease

Dementia affects around 30 million people and death among Alzheimer's has doubled and imposes a huge health care burden. There is no medicine known to reverse the progression of the disease.

Rare Diseases

Rare diseases collectively affect 6 to 8% of the world population; half are children. Of the 7,000 rare diseases, treatment is available for only 5%. There is great disparity in access to orphan medication amongst the countries of the world.

6. Strategies to Overcome Challenges [6]

To strengthen India's research and innovation eco system – financing, infrastructure, supporting policies and regulations is needed. To foster industry-ready talent, there are several government and private national and international initiatives. Clinical research – to augment capability there is a need for a research-oriented environment. ICMR online research methodology course is compulsory for post-graduates. ICMR also has an online course on ethics, it also provides research fellowships for students. Collaborations between medical colleges and established research institutes, expanding the pool of qualified clinical researchers, managing time effectively between research and clinical commitments and making provision for research administrative support to handle activities such as institutional agreements, patient approvals etc. are needed.

Start-ups: Boosting the Innovation Momentum

India with around 50,000 start-ups is the third largest start-up economy in the world. They are working across a range of innovative solutions for patient life cycle (disease management, treatment, diagnosis, telemedicine, remote monitoring) and product value chain (R&D, advanced drug technology platform, novel antibodies, 3D-cell Culture technology etc.). A survey of 60 life sciences and health care set-ups highlighted funding, innovation, market potential and government support as critical for growth. The government has taken several initiatives to tackle these challenges. Department of Science & Technology, Biotechnology, Council of Science & Industrial Research (CSIR) and Biotechnology Industry Research Assistance Council (BIRAC) are providing funds for mentoring and infrastructure. However, collaboration across departments and with ICMR is needed.

Indian Pharma

Indian pharma is investing relatively less in R&D (USD 0.15 billion from top 10 Indian compared to 8.17 billion top 10 US life sciences). The focus is on generics and bio-similar R&D. Globally, pharma companies are challenged by strained healthcare budgets, patent expiration, increased regulatory scrutiny and decreasing R&D productivity. Big pharma is sourcing innovation externally through acquisitions. Collaborations with smaller companies, and academia such as Pfizer and Moderna COVID-19 vaccines were conceptualized by small Biotech companies which incubate, invest, mentor and/or partner with entrepreneurs who devise winning ideas. This is an opportunity for young innovators. Collaborative efforts of a few physicins and scientists resulted in development of Liposomal Amphotericin, a drug delivery system which is marketed, used for systemic fungal infection in immunocompromised patients of Kala Azar. It has recently been found useful for treatment of Mucor Mycosis in Covid-19 patients [7,8]

Access to Data for Research and Innovation

With data protection and sharing, there are considerable opportunities for big data from different sources such as patient registries, historical clinical trial data, epidemiological databases and the recently launched Digital Health Mission (NDHM). Internationally, public-private partnership, artificial intelligence is being developed which can quickly and accurately predict promising compounds for development.

7. What is New?

Sources of Drugs

Natural Products

In the past, in several countries plants were a major source of drugs. Single active substances have been identified from plants (for example Quinine, Aspirin and Artemisinin). For several of these, chemical synthesis has been possible and some analogues of originals have been developed.

Despite the advent of combinatorial chemistry, high throughput screening impact of natural products on drug discovery is high. Natural products (plants, microorganisms, animals) derived drugs form 28% of all chemical entities. In cancer therapy, out of 175 molecules, 85 are from natural sources. For several plants especially those used in traditional medicine, extracts have been found to be more effective than purified single chemicals. At times a mixture has been found to be safer than a single plant. These have been regulated through various rules.

In India, Traditional medicines and drugs are regulated under AYUSH rules. While Phytopharmaceuticals are enriched standardized extract of plants with specific therapeutic claims which are regulated under the Drugs and Cosmetics Act, Nutraceuticals and dietary supplements are food-derived ingredients that offer health benefits. but terminology and regulations differ in different countries and include terms like functional foods and herbal medicines, regulated under FSSAI in India.

Computer Calculated Compounds/Use of Artificial Intelligence (AI) to Discover Drugs [9]

An estimated USD 2.6 billion is required for developing a new drug, most of which is due to 9 out of 10 candidates failing to reach the market. It is envisaged that AI and machine learning will help in quicker, cheaper and more effective drug discovery. On 12th June 2007, a robot called Adam identified the functions of yeast gene, when checked 9 out of 19 were new, and only one was wrong. Robot scientists using AI can test more compounds with accuracy, reproducibility and exhaustive searchable record keeping.

Medicinal Chemistry [10]

Medicinal chemists and pharmacologists with some creativity and intuition design synthesize Tests and try on animal model for effects and new chemicals. Now chemists are able to generate with rational focus libraries of compounds in a fraction of time using combinatorial chemistry and test it in vitro in high throughput screening. New graphics software such as Spotfire can facilitate the retrieval and analysis of data.

Molecular Biology

With the molecular genetics revolution, molecularly defined biological targets such as enzymes, receptors and transporters are available. Absorption metabolism can be tested in vitro using recombinant cytochrome P450 enzymes, and permeability and transporters assays are available, partly solving the problem of rat to human variation. In vitro toxicity screens are also available like tests for hERG (drugs that block this channel can cause prolongation of Q-T interval and ventricular fibrillation and death). Today, a structure-activity relationship can be much better worked out.

8. Clinical Trials Design and Analysis [11]

The classical randomized double-blind parallel-group (or cross over) design for a clinical trial is the gold standard. It is robust, easy to perform, interpret and suitable for assessing the efficacy of new drugs. However, it has disadvantages of high cost, large sample size, long study durations, inability (lack of power) to evaluate efficacy in sub-groups and is ethically questionable at times.

Alternatives that protect against bias and confounding have been developed in recent years. Pragmatic trials in a "real world" setting, effectiveness trials (large numbers, few exclusions, practically useful results), cluster trials (treatments allocated randomly to groups), adaptive design and master protocols are some examples. Unlike conventional trials adaptive design allows alteration of protocols, changing study population, sample size, study drugs etc. in preplanned decision rules.

The master protocol uses one protocol. In an umbrella trial, multiple targeted therapies are studied in a single disease, In a basket trial, one targeted therapy is studied in multiple diseases or disease subtypes. In platform trials, multiple therapies are studied in a single disease with a decision algorithm to enter or leave (e.g. recovery trial of COVID drugs). There are other issues with clinical trials viz. difficulties in recruitment, retention, managing and monitoring patients, contributing to high cost and trial failures. Artificial Intelligence, algorithms and electronic data reduce human error, allow continuous aggregation, coding, storage, management, saving time and enabling decisions.

9. Conclusions

Drug discovery and development is teamwork. COVID-19 has shown that rapid response, development of a vaccine and repurposing of drugs is possible for global needs with concerted efforts, use of technology and funding. Expanding knowledge base of diseases, aetiology, spread, and effect on the human body and society holds great promise for the discovery of important new medicines to tackle unmet needs, especially bearing in mind access and availability. From basic science to preclinical and clinical research there is a huge opportunity that young students today can seize and contribute to drug discovery development and health care.

References

1. Ng R. History of drug discovery and development in drugs. From discovery to approval, 2nd edn. 2009,391-397. John Wiley & sons Inc.
2. Rebecca A. History of the Pharmaceutical industry, pharmaphorum.com/r-d/a_history_of the pharmaceutical industry / Sept 1. 2020
3. Rago L, Santoso B. Drug and Regulations, history, present and future, in Drug benefits and risks. International textbook of clinical pharmacology. revised 2nd edition ed van Boxtel CJ, V Santosa B, Edwards i.e. 2008, IOS press and Upsala monitoring centre. 2008, chapter 6, 65-67.
4. US FDA guidelines
5. Rani KGA, Hamad NA, Zaher DM, Sieburth SM, &others. Drug development post Covid19 pandemic toward a better system to meet current and future global challenges. Expert opinion on drug discovery. https://dri.org/10.1080/17460441. 2021.886422.
6. Indian Pharmaceutical Industry 2021. Future in now. Earnst and Young.
7. Fleming N. Computer calculated Compounds. Nature, 2018; 557: 885, 855-857.
8. LLG Lowe III. JA. The role of the medicinal chemist in drug discovery – then and now. Nature reviews. Drug Discovery. 2004;3:853-861.
9. Ajmera Y, Singhal S, Dwivedi SN, Dey AB. The changing perspective of clinical trial design. Perspectives in Clinical Research, 2021,12,66-70.
10. Kshirsagar NA, Pandya SK, Kirodian BG, Sanath, S. Liposomal drug delivery system from laboratory to clinic. JPGM,2005;51(1): s 5-s15
11. Jadhav M, Jadhav P., Shinde V, Kadam K, Kshirsagar N, Liposomal Amphotericin B for the Treatment of Cryptococcal Meningitis in HIV/AIDS Patients in India-A Pilot Pharmacokinetic Study, Clin Pharmacol Drug Dev. 2013 Jan;2(1):48-52. doi: 10.1002/cpdd.6. Epub 2013 Feb 25

CHAPTER

18 Vaccines Against Infectious Diseases

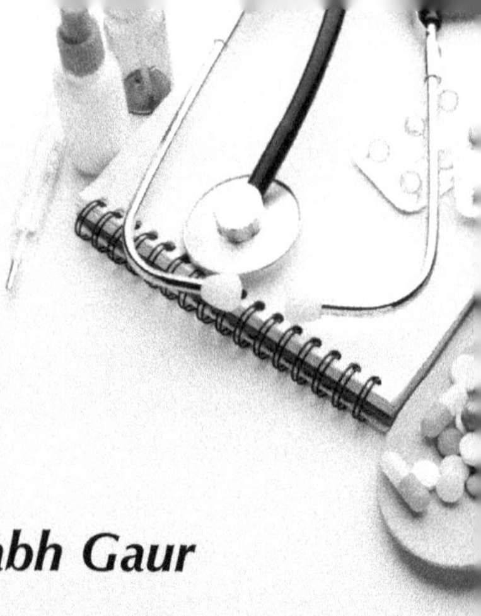

Narendra Chirmule and Amitabh Gaur

1. Introduction

In the last six decades [1], Vaccines have transformed the management of public health in the world. More than thirty vaccines against various infectious diseases have been approved and ~240 vaccines are in various stages of development [2]. The National health policies that provide vaccines to newborn children, adolescents, adults and the elderly have saved millions of lives. More than 2 million lives are saved each year by vaccinations, which have resulted in the reduction of Infant Mortality from 93 deaths per 1,000 live births in 1990 to 39 in 2018. In India, the National Vaccination Program statistics indicate that ~61% of infants have received vaccines. Several operational challenges are attributed to the lower rates. A detailed historical perspective of vaccination in India has been reviewed previously [3]. In the last decade, the Indian Pharmaceutical Companies have become the largest vaccine manufacturing units in the world, led by companies such as Serum Institute, Bharat Biotech, Biological E, Zydus-Cadilla and Shanta Biotech (now Sanofi). Regulatory guidelines of the Drugs and Cosmetics Act of 1945 and the updated gazettes, which require clinical trials, quality manufacturing processes and Pharmacovigilance Processes have enabled the development of safe and effective vaccines [4]. These advances in drug development, manufacturing and supply chain distribution have made it possible to vaccinate more than 1.2 billion people against COVID-19 in a relatively short time frame of six months in India. **Table 18.1** lists the bacterial and viral vaccines that have been approved in India and are a part of the National Immunization Schedule.

The aim of this write-up is to describe advances in design, development and regulatory aspects of the development of safe and effective vaccines. The factors that play a role in developing vaccines more efficiently could make use of:

(a) Multi-omics Data Analysis for Pharmacology,
(b) Flexible and Modular Manufacturing Processes,
(c) Predictive Toxicology,
(d) Adaptive Clinical Trial Designs,
(e) Post-approval Monitoring of Vaccine Effectiveness.

2. Vaccine Development - Key Immunological Concepts

Original Antigenic Sin

Initial exposure to an antigen primes the immune system by creating memory immune cells, which biases the immune response in favor of the first antigen and its determinants [5]. This imprinting of the immune system could help in rapidly mounting a robust immune response when cross-reactive epitopes are presented later. Alternatively, the presence of such bias in favor of certain epitopes may lead to a competitive state where the immune response to novel epitopes may get obscured leaving the organism in a more susceptible state to a new infection. Both kinds of effects have been reported in Influenza and Coronavirus Infections. In instances where the shared epitope results in a less efficacious vaccine, it may be advisable to remove those parts from the vaccine design.

Immune Memory and Clinical Correlate of Protection

During the clinical evaluation phase of any candidate vaccine, it is useful to develop a correlate of clinical protection. A bio-marker or analyte that could be measured reliably and serve as a surrogate for clinical protection would help in determining the efficacy of a vaccine candidate. Recently, in the case of the seven SARS-CoV-2 vaccines, the relationship of antibody levels with efficacy was examined. The data showed significant correlation between the levels of virus-neutralizing antibodies and vaccine efficacy. Similar correlation results were also seen between the levels of Spike protein-binding antibodies and vaccine efficacy. An agreed upon assay method fortified with standards of measurement and reporting units go a long way in developing such correlates of efficacy for any new set of vaccines being developed for a pathogen [6].

Antibody-Dependent Enhancement

The phenomenon of Antibody-Dependent Enhancement (ADE) across viruses and within different strains of the same virus presents an interesting challenge while designing vaccines. Flaviviruses like Dengue and Zika are prevalent in the same geographic regions and pre-existing immunity to one virus can affect the progression of the disease caused by another virus [7]. Antibodies to the Dengue virus from prior infection can cause ADE of Zika infection. Similar observations have been made in the case of Dengue infections wherein pre-existing antibodies to one strain of the virus leads to a more serious disease upon subsequent infection with another strain of the virus [8]. This phenomenon of ADE has affected the development and deployment of a Dengue vaccine. Future vaccine designs will have to consider how ADE can affect the success of their vaccine.

3. Vaccine Development

Development of vaccines requires a systematic approach that involves:

i. Understanding the Mechanism of Protection,
ii. A Manufacturing Process,

iii. Pharmacology,
iv. Toxicology,
v. Clinical trials to determine the safety and efficacy of the vaccine against the target pathogen.

We will utilize the examples of vaccines developed against SARS-CoV-2 to illustrate the complexities and challenges in vaccine development. **Figure 18.1** shows the key steps involved in vaccine development.

First, during the discovery phase, there needs to be a detailed knowledge of the mechanism of action and biology of the disease pathogenesis, epidemiology and disease spread in various geographies, the nature of the pathogen structure and its genetic variations, and clinical characteristics of the disease. All these aspects must be well known for effective and rational vaccine design. The goal of the vaccine is to prime the immune response and generate immune memory to facilitate adequate control of the pathogen when it infects naturally and in turn prevent clinical disease but not necessarily infection. In most cases, the efficacy and effectiveness of a vaccine can be improved significantly by addition of adjuvants. Advances in various molecular, biochemical and chemical technologies have enabled the design of novel vaccine platforms. These range from live-attenuated and inactivated pathogens to viral vectors, recombinant proteins, purified carbohydrates/lipids, DNA and most recently mRNA. Over the past several decades, with the advent of multi-omics data analysis to inform biological processes, the philosophy of identifying optimal vaccine candidates has transitioned from "shots-at-goal" approach to "pick-the-winner" approach.

The next step in vaccine development is to design a manufacturing process to produce the vaccine. The design of the process is initiated by defining a Target Product Profile (TPP) and Critical Quality Attributes (CQA) of the vaccine product. A battery of analytical methods ranging from physico-chemical to functional assays, are required to characterize the primary, secondary and tertiary structure of the vaccine components. Manufacturing under the regulations of Good Manufacturing Process (GMP) and using the principles of Quality-by-Design (QbD) are essential components of developing high-quality vaccines.

Animal models that closely mimic human disease are utilized to establish proof-of-principle in preclinical studies. These toxicology studies are performed to determine the Maximum Tolerated Dose (MTD) when unacceptable toxicities are observed or to record No Observed Effect Levels (NOEL) when no significant toxicities are observed. Although studies in animal models do not always predict the immune response in humans, they are used to study the pharmacological effects of the vaccine to determine optimal dose, immunization frequencies, potency, ability to induce long-term memory and most importantly efficacy in pathogen-challenge studies.

Finally, clinical trials are always required to provide the evidence of immunogenicity, safety and efficacy. In this respect, Phase I, Phase II and Phase III clinical trials are performed in sequence to determine the safety, optimal dose and overall safety, and efficacy of the vaccine, respectively. Recent advances in clinical trial design have demonstrated the advantages of adaptive clinical trial design in subjecting the least number of human subjects to clinical testing and ensuring optimal safety and efficacy endpoints.

The regulatory pathways of vaccine development from submission of the Investigational New Drug/Product (IND) Application to the approval of the Biological Licensing Application (BLA) are described in the Central Drugs Standard Control Organization (CDSCO) and Ministry of Health website. The increased collaborations between international agencies and philanthropic institutions such as International Council for Harmonization (ICH), World Health Organization (WHO), Gavi, The Vaccine Alliance, Gates Foundation and International Aids Vaccine Initiative (IAVI) have provided a systematic approach to the regulatory pathways.

After approval of a safe and effective vaccine, large numbers of people are vaccinated. Studying the control of the disease spread in populations provides the readout of vaccine effectiveness. When sufficient population is immunized, it has maximal impact on unimmunized individuals in the form of Herd Immunity. However, this requires detailed understanding of demography, age of maximal disease susceptibility and social and biological factors influencing pathogen transmission and replication.

4. Vaccines Approved or in Development in the Last Five Years

Malaria

Malaria, a tropical disease caused by a Protozoan Parasite, has affected human health since ancient times. Numerous measures to control the spread of the disease by controlling its vector—the Anopheles Mosquito—have had variable levels of impact. With over 220 million cases globally from 89 different countries (estimated in 2019), this disease has enormous socio-economic burden on societies where it is endemic. The quest for an effective vaccine has been going on for the last several decades. Currently, about 20 different vaccine candidates are at various stages of clinical evaluation [9]. Recently (2021), a WHO panel approved the first malaria vaccine for reducing *P. Falciparum*-induced clinical vents in children in Africa. Mosquirix®, the Pre-Erythrocytic *P. Falciparum* RTS, S/AS01E vaccine needs to be given 3-4 times and is about 30%–40% effective in controlling the disease. Despite this, the approval to Mosquirix® reinforces the promise of prophylactic vaccines in controlling parasitic diseases.

Dengue

Dengue, a member of the Flaviviridae family, is one of the most frequently transmitted viruses by a vector [10]. It causes debilitating disease in a large part of the global population, with about 400 million individuals affected by the disease annually. A large proportion of this population is in India. Four serotypes of the Dengue virus are transmitted by the

Aedes Genus mosquitoes. Over half a dozen vaccines are in various stages of development including Dengvaxia® that has received approval from the United States Food and Drugs Administration (USFDA) and other agencies. Generating a balanced immune response against all the four serotypes seems to be an important requirement to avoid causing more severe disease upon subsequent re-infection with another strain of the virus, presumably due to ADE. Dengvaxia® is a live, attenuated Tetravalent recombinant vaccine wherein Yellow Fever Virus enveloped protein encoding genes were replaced with envelope genes of the four Dengue serotypes. The vaccine is currently recommended for pre-exposed young population and is contraindicated for naïve populations. Vaccines following other approaches like recombinant attenuated live virus and Tetravalent Virus-Like Particles (VLPs) are also being developed for the effective control of Dengue [11].

Chikungunya

Arthritogenic Alphaviruses comprise a group of enveloped RNA viruses that are transmitted to humans by mosquitoes. [12] These viruses cause a debilitating, acute and chronic Musculoskeletal Disease, which is prevalent in various parts of the world including India. Chikungunya, Ross River, Mayaro and O'nyong'nyong are some of the emerging Alphaviruses that cause Arthritogenic Disease following infection. Chikungunya, a *Togaviridae* virus transmitted by the *Aedes Aegypti* Mosquito, occurs in various parts of the world including India and poses health risk with high morbidity in infected individuals. Multiple vaccine candidates against Chikungunya are being evaluated in clinical hearings. Valneva, a French vaccine company, has reported positive results from a pivotal Phase-III clinical trial of a vaccine candidate, which is live attenuated virus to be administered in a single dose [13]. Another potential vaccine, a Chikungunya Virus Like Particle (CHIKV VLP) developed by the NIAID and Emergent BioSolutions has been shown to generate high levels of neutralizing antibodies in Phase-II clinical trials and is currently being investigated in a Phase-III clinical trial [14].

Zika

Zika virus (ZIKV) is an arbovirus belonging to the Flaviviridae family. It has made its appearance in India in the past few years. In addition to the Vector-Borne Transmission, mixing of blood and other bodily fluids results in the transmission of ZIKV. Transplacental transmission of the virus in pregnant women may result in Congenital Zika Syndrome, manifesting as Fetal/Newborn Microcephaly, other congenital malformations and complications in pregnancy, including miscarriage. In some adults, symptoms of Guillain-Barre's Syndrome have appeared following infection with ZIKV. Dozens of experimental anti Zika vaccines are being tested at preclinical stages employing a host of technological platforms including the well-recognized VLP technology as effective immunogens [15]. A couple of DNA vaccines are in phase-II clinical evaluation and have so far not demonstrated any ADE complications relating to concomitant Flaviviral infections [16].

Nipah

Nipah and Hendra viruses are members of the Genus *Henipavirus* and family Paramyxovirus. These viruses can cause serious Neurological and Respiratory Diseases in humans with high rate of fatality ranging from 40% to 90%. These viruses have jumped through different species. As per records about 25 years ago, the viruses jumped from *Pteropus* Bats (Flying Foxes) to Horses and then to multiple other animals and into humans. Isolated instances of the Nipah virus (NiV) infection have occurred in India, with the most recent one happening in Kerala in 2018 that claimed the lives of 22 of the 23 infected individuals. Encephalitis, Meningitis and other symptoms may appear even up to 10 years following the viral infection because of re-emergence of the virus in the Central Nervous System. NiV-B (Bangladesh isolate), HeV and others are classified as a BSL-4 category-C pathogens with transmission from animals to humans and human to humans recorded in the past decade [17].

Over ten different studies have evaluated various vaccines against Nipah (NiV) and HeV, including Vaccinia vector expressing NiV G and F proteins, VLPs, mRNA and recombinant protein subunits in several different animal models. The African Green Monkey (AGM) model has been widely accepted as an animal model that replicates the human NiV disease quite closely. The Hendra Virus soluble G Protein (HeV-sG) recombinant protein subunit vaccine was recently shown to be highly effective in the AGM model. This vaccine candidate induced neutralizing antibodies that controlled viremia and more significantly protected the animals from live challenge with a lethal dose of the NiV-B. The HeV-sG subunit vaccine has been approved for equine use and is currently being tested in Phase-I clinical trials. It is on way to further evaluation against NiV infection.

Influenza

Influenza is caused by Influenza A and B Viruses. Most common modes of transmission are via Respiratory Droplets from one person to another or via Fomites. The influenza virus surface proteins go through antigenic drift as a consequence of accumulating mutations in the genes encoding these proteins. In addition, the A strain goes through antigenic shift with entirely new determinants appearing on the surface protein because of shuffling and rearrangement of genes between human and animal influenza viruses. Both these phenomena reduce the effectiveness of any pre-existing immunity, either acquired naturally or through immunization. Therefore, to combat the prevalent strain of the influenza virus, a new vaccine must be designed each season. Approved vaccines in use in wealthy countries are either a Trivalent vaccine (Two influenza A strains [H1N1 & H3N2] and one Influenza B strain) or a Tetravalent vaccine that includes two Influenza B strains (Victoria & Yamagata).

These vaccines are fine-tuned for the northern and southern hemispheres based upon the data on the circulating strains from the WHO Global Influenza Surveillance Response System (GISRS). Manufacturers prepare variations of Trivalent - inactivated and live attenuated and Tetravalent - inactivated and live attenuated vaccines and each formulation is tested on target groups for safety and efficacy [18]. Whether middle income or low income countries would benefit from Influenza vaccines is debated in the context of cost and benefit to the society and economy.

In an interesting finding of cross-benefits of influenza vaccine, a recent retrospective study of about 75,000 subjects from over 50 health centers revealed benefits of influenza vaccine to recipients who later became infected with the SARS-CoV-2 virus [19]. Significant reduction in events such as sepsis, Deep Vein Thrombosis (DVT), Emergency Room and Intensive Care Unit admissions pointed towards potential benefits of influenza vaccine that should be explored.

5. Lessons Learned from Vaccine Development

The lessons learned from the understanding of immune responses to infectious diseases and vaccine development to prevent their spread have been summarized below. These parameters can be utilized for vaccine development in the future.

Criteria for a Successful Vaccine

i. It should stimulate antibody responses and the titer of neutralizing antibodies should be ~2560 lasting for more than one year.
ii. It should stimulate a memory CD4 and CD8 T- and B-cells response.
iii. It should have a large effect size in a population that can enable Herd Immunity, e.g., >70%.
iv. It should render protection to children, pregnant women, older adults and patients with comorbidities, all of whom may have sub-optimal immune responses.
v. It should be safe and not result in acute hypersensitivity reactions. The occurrence of such events should be <0.1% subjects.
vi. It should have a formulation that makes the vaccine stable in extreme temperatures and distribution conditions.
vii. It should induce mucosal immunity, i.e., Immunity in the Oral-Respiratory Tract.

Anticipated Major Adverse Events from a Sub-Optimal Vaccine

Based on experiences with previous vaccines, we are providing possible Adverse Events that could occur with a sub-optimal COVID-19 vaccine. The list below provides potential aspects about the vaccine.

i. It may elicit an acute hypersensitivity shock due to antigens, impurities or formulation.
ii. It may activate cross-reaction to self-proteins resulting in Autoimmunity.
iii. It may induce local injection site reactions.

iv. It may result in activation of ADE of SARS-CoV-2 through interaction with Fc receptors.
v. It may induce activation of cells that upregulate ACE-2 or TMPRSS2 receptors, which in turn may result in creating a new reservoir of highly-infectable cells in vaccinated individuals.
vi. It may result in a weak immune response and not provide adequate levels of Herd Immunity, enabling spread of the virus in the community.
vi. It may exacerbate comorbidities such as Diabetes and Heart Disease.

The criteria and potential adverse effects listed above can be used to define the requirements of vaccines in a Target Product Profile (TPP), where the specifications can assist in designing appropriate vaccine antigens, adjuvants, immunization schedules and methods of measurement of efficacy, safety and effectiveness.

6. Vaccine against SARS-CoV-2 (COVID-19)

Immunopathogenesis of COVID-19

SARS-CoV-2 infects individuals through the Nasopharyngeal Pathway. This infection is the cause of all subsequent effects. The Viral Load is measured by Reverse-Transcriptase Quantitative Polymerase Chain Reaction (RT-qPCR), which detects the viral RNA from Nasopharyngeal Swabs. The test relies on Synthesis of cDNA from viral RNA and multiple cycles of amplification to produce detectable amounts of DNA in the mixed Nucleic acid sample. Viral Load in patients is dependent on various factors including the number of ACE2 and TMPRSS2 receptors, comorbidities, cytokines, the number of viral particles in the infection, and the overall immune health status. Viral Loads have been demonstrated to have a direct correlation with disease severity and mortality in COVID-19.

High Viral Loads evoke defensive mechanisms that can induce inflammation. This subsequently leads to Dysregulated innate immune response that could result in a Cytokine Storm characterized by fever-inducing levels of cytokines such as IL6, IFN, IL1 and CXCL-10 [20]. Interestingly, CXCL-10 was also found to be indicative of severe outcomes in patients affected by the SARS-CoV-1 outbreak in 2002 [21]. Cytokine Storm has been implicated in contributing to Pulmonary Immunopathology, leading to severe clinical disease and mortality. Laboratory-based parameters indicating inflammation in the serum, such as D-Dimer and Ferritin, have been shown to lead to a reduction in blood oxygen saturation levels, reflecting Inadequate Oxygenation in the lungs [22].

Generally, neutralizing antibodies bind to specific surface receptors on infectious agents such as viruses and toxins, reducing or eliminating their ability to exert harmful effects on the cells. SARS-CoV-2–infected individuals generate a robust and long-lasting neutralizing antibody response. and plasma from convalescent COVID-19 patients has been used for treatment of severe disease. Monoclonal antibodies derived from recovering patients are currently used to treat COVID-19 patients.

Vaccines

To curb the global COVID-19 pandemic, a safe and effective vaccine which is reliable, effective, permanent and accessible to a large population is a critical tool in the arsenal of public health. Since the virus is mutating at a high rate, which can make vaccines ineffective, it is important to have a process to create a secure and reliable vaccine in advance for future outbreaks of SARS-CoV-2 variants. Most approaches for developing COVID-19 vaccines rely on the ability to produce antibodies that neutralize the Spike protein by binding to the Receptor-Binding Domain (RBD). Various candidate vaccines have been developed using platforms such as viral vector vaccines, nucleic acid-based (RNA/DNA) vaccines, purified viral proteins and live vaccines. The end point of the COVID-19 pandemic is protection against severe disease and mortality and eventually Herd Immunity [12, 23]. This outcome can be achieved only after widespread availability of an effective vaccine. Many of these vaccines have been developed and approved in unprecedented timelines.

There are over 330 different vaccine candidates under development to prevent or ameliorate COVID-19 [24]. Included in this list are *Pan* Corona virus vaccine candidates with the potential of neutralizing multiple strains and variants including those that may emerge later. The Spike Ferritin Nanoparticle (SpFN) is one such possible platform. The SpFN approach would allow for up to two dozen different Spike proteins to be displayed on one Nano Particle covering a broader swath of variants of the viral strains [25].

We have summarized the steps involved in the SARS-CoV-2 vaccine development process, which have enabled these vaccines to be made available in 12-18 months, which usually takes decades. Using a detailed risk-analysis process, we have listed the steps in the process that could be utilized for improving the efficiency of vaccine development for other pathogens in the future. Some of these factors for the ability to develop these vaccines in record time include:

1. *Genome Sequences of the virus were elucidated and shared in February 2020.*
2. *Companies collaborated with each other. For example, Pfizer and BioNTech;and, AstraZeneca, Oxford and Serum Institute of India.*
3. *Governments provided financial support. For example, the USA Government funded Moderna.*
4. *Findings were published fast and were free to access. These were mostly in pre-print manner in MedRxiv/BioRxiv Platforms.*
5. *Regulatory Authorities provided guidance on process and review.*
6. *Advances in Technologies such as Multi-omics, Machine-Learning based Modeling and Cryo-EM Structures helped in understanding the mechanism of the Viral Life Cycle and Immuno-Pathogenesis.*
7. *At-risk Manufacturing, scale-up and Supply Chain Management were planned and executed much before efficacy and safety results were obtained.*

COVID-19 saw an upsurge in funding where efforts led by Coalition for Epidemic Preparedness Innovations (CEPI) and Operation Warp Speed brought unprecedented levels of multiple private and public funds together minimizing the risk to vaccine developers and encouraging them to conduct cost-intensive large studies in parallel. The three phases of trials were conducted in a manner where one phase overlapped with another to expedite the evaluation.

The National Institute of Virology/Indian Council of Medical Research collaboration with a private sector player, Bharat Biotech, is another example of synergizing private and public resources to develop a vaccine (Covaxin) in record time.

Designing the Vaccine

The initial step of a viral life cycle involves binding of the Spike protein RBD to the ACE2 and TMPRSS2 receptors on cells. In the first months of the pandemic, it was experimentally demonstrated that antibodies directed against the RBD of Spike could effectively block viral entry and neutralize the virus. This finding reduced the time required for identifying the dominant protective antigen from several years to a few months. Further, as this information was shared immediately, several vaccine designers developed the vaccine on various platforms. **Table 18.3** shows the various vaccine platforms expressing the Spike protein and their potential to induce cell-mediated and Humoral immune responses. Majority of these platforms have utilized the Spike protein or the RBD of the Spike protein to develop vaccines. Some of these platforms were mRNA, DNA, Adenoviral vectors and protein-based platforms. In addition, Killed-Whole-Virus vaccines were developed by Bharat Biotech and approved for emergency use. The data for the "validation" of the use of Spike protein for inducing neutralizing antibodies and T-cell responses to elicit long-term protective immunity is being generated.

Efficacy Versus Effectiveness

Efficacy of vaccines is evaluated in clinical rials using statistically powered studies, which compare vaccinated subjects with placebo- or control-vaccine administered subjects, which were carefully chosen to be part of the study through precisely defined inclusion and exclusion criteria. For example, initial trials include healthy subjects aged 18-55 years from defined geographies and have the wherewithal to participate in long-term studies. Subjects are included only after a thorough Informed Consent Approval Process. Vaccines against SARS-CoV-2 have demonstrated *Efficacy* ranging from 80% to 95% against preventing severe disease and death. There have been some vaccines with lower than 80% Efficacy. Extensive systems-immunology investigative studies have enabled comprehensive characterization of cellular and molecular networks that drive antigen-specific immune responses. All the vaccines approved for emergency use induce binding and neutralizing antibodies after primary vaccination, which are boosted after second and third doses. The vaccines have been shown to induce antibodies against RBD, which elicit neutralizing activity against multiple strains of SARS-CoV-2, from Alpha to Delta, with varying efficacy to block virus entry. Most reports have indicated effectiveness of the vaccines to limit severe disease and hospitalization.

Thus, despite induction of systemic neutralizing antibodies, subjects exposed to the virus can be infected through the Naso-Pharyngeal Route. It is not surprising since these vaccines, which are administered Sub-cutaneously or Intra-Dermally, may not result in a robust Mucosal immune response. Vaccines that can be administered through the Intra Nasal Route may be more effective in controlling the primary viral infection. Several clinical trials are currently underway to examine this hypothesis. Vaccines also induce specific T-cell responses, which are detectable after a second dose. Both CD4 and CD8 T-cells, which secrete IFNγ, have been reported indicating the presence of Th1-type response. Pre-existing IFNγ-secreting T-cells have been reported even at baseline, indicating exposure to other related viruses that exhibit cross reactivity.

Effectiveness of Vaccines

The effectiveness of the vaccines is evaluated in real-world settings. The vaccine is administered to a large number (hundreds of thousands and even millions) of subjects. There is no "Control Arm" in effectiveness studies. These subjects can have a wide range of underlying heath concerns. They can be from various geographies and of different races, gender, and may include several other variables. The effectiveness is generally evaluated by measuring the rate of severe disease occurring among vaccinated populations compared to non-vaccinated populations in similar geographies. It is interesting to note that most of the SARS-CoV-2 vaccines have reported >90% effectiveness when large number of subjects were studied. This observation indicated the success of vaccines to prevent the spread of the virus. Longer-term effectiveness against homologous strains of the virus and more importantly, heterologous mutated strains such as Delta and Omicron, remains to be established.

Rationale for Booster

Vaccines using mRNA-encoded Spike proteins have been effective at inducing robust immune response and rendering protection against COVID-19. At six months post vaccination, antibodies to the Spike protein and neutralizing antibodies to RBD reactive to four variants remained above pre- vaccination levels. Further, memory B- and T-cells capable of reactivation and rapid production of antibodies following exposure to recall antigens from four different variants of concern (VOCs; Wild Type, Alpha, Beta, Delta) were observed. The long-lasting (6 month) induction of memory B- and T-cells following initial vaccination and their reactivation upon introduction of recall antigens points towards the utility of another shot of the vaccine at that time point to boost the immune response to SARS-CoV-2 variants and extend protection against COVID-19. In addition, inclusion of epitopes from emerging variants like Omicron in a booster may provide broader protection. Currently, such bivalent boosters are being evaluated for improved efficacy against novel variants.

7. Summary

Vaccines are central to developing affordable healthcare policies. Over the past century, several dozen vaccines against infectious diseases have been empirically developed. The goal of a majority of the vaccines against infectious diseases has been to target dominant antigens of pathogens that can induce long term protection against Homologous and Heterologous Strains of the pathogen. In this review we have outlined the various aspects of vaccine development from discovery, process development pharmacology, toxicology and clinical trials in the India context. We have listed the recent advances in vaccine development for various infectious diseases exemplified by rapid development of vaccine against SAR-DcO2 (COVID-10). The major criteria for Efficacy and Safety Assessment which have been highlighted may be useful for future vaccine development.

Vaccine development in India is at a critical juncture with a potential to have an exponential impact on novel vaccines against the most difficult-to-treat infectious diseases. Significant improvements in the vaccine development process could be achieved by:

i. Enabling Affordable Infrastructure,
ii. Enhancing the Education Process in Biotechnology to align it with requirements of the industry,
iii. Enabling Discovery Research and Innovation of Processes,
iv. Fostering Collaboration between Academia and Industry.

Table 18.1: Vaccines approved in India under the National Universal Immunization Program

Bacterial	BCG, Diphtheria, Pertussis, Tetanus Toxoid, Hemophilus Influenzae Type-B (HiB), Streptococcus Pneumoniae, Meningococcus
Viral	Oral Polio, Measles, Mumps, Rubella, Hepatitis B (Hep-B), Japanese Encephalitis Virus (JEV), Rabies Rotavirus, Human Papilloma Virus (HPV), Annual Influenza
	Combination Vaccines
	2020-2021 Several COVID-19 Vaccines.

The list of vaccines has been obtained from the National Health Mission (NHM) website (https://nhm.gov.in), which updates the information regularly.

"NHM has launched Mission Indradhanush (MI), which aims at increasing the full immunization coverage for children to 90%. Under this drive, focus is given on pockets of low immunization coverage and hard to reach areas where the proportion of unvaccinated and partially vaccinated children is highest. A total of six phases of MI have been completed covering 554 districts across the country. It was also identified as one of the flagship schemes under the Gram Swaraj Abhiyan (16,850 villages across 541 districts) and Extended Gram Swaraj Abhiyan (48,929 villages across 117 aspirational districts). While the first two phases of MI resulted in 6.7% increase in full immunization coverage in a year, a recent survey conducted in 190 districts covered in Intensified MI (5th phase) shows 18.5% increase in full immunization coverage as compared to NFHS-4 survey conducted in 2015-16."

Table 18.2: Common Technology Platforms for Vaccine Development

Platform	Example of Approved or In-Development Vaccines
DNA	Hep-B
mRNA	SARS-CoV-2; Hep-C
Viral Vector	SARS-CoV-2
Inactivated Virus	Influenza, Polio, Pertussis, Rabies, JEV, SARS-CoV-2
Live Attenuated	Small-Pox, Influenza Tetravalent, Rotavirus, Varicella
Subunit Protein	Tetanus, SARS-CoV-2
VLPs	HBV, HAV, HEV, HPV, Influenza, Dengue

Table 18.3: COVID-19 Vaccines: Summary of Efficacy and Effectiveness

Platform	Company	Antigen	Efficacy	Effectiveness
mRNA	Pfizer	Spike RBD	95%	88%
mRNA	Moderna	Spike RBD	94%	88%
Chimp-Adenovirus	Oxford/AZ/Serum	Spike	72%	70%
Human-Adenovirus	Gamaleya Institute	Spike	85%	NA
Inactivated Whole Virus	Bharat Biotech	All Viral Proteins	85%	78%
Protein	Novavax	Spike	90%	90%
Adenovirus 26	Janssen	Spike	68%	70%
mRNA	CureVAC	Spike	47%	NA

The percentage numbers are derived from summaries of several reports. Efficacy is derived by comparing vaccinated and placebo arms of a statistically controlled clinical trial. Effectiveness is derived from evaluating the incidence of severe infections in vaccinated versus non-vaccinated groups in a population.

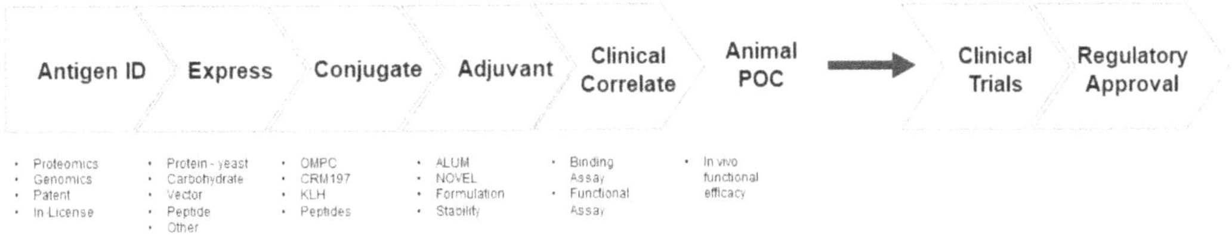

Figure 18.1: The Pathway of Development of Vaccines.

Acknowledgements

We thank Vihang Ghalsasi for detailed copy-editing.

References

1. Piot, P., et al., *Immunization: vital progress, unfinished agenda.* Nature, 2019. **575**(7781): p. 119-129.
2. Pollard, A.J. and E.M. Bijker, *A guide to vaccinology: from basic principles to new developments.* Nat Rev Immunol, 2021. **21**(2): p. 83-100.
3. Lahariya, C., *A brief history of vaccines & vaccination in India.* Indian J Med Res, 2014. **139**(4): p. 491-511.
4. Stern, P.L., *Key steps in vaccine development.* Ann Allergy Asthma Immunol, 2020. **125**(1): p. 17-27.
5. Pulendran, B. and M.M. Davis, *The science and medicine of human immunology.* Science, 2020. **369**(6511).
6. Fauci, A., *Victories against AIDS have lessons for COVID-19.* Nature, 2021. **600**(7887): p. 9.
7. Weaver, S.C., et al., *Zika, Chikungunya, and Other Emerging Vector-Borne Viral Diseases.* Annu Rev Med, 2018. **69**: p. 395-408.
8. Bardina, S.V., et al., *Enhancement of Zika virus pathogenesis by preexisting antiflavivirus immunity.* Science, 2017. **356**(6334): p. 175-180.
9. Duffy, P.E. and J. Patrick Gorres, *Malaria vaccines since 2000: progress, priorities, products.* NPJ Vaccines, 2020. **5**(1): p. 48.
10. Park, J., J. Kim, and Y.S. Jang, *Current status and perspectives on vaccine development against dengue virus infection.* J Microbiol, 2022. **60**(3): p. 247-254.
11. Ramasamy, V., et al., *A tetravalent virus-like particle vaccine designed to display domain III of dengue envelope proteins induces multi-serotype neutralizing antibodies in mice and macaques which confer protection against antibody dependent enhancement in AG129 mice.* PLoS Negl Trop Dis, 2018. **12**(1): p. e0006191.
12. Chen, G.L., et al., *Effect of a Chikungunya Virus-Like Particle Vaccine on Safety and Tolerability Outcomes: A Randomized Clinical Trial.* Jama, 2020. **323**(14): p. 1369-1377.
13. McMahon, R., et al. *Progress of clinical development of a live-attenuated single shot chikungunya vaccine candidate.* 2021 11 June 2022]; Available from: https://valneva.com/wp-content/uploads/2022/04/VAL_Poster_Chikungunya_841x1189_0422_V3.pdf.
14. Biosolutions, E. *Emergent BioSolutions Announces initiation of Pivotal Phase 3 Study Evaluating the Safety and Immunogenicity of Its Single-Dose Chikungunya Vaccine Candidate,*

CHIKV VLP. 2021 11 June 2022]; Available from: https://www.globenewswire.com/news-release/2021/10/15/2314890/33240/en/Emergent-BioSolutions-Announces-Initiation-of-Pivotal-Phase-3-Study-Evaluating-the-Safety-and-Immunogenicity-of-Its-Single-Dose-Chikungunya-Vaccine-Candidate-CHIKV-VLP.html.

15. Cimica, V., et al., *Current development of Zika virus vaccines with special emphasis on virus-like particle technology.* Expert Rev Vaccines, 2021. **20**(11): p. 1483-1498.
16. Gaudinski, M.R., et al., *Safety, tolerability, and immunogenicity of two Zika virus DNA vaccine candidates in healthy adults: randomised, open-label, phase 1 clinical trials.* Lancet, 2018. **391**(10120): p. 552-562.
17. Geisbert, T.W., et al., *A single dose investigational subunit vaccine for human use against Nipah virus and Hendra virus.* NPJ Vaccines, 2021. **6**(1): p. 23.
18. Stierwalt, S., *How Are Seasonal Flu Vaccines Made?* Scientific American, 2016.
19. Taghioff, S.M., et al., *Examining the potential benefits of the influenza vaccine against SARS-CoV-2: A retrospective cohort analysis of 74,754 patients.* PLoS One, 2021. **16**(8): p. e0255541.
20. Grifoni, A., et al., *Targets of T Cell Responses to SARS-CoV-2 Coronavirus in Humans with COVID-19 Disease and Unexposed Individuals.* Cell, 2020. **181**(7): p. 1489-1501.e15.
21. Ernst, D., et al., *Bead Based Flow Cytometric Assays: A Multiplex Assay Platform with Applications in Diagnostic Microbiology*
In: Advanced Techniques in Diagnostic Microbiology, Eds: Y.W. Tang and C.W. Stratton
Springer, Y.W. Tang and C.W. Stratton, Editors. 2006. p. 427-443.
22. Chirmule, N., et al., *Predicting the Severity of Disease Progression in COVID-19 at the Individual and Population Level: A Mathematical Model.* Clin Exp Pharmacol, 2021. **11**(5).
23. Earle, K.A., et al., *Evidence for antibody as a protective correlate for COVID-19 vaccines.* Vaccine, 2021. **39**(32): p. 4423-4428.
24. Krammer, F., *SARS-CoV-2 vaccines in development.* Nature, 2020. **586**(7830): p. 516-527.
25. Joyce, M.G., et al., *SARS-CoV-2 ferritin nanoparticle vaccines elicit broad SARS coronavirus immunogenicity.* Cell Rep, 2021. **37**(12): p. 110143.

CHAPTER

19 Indian Regulatory Scenario in Drug and Vaccine Development

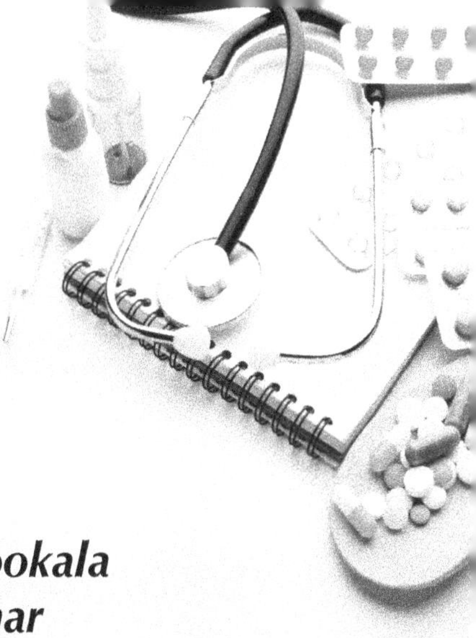

Vikram Gota, Manjunath Nookala Krishnamurthy, Sharath Kumar

1. Brief history

Providing access to safe, effective and quality medication to people is the major task before any government. Discrete laws are required to regulate the manufacture, sale, distribution, import, and clinical research of drugs. Previously, during the British rule, drugs were imported from other countries as hardly any drug was manufactured locally. In consequence during the 20th century, many spurious and adulterated drugs entered the market (Gigantic Quinine Fraud – where under-strength quinine was dispensed). Subsequently, based on the Drug Inquiry Committee's (the Chopra Committee) recommendations The Drug 'Bill' came into force. This later got amended to the Drugs and Cosmetics Act 1940 and the Drugs and Cosmetic Rules of 1945. This also resulted in the establishment of the Central Drugs Standard Control Organization (CDSCO), headed by the Drugs Controller General (India) (DCG (I)). The Act has contents framed as Chapters, Rules, and Schedules. It got amended from time to time. Two statutory boards and a committee have been framed under Chapter 2 of this act. The Drugs Technical Advisory Board (DTAB) advises the central and state governments on technical drug matters and on making rules. The Drug Consultative Committee (DCC) along with the central and state governments and the DTAB ensure that drug control measures are enforced throughout India.

Process patent came after the recommendation of Justice Rajagopala Ayyangar Committee report, as western firms feared in introducing their novel products in India. Consequently, India signed an agreement on the Trade-Related aspects of Intellectual Property Rights (TRIPS), which put an obligation to provide patent protection for pharmaceutical products. Later, Schedule Y was amended in the act. Recognizing the importance of guidelines and requirements for clinical trials, the government developed ethical and regulatory guidelines. Under this in 2000 and 2001, ICMR issued the ethical guidelines for Biomedical Research on Human Subjects and CDSCO released the Indian Good Clinical Practice (GCP) guidelines, respectively. CDSCO made revisions to Schedule Y, including definitions for Phase I-IV trials, elimination of Phase Lag, responsibilities of investigators and sponsors were updated and requirements for notifying changes in protocol were made. CDSCO introduced fast-tracking of clinical trials in 2006, at par with the US, Britain, Canada, Germany, South Africa, Switzerland, Australia, Japan and countries in the European Medicines Agency eligible for the same, taking no more than 2-4 weeks. In addition, trials conducted in countries with competent, mature regulatory systems, approval takes 12 weeks once an application is considered.

Guidelines have been set-up for a work- flow that initiates from obtaining a written permission from IEC and DCG (I). Various regulatory bodies, their function in the drug development process, import of drugs and waivers have been discussed below.

2. Regulatory Bodies and Their Functions

Various regulatory bodies and their functions have been mentioned in table 19.1

Table 19.1: Regulatory bodies and their functions

Regulatory body	Functions
CDSCO	• Clinical trial review and approval • Permission to test new drugs • Import of registration and licensing • Amendments to the D & C Act and Rules • Withdrawal of approval of drugs and cosmetics • Grant of export licenses • Oversight and market surveillance through the centre's inspectorate
ICMR	• For formulation, coordination and promotion of bio-medical research • Conduct, coordinate and implement medical research for the benefit of the society • Translating medical innovations into products/processes and introducing them into the public health system
AYUSH department	• Upgrading the educational standard of the Indian Systems of Medicine and Homoeopathy colleges in the country • Strengthening current research institutions and to ensuring time-bound research programs on identified diseases for which these systems have an effective therapy. • Designing schemes for cultivating, promoting, and regenerating medicinal plants that are used in these systems • Develop pharmacopoeial standards for Indian Systems of Medicine and Homoeopathy drugs.

Regulatory body	Functions
DBT	• Promoting large scale use of Biotechnology • Supporting R&D and manufacturing in Biology • Promoting University-Industry collaboration • Identifying and establishing Centres of Excellence for R&D • Serving as Nodal Point for specific International Collaborations • Establishing infrastructure facilities to support R&D and production • Evolving Bio Safety Guidelines, manufacture and application of cell-based vaccines
RCGM	• To frame regulations for the institutions involved in rDNA research activities • To review the on-going research involving hazardous microorganisms • To visit the experimental site and ensure that the trial is being carried out as per the guidelines • To advice the custom authority on import of microorganism and GM products

CDSCO-Central Drugs Standard Control Organization,

ICMR-Indian Council of Medical Research,

AYUSH-Ayurveda, Yoga and Naturopathy, Unani, Siddha and Homeopathy,

DBT-Department of Biotechnology,

RCGM-Review Committee on Genetic Manipulation,

R&D-Research and Development,

rDNA-Recombinant DNA,

GM-Genetically Modified.

3. Drug Development Process

Screening and development

Screening

An unmet need in a disease process (without a suitable drug) allows the researchers to design a product that will result in a therapeutic effect in the underlying disease. The first step in drug development would be to identify and validate a target that is safe, effective, meets clinical and commercial criteria and is druggable. Following that, the hit identification and lead discovery phase yields a compound that exhibits the desired activity in a screen and whose activity is verified upon retesting. Lead compounds are obtained from primary and secondary screening. Compounds at this stage may be judged to have met the lead optimization phase's initial goals and are ready for final characterization before being declared pre-clinical candidates.

Pre-clinical research

Pre-clinical development connects in-vitro drug discovery to initiation of First-in-human trials. These can be designed to choose a lead candidate from several hits to select the optimal formulation to determine the route of administration, frequency and duration of exposure; and finally, to support the clinical trial design. To describe the pharmacokinetic profile and general safety, as well as to identify toxicity patterns rodent and non-rodent mammalian models are generally used. Toxicology and safety studies identify potential target organs for adverse effects and define the Therapeutic Index to determine the initial starting doses in clinical trials. The results of pre-clinical testing are examined and the decision to proceed to Phase-I trials is made.

Clinical Research Phase Studies

Phase-1

The primary goal of a Phase-I trial is to determine the safety and tolerability (Maximum Tolerated Dose) of an investigational new drug when it is first administered to humans (Non-therapeutic). These are normally conducted in healthy volunteers. However, cytotoxic drugs are usually studied in patients where investigators trained in clinical pharmacology with access to necessary facilities properly observe, examine and monitor the participants. Studies conducted in Phase-I also involve objectives like Pharmacokinetics, Pharmacodynamics, and early measurement of drug activity. Recommended dose for Phase-II trials are also determined.

Phase-2

The primary goal is to evaluate the efficacy of a drug for a specific indication or indications in patients with the condition under research, as well as treatment's common short-term adverse effects and risks. Phase-II studies should be undertaken in a small number of patients who are chosen based on a set of stringent criteria resulting in a homogeneous population. An important goal for this phase is to determine the dose and regimen for Phase-III trials. Objectives of Phase-II studies also include evaluation of potential study endpoints, therapeutic regimens (including concomitant medications) and target populations (e.g. Mild versus severe disease) for further studies in Phase-II or III.

Phase-3

The major goal of Phase-III study is to demonstrate or confirm therapeutic benefits. Phase-III studies are meant to corroborate the preliminary data gathered in Phase II studies. These studies should be designed to give a solid foundation for obtaining marketing approval. These also look into the dose-response relationships in different stages of disease, as well as the drug's safety and efficacy in combination with other drugs. Trials with extended exposure to the drug are typically undertaken in Phase-III trials.

Phase-4

Phase-IV or post marketing trials of new drugs are conducted after the drug has been approved for indication of interest. These trials go beyond demonstrating the drug's safety, efficacy and dose definition. Such trials might not have been considered essential at the time of the new drug approval due to various reasons such as limitation in terms of patient exposure, duration of treatment during clinical development of the drug, need for early introduction of the new drug in the interest of patients etc. Additionally, these trials include drug-drug interaction, dose response or safety studies and the trials design to support use under the approved indication such as mortality or morbidity studies, epidemiological studies, and so on.

4. Role of Regulatory Bodies in the Process of Drug Development

a. Drug

i. ***In-vitro studies – Screening and development of a promising drug:***
Regulatory bodies do not have any specified role in in-vitro studies.

ii. ***In-vivo studies – Preclinical drug development:***

Pre-clinical studies act as an interphase between in-vitro studies and clinical trials. Committee for the Purpose of Control and Supervision of Experiments on Animals (CPCSEA) under the Government of India monitors animal experiments through the Ethics Committees set up in respective institutions.

iii. ***Clinical trials:***

Conduct of clinical trials is regulated by CDSCO – DCGI along with different bodies depending upon the nature of the Investigational New Drug (IND) or the trial. Before a drug is transported or distributed across states, the Current Federal Law requires that the drug be the subject of an approved marketing application and must also seek an exemption from that legal requirement for which IND is the means through which the sponsor technically obtains this. During the new drug's early pre-clinical development, the sponsor's main goal is to determine if the product is practically safe for initial use in humans and if the compound exhibits pharmacological activity that justifies commercial development, which is identified as a feasible candidate for further development, the sponsor then focuses on the collection of data and information necessary to establish that the product will be safe in humans when used in limited, early-stage clinical studies.

When the manufacturer has screened the new molecule for pharmacological activity and acute toxicity potential in animals and wants to test its diagnostic or therapeutic potential in humans, the role of CDSCO-DCGI begins. Grant of permission to conduct the clinical trial of a new drug or investigational new drug as part of discovery, research and manufacture in India and to conduct a clinical trial of a new drug already approved outside India will follow the same process as the grant of permission to IND. Flow-chart representing the work-flow to apply for an IND has been mentioned in Figure 19.1.

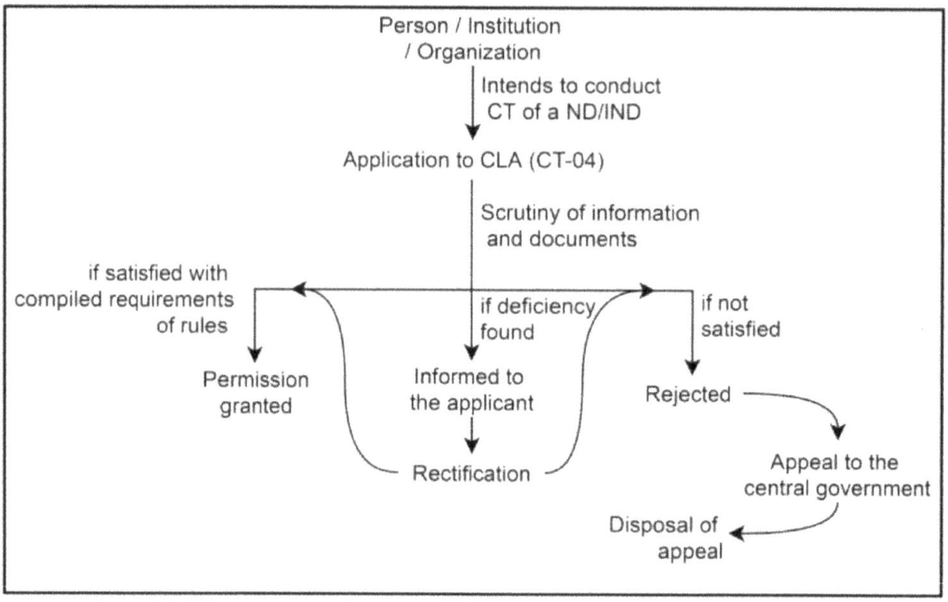

Figure 19.1: Flowchart representing the Workflow to apply for an IND

Marketing Authorization

Post phase-III trials, the New Drug Application (NDA) is submitted to the regulatory authority (CDSCO) for marketing authorization. The NDA is reviewed and the Marketing Authorization Holders (MAH) are granted permission to market the drug throughout the country.

iv. ***Phase-IV studies/Post-marketing Surveillance (PMS):***

The regulatory authority may order the MAH for conducting a Phase-IV study, if they believe that the drug might show rare adverse drug reactions and long-term adverse effects once marketed, as Phase-III studies have less external validity. A Phase-IV study may also be required for drugs approved and marketed outside India.

b. Cell Therapy

Clinical trials of Stem cells and cell-based 'products' are regulated similarly to Drugs. ICMR has published guidelines for research related SCCPs as the National Guideline for Stem Cell research in 2017. These guidelines elaborate on restricted, prohibited and permitted research along with minimal, substantial and major manipulation. These guidelines also elaborate on indications that do not require prior approval such as Stem cell Transplantation which are mentioned in Annexure III of the ICMR guidelines. CMC, pre-clinical and clinical trial data on safety & efficacy are submitted for approval of stem cell and cell-based products which are evaluated by an Expert Committee (CBBTDEC). There are also other screening committees involved in the approval of SCCP in India - Technical and Apex committees which mainly focus on import/marketing authorization. Indigenous manufacturers/applicants are required to obtain market authorization from DCGI in Form 46 and manufacturing license in Form 28 from the State Licensing Authority, where importers are required to obtain market authorization from DCG (I) in Form 45 before obtaining Registration Certificate in Form 41 and import license in Form 10. Flowchart representing the workflow to apply for an SCCP import and manufacture authorization in India has been mentioned in Figure 19.2. (NGSCR 2017)

c. Vaccines

According to the New Drugs and Clinical Trials Rules 2019, vaccines are also considered new drugs and the conduct of non-clinical and clinical studies and approval are similar to drugs as stated above. Manufacturers are required to obtain manufacturing permission from CDSCO under the New Drugs and Clinical Trials Rules, 2019, before licensing the product under the Drugs and Cosmetics Rules, 1945. The Manufacturing License for such products is granted after joint evaluation and inspection by the concerned State Licensing Authority & CDSCO. The DCG (I) approves vaccines introduced in the country, grants permission to conduct clinical trials, registers and controls the quality of imported vaccines and lays down standards for updating Indian Pharmacopoeia. It also approves licenses as the Central License Approving Authority (CLAA) for the manufacture of vaccines, coordinates the activities of the States and advises them on matters relating to uniform administration of the Act and Rules.

The Second Amendment was done by the Indian Union Government after consultation with the Drugs Technical Advisory Board in 2019. The Medical Device Rules classify medical devices based upon the intended purpose, invasiveness and duration of implantation of the device. There is a need for clinical trial for each of the classified types of the medical device. A sponsor cannot investigate it without approval from CDSCO (Central Drugs Standard Control Organization) and the Institutional Ethics Committee which is required even for a medical device that claims to have substantial equivalence to a predicate device. Every study must be compulsorily enrolled in the

The Central Drugs Laboratory (CDL), Kasauli performs lot release for all imported vaccines as well as locally produced vaccines. However, vaccines, unlike chemical drugs, are a complex heterogeneous class of medical products. Hence, specific consideration in the development of Chemistry, Manufacturing and Controls (CMC) data, non-clinical data and clinical data provide a clear understanding of the regulatory landscape for their development and approval in a scientific manner. It requires additional approvals from Genetic Engineering Approval Council, Guidelines on the Recombinant Technologies under

DBT, Ethical Guidelines under ICMR and from five competent authorities i.e. Institutional Bio-Safety Committees (IBSC), Ethics Committee, Review Committee of Genetic Manipulation (RCGM), State Biotechnology Coordination Committee (SBCC) and District Level Committee (DLC) for handling of various aspects of the rules. The manufacture and distribution of biological products for human use are regulated under the following two statutory authorities:

i. Drugs Controller General of India (DCGI)
ii. Genetic Engineering Approval Committee (GEAC)

Depending on the type of vaccine (live or killed) the approval or waiver from GEAC is sorted for all vaccine trials conducted in India. The ownership of a vaccine developed in India will be crucial in having an affordable vaccine for public health use. As per the National Vaccine Policy 2011, under scope for improvements in the quality assessments of vaccine research and development, the need for developing pre-qualification standards which are in alignment with WHO-UNICEF standards and Single window system to prevent any unnecessary delays in regulatory clearances were highlighted. Yet, not a significant advancement has been observed even after a decade. (Data source - Regulatory guidelines for the development of vaccines with special consideration for COVID-19 vaccine, dated 20/9/2020 and National Vaccine Policy 2011).

d. Devices

To come up with the right diagnosis of a Patient's medical condition, access to medical devices is vital. In India, devices were also put under the category of new drugs, biologicals and vaccines for which clinical trials were guided by the same regulations, i.e. Schedule Y of the Drug & Cosmetics Rules, 1945. Unwilling to accept these rules by the manufacturers resulted in a very small number of clinical trials for medical devices in India. The Drugs and Cosmetics Rules, 1945, were reframed for medical devices as Medical Devices Rules, 2017, which became effective from January 1, 2018 (included in-vitro diagnostic kits, surgical dressing, mechanical contraceptives and others).

The Second Amendment was done by the Indian Union Government after consultation with the Drugs Technical Advisory Board in 2019. The Medical Device Rules classify medical devices based upon the intended purpose, invasiveness and duration of implantation of the device. There is a need for clinical trial for each of the classified types of the medical device. A sponsor cannot investigate it without approval from CDSCO (Central Drugs Standard Control Organization) and the Institutional Ethics Committee which is required even for a medical device that claims to have substantial equivalence to a predicate device. Every study must be compulsorily enrolled in the Clinical Trial Registry of India before the enrollment starts and the status of the study must be submitted annually to CDSCO by the sponsor.

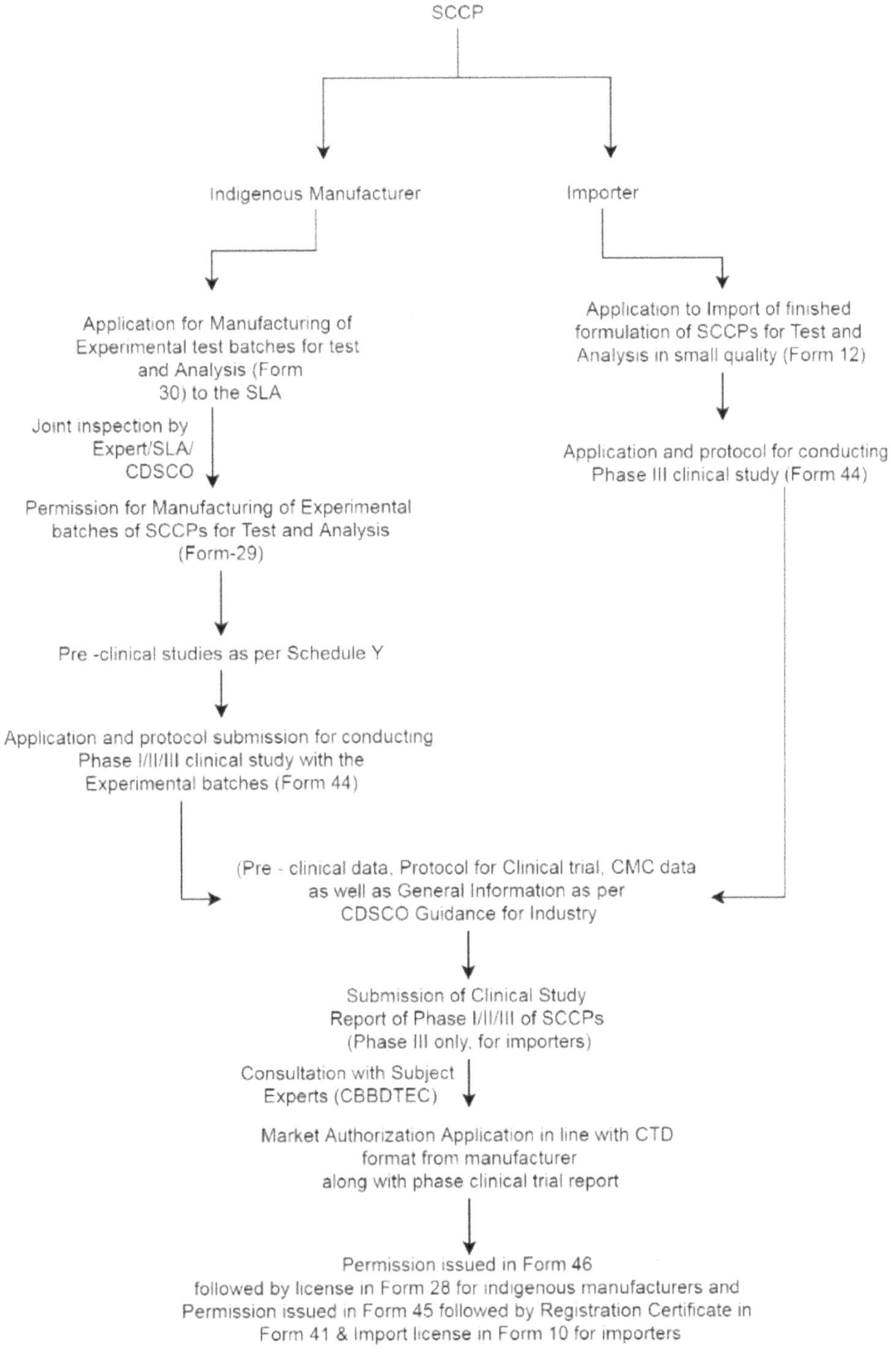

Figure 19.2: Flowchart representing the workflow to apply for an SCCP import and manufacture authorization in India.

SCCP-Stem Cell and Cell-Based Products, SLA-Service Level Agreements, CBBDTEC-Cellular Biology Based Therapeutic Drug Evaluation Committee, CTD-Common Technical Document

e. Alternative medicines

In India, the Department of AYUSH controls the ASU (Ayurveda, Siddha, or Unani) drugs. The design, conduct, termination, audit, analysis, reporting and documentation of the systematic studies involving human subjects for determining the safety and efficacy of ASU drugs is monitored by the GCP-ASU guidelines and regulatory requirements are prescribed in the Rule 158-B of the Drugs & Cosmetics Act 1945. Though clinical trials were initially mandatory, according to the new order issued in 2019, pilot studies as per D&C Act, 1940 would be sufficient for obtaining licenses and quality and efficiency of these drugs will be examined by DDC (Ayurveda)/SLA, (GCP Guidelines for Clinical Trials in ASU drugs – Department of AYUSH, MOHFW, GOI; The Drugs and Cosmetics Act and Rules, as amended up to 31st December 2016).

f. Phytopharmaceuticals

CDSCO regulates the phytopharmaceuticals. The regulatory process for a phytopharmaceutical is similar to the new drugs. The newly added Appendix I-B in Schedule Y describes the data of the phytopharmaceutical to be submitted along with the application to conduct the clinical trial or for its import or manufacture. For regulatory requirements of the NDA of the phytopharmaceutical, new drug-safety standards, pharmacological information, human studies and confirmatory clinical trials are essential. Approval from regulatory agencies required for various types of drugs have been mentioned in Table 19.2.

Table 19.2: Drugs and their respective regulatory agencies.

Sl. No.	Drug type	Regulatory Agencies
1.	Phytopharmaceuticals	• Department of AYUSH • CDSCO
2.	Gene therapy	• CDSCO • RDAC • RCGM • GEAC • IBSC
3.	Immunotherapy trials	• CDSCO • NAC-SCRT • RCGM
4.	Biologics& Similar biologics	• CDSCO • RCGM • GEAC • IBSC
5.	Vaccine trials	• CDSCO • GEAC • RCGM

Sl. No.	Drug type	Regulatory Agencies
6.	New Chemical Entity (NCE)	• CDSCO
7.	Cell therapy	• CDSCO • NAC-SCRT • DBT • ICMR
8.	AYUSH drugs	• Department of AYUSH

CDSCO–Central Drug Standard Control Organization,
RDAC–rDNA Advisory Committee,
RCGM–Review Committee on Genetic Manipulation,
GEAC–Genetic Engineering Appraisal Committee,
IBSC–Institutional Biosafety Committee,
NAC-SCRT–National Apex Committee for Stem Cell Research and Therapy,
DBT–Department of Biotechnology,
ICMR–Indian Council of Medical Research

5. Import of Drugs

Phase-I data (produced outside India) must be submitted with the application to the Central Licensing Authority for the import of a new medicine discovered or developed in a country other than India. After submission of this data, permission may be granted to repeat Phase-I trials in India or to conduct Phase-II trials and subsequently, Phase-III trial concurrently with other global trials for that drug. For new drugs approved outside India, Phase-III studies may be required if scientifically and ethically appropriate, primarily to generate evidence of efficacy and safety of the drug in the Indian patients when used as indicated in prescribing information. The Central Licensing Authority needs a bioequivalence study before conducting Phase-III investigations in Indian participants (Bridging studies).

6. Waivers

Waiver for requirements of non-clinical and clinical data

In case of drugs intended for life-threatening or serious disease conditions or rare diseases, or drugs to be used in the diseases of specific relevance to the Indian situation or unmet medical need in India, disaster or special defense use (drugs for combating chemical, nuclear, biological infliction etc), the non-clinical and clinical data may be waived off. However, depending on the nature of the new drugs, proposed indication and other factors such as relaxation, abbreviations, omission or deferment of data will be reviewed on a case-by-case basis.

Waiver for requirements of clinical trials

Clinical trials may be waived in the case of new drugs which are approved and used in other countries for several years. Multiple situations exist for obtaining a local clinical trial waiver for the approval of a new drug. If the drug is already approved in countries specified by the CLA (U.S., Britain, Switzerland, Australia, Canada, Germany, South Africa, Japan and European Union), if there have been no major unexpected serious adverse events reported, there is no difference in the Indian population of the gene involved in the metabolism of the new drug or any factor affecting pharmacokinetics, pharmacodynamics, safety or efficacy of the new drug and the applicant has given written undertaking to conduct Phase-IV clinical trials to establish safety and effectiveness of the new drug as per design approved by the CLA.

Waiver for requirement of local Phase IV clinical trial

For a new drug that is indicated in life threatening or serious diseases that are particularly relevant to the Indian health scenario or for a condition that is an unmet need in India (Multidrug-resistant Tuberculosis, Hepatitis-C etc.) or rare diseases for which drugs are not available or are available at a high cost or if it is an orphan drug.

Additional Reading

1. Blass BE. Basic Principles of Drug Discovery and Development. Boston: Academic Press; 2015. 582 p.
2. The Drug Development Process. FDA; 2020
3. Ethical Guidelines For Biomedical Research on Human Participants
4. Friedman LM, Furberg CD, DeMets DL. Fundamentals of Clinical Trials. Springer Science & Business Media; 2010. 456 p
5. General Guidelines for Methodologies on Research and Evaluation of Traditional Medicine, World Health Organization 2000
6. Good Clinical Practice Guidelines for Clinical trials in Ayurveda, Siddha, Unani (ASU) Medicine
7. Guideline For Good Clinical Practice, E6(R1), International Conference On Harmonisation of Technical Requirements For Registration of Pharmaceuticals for Human Use
8. New Drugs CT Rules 2019
9. National Guidelines for Stem Cell Research, 2017
10. National Vaccine Policy 2011
11. Regulatory guidelines for the development of vaccines with special consideration for COVID-19 vaccine
12. Medical Devices Rules, 2017
13. General guidelines for drug development of Ayurvedic formulations, 2018

CHAPTER

20 Power of Powerful Presentation

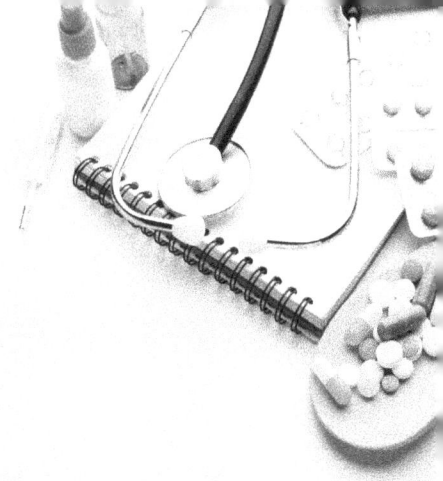

Suresh Chari

"The human mind is a wonderful thing.
It operates from the moment you are born until
the time you get up to make a presentation"

1. Introduction

I remember a certain surgery postgraduate student Dr Sagar, who had secured a great rank in his PG entrance exam. In his first year of Residency he showed excellent surgical skills and was brilliant in his academics. He was excited when he was involved in a classical clinical case. Then came the trauma when he was asked to present this case in the clinical meeting of the institute. His guide, Dr Sudhir came to me and said "Suresh Sir, I am worried about this PG student of mine who no doubt is a brilliant student, but of late very nervous since he has been asked to make a presentation". He continued, "his PPT`s are good but when I heard him yesterday he was visibly shaking and fumbling with the words. You are regularly involved with speaking skills, please do something".

I smiled and said, "Sudhir, these are very common symptoms and such butterflies are experienced by everyone, only the size and quantum differs from people to people. don`t you worry, presentation is a skill and if it's a skill it can be learnt. Sachin Tendulkar, the great cricket legend, was not born with a bat in his hand. He learnt this skill the hard way. Give me a week with this PG student, send him to our Communication Skills Lab and let's see what can be done." Sure enough, when the day came Sagar did a fairly good job and this is what he had to say, "Sir, thanks for your guidance and support. If not anything else, my confidence was good, next time it will be better".

2. Presentation

Presentation is a skill and it can be learnt. To have academic knowledge is one thing and to have the skill to deliver that knowledge in front of colleagues and experts either in house or in a conference is another. But as I have said earlier, if it's a skill it can be learnt

---

Editor's comments: This article deviates in style from the rest of this book. However, its contents are very informative and will be useful for young researchers

and mastered slowly. The art of making a powerful presentation is coachable and every time you get up to make a presentation you can see success when you look in the eyes of your audience. You enjoy doing this again and again and it just grows on you. And then it becomes a habit and people just love to listen to you.

In the following pages I am sharing my experience from the several public speaking and presentation skills workshops that I have conducted for youth and adults. These are just tips to make your presentation powerful. However, it's how you practice them and put your own creativity that makes it all the more powerful. But the principles remain the same whether you are a CEO or a student or a faculty making a presentation in a conference or a public function.

3. Butterflies in the Stomach

All of us have felt the Butterflies in our stomach, the first time we went on any platform for a Presentation. During a survey conducted on the **ten worst human fears in USA,** following was the result:

10. Dogs
09. Loneliness
08. Flying
07. Death
06. Sickness
05. Deep Water
04. Financial Problems
03. Insects & Bugs
02. Heights
01. Speaking Before an Audience

The least feared were dogs and most when they got up to speak in front of an audience which just goes to show that Stage Fight is natural and everyone experiences it at one time or the other.

4. Stage Fright

Have you experienced the symptoms of rapid heartbeat, trembling knees, quivering voice, fluttering stomach, blurring eyes, sweating hands, dryness of mouth, fast breathing, mind going blank, voice cracking, flop sweat (one small drop of sweat that drains down your vertebral column) and all these leading to embarrassment-panic-shame-humiliation-terror. If you have experienced any of the above, don`t worry, these are natural common symptoms.

Reasons for such Fright is the Fear of......

1. Failure: What if I fail, if the electricity goes off, slides stops working?
2. Ridicule/Humiliation: What if someone laughs?
3. Presence of some persons: Such as Boss, Peers, known or unknown

4. Criticism
5. Incompetence of Language
6. Exposure of thoughts, emotions
7. Loss of Relationships
8. Concern of Consequence
9. Own Voice
10. Crowd-People
11. Competition
12. Lack of Knowledge

5. Steps to Control Stage Fear

1. Choose a subject that you strongly wish to discuss with your listeners.
2. Prepare and practice thoroughly.
3. Recognize that you are not alone in suffering from Stage Fears.
4. Realize that you appear more confident than you feel.
5. Understand that with experience your Stage Fear will reduce.
6. Know that the audience wants you to perform well.
7. Remember there will always be a next time.

6. Important Steps while Making a Presentation

(a) Audience Analysis
(b) Audience Analysis Guidesheet
(c) Designing and Organizing the Contents
(d) Adding Style to the Presentation
(e) Evaluating or Looking for Feedback

(A) Audience Analysis

The **most important step** for a powerful presentation is analysis of the audience. Before you sit and assemble your contents you should be able to get answer to the five W`s, that will decide the final H (how).

FIVE WIVES (W`s) & ONE HUSBAND (H):

1. WHO are these people? What is their level? What is their gender and age? Which language do most of them understand? How many are they (Number)? What is their Attitude towards you? Which Subject do you wish to speak on?

2. WHAT kind of presentation or speech are you giving: Entertaining, Informative, Motivational, Introduction, Welcome, Farewell, Thanks Giving, Winners or Losers Speech, Conveying good or bad News etc.

3. WHEN, what time of the day is your Presentation? Is it before breakfast, Pre-lunch, Post-lunch, evening just before the cocktails and dinner or during the dinner? Also, what is the duration of your speech? How much time have you been given by the organizers?

4. WHERE, What is the location & ambience/surroundings? Is it a closed auditorium with our without aircon? An open area, lawn or garden with lot of distractions? Or, Is it in a State-of-the-Art Conference Hall with excellent acoustics?

5. Finally, WHY? Why have you been chosen to speak? Is it because you are an Expert? Or, Is it a competition of sorts? And, Why now, Is there a special occasion?

Once you seek answers for these five W`s then you can sit back and decide the HOW, the H.

Your designing of the presentation largely depends on your Audience Analysis. You must have realized that if "WHO" changes "HOW" will change. Your content and skill will differ depending on whether you are speaking in front of Peers or Seniors or a mixed group or on-Professionals or they are more knowledgeable than you about the subject or less knowledgeable or college students or school children or slum dwellers or complete professionals. If a Presentation fails, it's almost always because the speaker didn't frame it correctly in accordance with the need of the audience or just misjudged the Audience's level of interest or knowledge.

(B) Audience Analysis Guidesheet

1. How many people do I expect in the Audience?
2. Is the knowledge level of all the members diverse or about the same?
3. What is their knowledge of the content area?
   High/Same/Less/None/Varied/Not sure?
4. What will impress this audience?
   Technical/Statistical/Cost/Figures/History/Generalizations/Demonstrations?
5. Will different members of the audience be impressed with different things?
6. What is the audience's attitude towards the subject?
   Positive/Neutral/Negative/Not sure?
7. What is the audiences' attitude towards you as a speaker?
   Credible/Knowledgeable/No Opinion/Not sure?
8. What is the audiences' attitude towards the organization you represent? Reliable/Average/Not sure?
9. What will be the audiences' disposition at the time of the Presentation? Listened to many/Sitting at one place for a long time/Easy to grab attention/Early item hence fresh?
10. What is the audience's status compared to mine Superior/Junior/Same/Mixed/Not sure?

Hence personally, I give a lot of importance and spend a lot of time in analyzing my audience before I sit and design my Presentation.

(C) *Designing and Organizing the Contents*

There's no way you can give a good talk unless you have something worth talking about. Conceptualizing and framing what you want to say is the most vital part of your preparation.

While designing the HOW, you should divide the Presentation into three parts:
The opening (15%),
The body (75%), and
The closing (10%),

All this takes the audience through a Journey.

i The Opening:

The beginning of your presentation is crucial.
You need to grab your audience`s attention and hold it!
A good opening is the key before you launch yourself into the main content area. The initial moments set the induction and connect you with the audience. How much time you spend on the opening is decided by the total time allotted to you, but not more than 12-15%. I have personally realized that many times it is important to sit through the talk of the earlier speaker and in your opening pick up from where he/she left off.

Exciting openings are recommended in post-lunch sessions or if you feel the audience has slept through the previous session even in an academic presentation. In any case, a solid start is a Launch Pad for your presentation in the subsequent minutes. If you start by using jargon or get too technical, you will lose your audience. Once you lose your audience it is very difficult to bring them back. The most Powerful Presenters do a superb job of very quickly introducing the topic, explaining why they care so deeply about it and convincing the audience that they should do so too.

An opening should announce that you have arrived!

- They are also called Icebreakers, De Freezers or Acclimatizers.
- They are Attention Getters and should arouse interest.
- They could be illustrations, couplets, questions, exhibits, shocking facts, story smile.
- They may start with Salutations (Addressing the people on the dais and off the dais)

ii The Body

To make the purpose of the speech explicit and clear is the basic task of the body of the presentation. No hard and fast rules may be given for the arrangement of ideas and construction of the speech body, since each speech presents its own problems. For an effective communication, simple and logical development of the speech is a must:

- Arrange the main points logically with data support
- Think-Observe-Read-Converse-Interview
- Meant to clear the purpose
- Use concrete examples, facts and figures
- Simple logical development to be completed within time
- Use creative appropriate humor. Use cue ards
- Avoid: abstract & generalized statements with too many technical words

If you want to make your presentation stand out from the rest, you have to focus on creating a well- designed, visually pleasing presentation filled with convincing data and a narrative structure that resonates.

Think about how you are going to share the facts and figures. If you are showing a trend or comparison, then a well-constructed Line Graph or Bar Chart may be all that's required to make your point. Be cautious when using Pie Charts though. It's not easy to make sense of abstract angles and it gets worse if there are a lot of segments.

Consider your use of text carefully. I recently saw a presentation of a faculty with 278 words on a single slide. Yes, I counted. And no, I'm still not sure what their message was. Maybe because I was busy counting!! Use text sparingly and use a large, clear ont. It can be useful for quotes or to emphasize a point that you've just made. Just remember that your audience can't read and listen to you at the same time, so always pause after revealing something on the screen.

Use animation with caution in a power point presentation. Academic presentations should not have cartoon characters dropping in and out of the slide every time you change the slide. Avoid showing all the text at the same time because when you speak about the first point, the audience is reading your last line. So the best thing is to use custom animation to reveal one line at a time. In any case **keep it simple**.

iii The Closing

The closing should be gradual not abrupt. You should avoid saying "I have nothing else to say, so I think I will stop now". It should be as logical as the body that should gradually merge with building a climax with time in mind.

Purpose of a Good Closing:

- Summarize and restate-outline the main points covered in the speech.
- Make a memorable statement that should be remembered for a long time.
- Appeal for action.
- Pay the audience a sincere compliment.

(D) Adding Style to the Presentation

Non-verbal cues can either make or break a good presentation. Remember the audience is not only reading with you and listening to what you are saying but are also actively involved in looking at you. **Anything that distracts the audience can be dangerous** since then the audience spends most of its time focusing on these distractions rather than your presentation.

In fact you are judged even before you begin to speak. No sooner is your name announced that all eyes are on you so take special care of yourself. Walk gracefully since you are under scrutiny.

Elements like Dress Sense (what you wear), Posture (how you stand and move), Gesture (movements of hands), Facial Expressions, Eye Contact, Language, Listening Cues and Voice Modulation could be support systems that could make your presentation exemplary or could be distracters taking the focus of the audience away from your presentation.

i ***Dress Sense:***

Dress to the occasion. Both you and the audience should feel comfortable with what you wear. There is nothing wrong in looking good and it is important, but avoid excess makeup and flashy dress for an academic or professional presentation. It's safe to wear formals. Dress that does not match with the occasion may distract the audience. Smart attire radiates confidence.

ii ***Posture:***

It is important how you stand and move. If it's a podium presentation your movements may be restricted, but when there is freedom to move then remember to make small but not brisk or fast movements. While standing its best to keep your feet several inches apart, body well balanced, non-rocking with a natural lean.

iii ***Gestures:***

Parking of the hand is always a problem. Some presenters have this habit of moving their hands in a peculiar manner or keeping their hands in the pockets or playing with the keys in their hands or pocket or using a particular word repeatedly. I have seen the audience busy counting the number of times a word or an action was repeated. Focus shifts from the presentation to the presenter.

Subtle movements of the hand while making a point and making the right gesture to emphasize the word gives power to the presentation. Gestures should be natural, easy and spontaneous and match with the thinking and the words that are spoken. Avoid too many, too large or too frequent busy movements of the hands so that it does not appear too dramatic. In short, avoid distracting mannerisms.

iv ***Facial Expressions:***

Facial expressions should be congruent with the spoken words. Smile when there is a touch of humor to be added. Firm expression when there is a serious matter to be stated. Even while thanking people, the face should reflect "Thank you". Face should be animated, alert, intelligent, pleasing, enthusiastic, smiling and relaxed.

v ***Eye Contact:***

Good Eye Contact makes every individual feel as if you are addressing him/her. Eye Contact makes the person feel more important. In fact a smart presenter uses eye contact for multiple purposes like feedback, gaining attention or increasing acceptance to bring back the non-attentive audience. In any case I strongly recommend you avoid a fixed gaze and when addressing a large gathering you should not follow a pattern but the eye movements should be random and sweeping.

vi ***Language:***

Although it is recommended to use a single language, my personal experience encourages the use of National and local language in bits and pieces. Simple language without jargon is largely accepted by the audience. Care should be taken to spell check all slides in your presentation and look for any grammatical mistakes.

vii ***Listening Cues:***

When a question is asked or someone is answering in the audience, take time and demonstrate good listening skills. This will encourage the audience to connect with you and respond better.

viii ***Modulation of Voice:***

All the above style skills are of no use without proper Voice Modulation which includes voice pitch, pace, pause & emphasis. I remember my school English teacher giving me paragraphs from speeches of eminent scholars and asking me to read them several times with a challenge that each time the modulation should be different. Power of powerful presentation strongly circles around how good your modulation is. When to raise your voice, which word to emphasize and letting your voice rise and fall at the appropriate moment. Speed should not be too fast or too slow, give intervals between words, ideas, sentences to enable the listeners to absorb, register, assimilate and also enable you to breathe. Modulation makes your voice appealing to the listeners and offers emotions in different shades to your presentation.

"They may forget what you said, but they will never forget how you made them feel."

Carl W Buechner

7. Evaluating or Looking for Feedback

I keep asking my participants, "Do you have a feedback partner?"

A careful look at the audience will informally tell you if your presentation has been successful or not, but you need to have formal feedback channels to evaluate your performance. After your presentation there will be several known and unknown persons who will come to you and say, "Sir, your Presentation today was too good, excellent, never heard before etc etc". But I would think twice before believing them. Some may be genuine, which we will be able to recognize only with experience. I strongly recommend cultivating or nurturing a feedback partner, someone who will give an honest critical criticism about the content & style. I know this is easier said than done. But surely this helps you in your next presentation.

"I am the most spontaneous speaker in the world because every word, every gesture, and every retort has been carefully rehearsed".

George Bernard Shaw

8. Mic: Devil or Friend?

1. Always use a Mic as it helps you throw your voice.
2. Use a collar mic since it leaves your hands free for gestures.
3. Take time to adjust the mic. Keep it below your lips and its midpoint in level with your chin. Check that the mic does not cover your face. Adjust yourself to the mic.
4. Distance approximately: One fist-full (depending on the quality of the mic)
5. Do not start till you are sure the mic system works well.
6. Do not shout but speak naturally into the mic.
7. Don't worry if your own voice sounds queer or changed.

9. Tips for a Powerful Presentation

1. Thoroughly analyze your audience
2. Use Simple unadulterated language
3. Avoid too much History, Statistics
4. Clarity of Thoughts before Presentation
5. Use Cue Cards. Avoid memorizing or reading

6. Don't be sarcastic, sentimental or exaggerated
7. Eat sparingly before your speech
8. Develop the habit of reading and discussing issues
9. Be on time
10. Do not start with an Apology
11. Do not Conclude Abruptly
12. Practice, Practice & Practice with your Feedback Partner.

There are always three speeches for every one that you actually gave:

The one you practiced

The one you gave

The one you wish you gave

Dale Carnegie

Index

Q

R

S

www.ingramcontent.com/pod-product-compliance
Lightning Source LLC
Chambersburg PA
CBHW041918180526
45172CB00013B/1327
* 9 7 8 1 6 3 6 4 0 8 1 4 9 *